T0228998

Intensive Care of the Cancer Patient

Guest Editors

STEPHEN M. PASTORES, MD, FACP, FCCP, FCCM
NEIL A. HALPERN, MD, FACP, FCCP, FCCM

CRITICAL CARE CLINICS

www.criticalcare.theclinics.com

January 2010 • Volume 26 • Number 1

SAUNDERS an imprint of ELSEVIER, Inc.

W.B. SAUNDERS COMPANY

A Division of Elsevier Inc.

Elsevier Inc. • 1600 John F. Kennedy Blvd., • Suite 1800 • Philadelphia, Pennsylvania 19103-2899

http://www.theclinics.com

CRITICAL CARE CLINICS Volume 26, Number 1
January 2010 ISSN 0749-0704, ISBN-13: 978-1-4377-1806-5

Editor: Patrick Manley
Developmental Editor: Donald Mumford

Critical Care Clinics (ISSN: 0749-0704) is published quarterly by Elsevier Inc., 360 Park Avenue South, New York, NY 10010-1710. Months of issue are January, April, July, and October. Business and Editorial Offices: 1600 John F. Kennedy Blvd., Suite 1800, Philadelphia, PA 19103-2899. Customer Service Office: 6277 Sea Harbor Drive, Orlando, FL 32887-4800. Periodicals postage paid at New York, NY and additional mailing offices. Subscription prices are $167.00 per year for US individuals, $395.00 per year for US institution, $83.00 per year for US students and residents, $206.00 per year for Canadian individuals, $490.00 per year for Canadian institutions, $240.00 per year for international individuals, $490.00 per year for international institutions and $121.00 per year for Canadian and foreign students/residents. To receive student/resident rate, orders must be accompanied by name of affiliated institution, date of term, and the *signature* of program/residency coordinator on institution letterhead. Orders will be billed at individual rate until proof of status is received. Foreign air speed delivery is included in all *Clinics* subscription prices. All prices are subject to change without notice. POSTMASTER: Send address changes to *Critical Care Clinics*, Elsevier Periodicals Customer Service, 11830 Westline Industrial Drive, St. Louis, MO 63146. **Customer Service: 1-800-654-2452 (US). From outside of the US, call 1-314-447-8871. Fax: 1-314-447-8029. E-mail: journalscustomerservice-usa@elsevier.com (for print support) or journalsonlinesupport-usa@elsevier.com (for online support).**

Reprints. For copies of 100 or more of articles in this publication, please contact the Commercial Reprints Department, Elsevier Inc., 360 Park Avenue South, New York, NY 10010-1710. Tel.: 212-633-3813; Fax: 212-462-1935; E-mail: reprints@elsevier.com.

Critical Care Clinics is also published in Spanish by Editorial Inter-Medica, Junin 917, 1er A, 1113, Buenos Aires, Argentina.

Critical Care Clinics is covered in *MEDLINE/PubMed (Index Medicus), EMBASE/Excerpta Medica, Current Concepts/ Clinical Medicine, ISI/BIOMED,* and *Chemical Abstracts.*

Printed and bound in the United Kingdom
Transferred to Digital Print 2011

Contributors

GUEST EDITORS

STEPHEN M. PASTORES, MD, FACP, FCCP, FCCM
Professor of Medicine, Department of Clinical Anesthesiology, Weill Medical College of Cornell University; Director, Critical Care Medicine Fellowship and Research Programs, Department of Anesthesiology and Critical Care Medicine, Memorial Sloan-Kettering Cancer Center, New York, New York

NEIL A. HALPERN, MD, FACP, FCCP, FCCM
Professor of Medicine and Anesthesiology, Weill Medical College of Cornell University; Chief, Critical Care Medicine Service, Department of Anesthesiology and Critical Care Medicine, Memorial Sloan-Kettering Cancer Center, New York, New York

AUTHORS

BEKELE AFESSA, MD
Associate Professor of Medicine, Division of Pulmonary and Critical Care Medicine, Mayo Clinic College of Medicine, Rochester, Minnesota

SANAM AHMED, MD
Fellow, Division of Critical Care Medicine, Department of Surgery, The Mount Sinai School of Medicine, New York, New York

ELIE AZOULAY, MD, PhD
Professor of Medicine, Service de Réanimation Médicale, Hôpital Saint-Louis, Paris, France

DEEPTI BEHL, MD
Clinical Instructor, Hematology and Oncology, Mayo Clinic College of Medicine, Rochester, Minnesota

DOMINIQUE D. BENOIT, MD, PhD
Department of Intensive Care Medicine, Medical Unit, Ghent University Hospital, Gent, Belgium

KAREN S. CARLSON, MD, PhD
Hematology-Oncology Fellow, Department of Medicine, New York Presbyterian Hospital of Weill Cornell Medical College, New York, New York

SANJAY CHAWLA, MD, FCCP
Assistant Professor of Medicine in Clinical Anesthesiology, Weill Cornell Medical College, New York, New York; Assistant Attending, Critical Care Medicine Service, Department of Anesthesiology and Critical Care Medicine, Memorial Sloan-Kettering Cancer Center, New York, New York

RHONDA D'AGOSTINO, ACNP-BC
Acute Care Nurse Practitioner Coordinator, Department of Anesthesiology and Critical Care Medicine, Memorial Sloan Kettering Cancer Center, New York; Critical Care Nurse Practitioner Program Coordinator, Memorial Sloan-Kettering Cancer Center, New York

PIETER O. DEPUYDT, MD, PhD
Attending Critical Care Physician, Department of Intensive Care Medicine, Ghent University Hospital, Belgium

MARIA T. DESANCHO, MD, MSc
Associate Professor of Clinical Medicine, Department of Medicine, New York Presbyterian Hospital of Weill Cornell Medical College, New York, New York

SUSAN GAETA, MD
Associate Medical Director and Assistant Professor of Critical Care Medicine, Department of Critical Care Medicine, University of Texas, MD Anderson Cancer Center, Houston, Texas

NEIL A. HALPERN, MD, FACP, FCCP, FCCM
Professor of Medicine and Anesthesiology, Weill Medical College of Cornell University; Chief, Critical Care Medicine Service, Department of Anesthesiology and Critical Care Medicine, Memorial Sloan-Kettering Cancer Center, New York, New York

ANDREA WAHNER HENDRICKSON, MD
Clinical Fellow, Hematology and Oncology, Mayo Clinic College of Medicine, Rochester, Minnesota

ERIC A. HOSTE, MD, PhD
Department of Intensive Care Medicine, Surgical Unit, Ghent University Hospital, Gent, Belgium

TIMOTHY J. MOYNIHAN, MD
Associate Professor, Department of Oncology, Mayo Clinic College of Medicine, Rochester, Minnesota

JOHN M. OROPELLO, MD
Professor of Surgery and Medicine, Division of Critical Care Medicine, Department of Surgery, The Mount Sinai School of Medicine, New York, New York

STEPHEN M. PASTORES, MD, FACP, FCCP, FCCM
Professor of Medicine, Department of Clinical Anesthesiology, Weill Medical College of Cornell University; Director, Critical Care Medicine Fellowship and Research Programs, Department of Anesthesiology and Critical Care Medicine, Memorial Sloan-Kettering Cancer Center, New York, New York

KRISTEN J. PRICE, MD
Professor and Chief of Critical Care Medicine and Medical Director of Respiratory Care, University of Texas, MD Anderson Cancer Center, Houston, Texas

MADHUSUDANAN RAMASWAMY, MD
Critical Care Medicine Fellow, Critical Care Medicine Service, Department of Anesthesiology and Critical Care Medicine, Memorial Sloan-Kettering Cancer Center, New York, New York

JORGE I.F. SALLUH, MD, PhD
Medical Director, Intensive Care Unit, Instituto Nacional de Câncer, Rio de Janeiro, Rio de Janeiro, Brazil

BRENDA K. SHELTON, MS, RN, CCRN, AOCN
Critical Care Nurse Specialist, The Sidney Kimmel Comprehensive Cancer Center at Johns Hopkins, Baltimore, Maryland

MÁRCIO SOARES, MD, PhD
Attending Critical Care Physician, Intensive Care Unit, Instituto Nacional de Câncer, Rio de Janeiro, Rio de Janeiro, Brazil

RAGHUKUMAR THIRUMALA, MD
Critical Care Medicine Fellow, Critical Care Medicine Service, Department of Anesthesiology and Critical Care Medicine, Memorial Sloan-Kettering Cancer Center, New York, New York

LOUIS P. VOIGT, MD, FCCP
Assistant Professor of Medicine in Clinical Anesthesiology, Weill Cornell Medical College; Assistant Attending Critical Care Physician, Critical Care Medicine Service, Department of Anesthesiology and Critical Care Medicine, Memorial Sloan-Kettering Cancer Center, New York, New York

Contents

Critical care for patients with cancer was once considered inappropriate
because of a perceived poor prognosis for their long-term survival. Three
decades of research has yielded evidence to support the use of critical
care resources for many patients with cancer. A methodical approach to
triage and evaluation of critically ill patients regardless of baseline medical
diagnosis, coupled with an appreciation for the likely prognosis of their
current cancer, is most likely to yield the fairest and most accurate appro-
priation of care. No clinical scoring system has emerged that accurately
defines the severity of illness and likelihood for survival in patients with
cancer. This article reviews the studies that have attempted to apply mortality prediction scales or scoring systems to these patients. Clinical judgment with incorporation of consensus opinions from the literature should
be used to develop admission or restriction criteria for intensive care of patients with cancer.

Acute respiratory failure (ARF) remains the major reason for admission to
the intensive care unit (ICU) in patients with cancer and is often associated
with high mortality, especially in those who require mechanical ventilation.
The diagnosis and management of ARF in patients who have cancer pose
unique challenges to the intensivist. This article reviews the most common
causes of ARF in patients with cancer and discusses recent advances in
the diagnostic and management approaches of these disorders. Timely diagnosis and treatment of reversible causes of respiratory failure, including
earlier use of noninvasive ventilation and judicious ventilator and fluid management in patients with acute lung injury, are essential to achieve an
optimal outcome. Close collaboration between oncologists and intensivists helps ensure that clear goals, including direction of treatment and
quality of life, are established for every patient with cancer who requires
mechanical ventilation for ARF.

Acute respiratory failure with the need for mechanical ventilation is a severe
and frequent complication, and a leading reason for admission to the
intensive care unit (ICU) in patients with malignancies. Nevertheless,

improvements in patient survival have been observed over the last decade. This article reviews the epidemiology of adult patients with malignancies requiring ventilatory support. Criteria used to assist decisions to admit a patient to the ICU and to select the initial ventilatory strategy are discussed.

Cancer and its treatments lead to profound suppression of innate and acquired immune function. In this population, bacterial infections are common and may rapidly lead to overwhelming sepsis and death. Furthermore, infections caused by viral and fungal pathogens should be considered in patients who have specific immune defects. As cancer therapies have become more aggressive the risk for infection has increased and many patients require intensive care support. Despite improvements in long-term survival, infections remain a common complication of cancer therapy and accounts for the majority of chemotherapy-associated deaths. By understanding the host defense impairments and likely pathogens clinicians will be better able to guide diagnosis and management of this unique population.

As life expectancy increases and advances in cancer treatment more often convert deadly conditions into more chronic diseases, the surgical intensivist can expect to be faced with greater numbers of oncology patients undergoing aggressive surgical treatments for curative intent, prolonging survival, or primarily palliation by alleviating obstruction, infection, bleeding, or pain. Cytoreductive surgery (CRS) and heated intraperitoneal chemotherapy (HIPEC) are a paradigm for the emerging field of multimodal aggressive oncological surgery. This article describes the CRS/HIPEC technique, and discusses the most common postoperative complications and critical care issues in these patients, including anastomotic leaks, intestinal perforation, abscesses, and intra-abdominal bleeding. The leading cause of mortality is sepsis leading to multiple organ failure, and such patients are at particularly higher risk due to the extensive CRS and HIPEC. The intensivist must be vigilant to ensure that source control is not overlooked. This process is a very difficult one, made even more challenging by the blunting of physiologic responses and the frequent absence of the classic acute abdomen.

Patients with solid and hematologic malignancies presenting with major bleeding or thrombotic complications, potentially life-ending events in a cancer patient's clinical course, usually require admission to an intensive care unit (ICU), making their diagnosis and management even more important for the intensivist. Given the significant advances in the diagnosis and treatment of almost all types of cancers in recent years, the intensivist is likely to encounter an ever-increasing number of cancer patients in the ICU setting with these complications. Abnormal hemostasis can occur as a consequence of both the pathology and treatment of cancer. Because cancer can have multiple effects on hemostatic equilibrium, treatment of these complications can be more complex than in the general population. This article reviews the physiology of coagulation and fibrinolysis, with special attention to those aspects that are most frequently altered in the setting of malignancy. The pathophysiology of bleeding and thrombotic complications specific to critically ill cancer patients are then detailed, and the diagnostic and therapeutic strategies are discussed. Special emphasis is placed on new cancer medications that have an effect on hemostasis, and on novel clotting and anticoagulant agents that are available to the intensivist for the management of these patients.

well as its duration should be in proportion with the patient's expected long-term prognosis and quality of life.

RELATED INTEREST

Anesthesiology Clinics Volume 27, Issue 4, December 2009
Sedation and Analgesia in the ICU
L. Fleisher, *Guest Editor*

THE CLINICS ARE NOW AVAILABLE ONLINE!
Access your subscription at:
www.theclinics.com

Preface

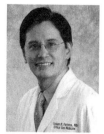 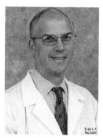

Stephen M. Pastores, MD,   Neil A. Halpern, MD,
FACP, FCCP, FCCM   FACP, FCCP, FCCM
Guest Editors

Providing critical care to patients with cancer was once considered inappropriate because their prognosis for long-term survival was perceived to be poor. Over the past few decades, however, significant strides have been made in reducing the overall mortality from cancer while simultaneously improving the quality of life of survivors. Recent evidence now supports the expanded use of critical care resources for selected patients with cancer and shows a modest increase in their survival rates in the intensive care unit (ICU). It is crucial for intensivists to be familiar with the progress in critical care of oncologic patients. The projected "numbers" for 2009—1,479,350 new cancer cases and 562,340 deaths from cancer in the United States—speak for themselves.

Many of these cancer patients will end up in our already crowded ICUs for cancer-related illnesses, treatment-associated side effects, or other underlying clinical problems that are not cancer-related. Distinguishing among these possibilities and prioritizing care in the ICU setting is quite challenging. Furthermore, the intensivist is faced with the added burdens associated with caring for the ICU patient with cancer. These include the endless array of possible oncologic treatment offerings; the increasingly complex nature of cancer protocols; the potentially unrealistic expectations on the part of the patient, family, and oncologist or oncologic surgeon; the frequently shifting goals of care between aggressive therapy and palliative care; and the emotional difficulties of addressing end-of-life issues.

In this issue of the *Clinics*, we have gathered an excellent group of practicing clinicians and investigators devoted to the care of the cancer patient. Our authors have strived to highlight the serious and life-threatening syndromes that occur in ICU patients with cancer and to underscore their diagnostic and management dilemmas. We hope the reader will gain insight into this unique and complicated group of critically ill patients.

Crit Care Clin 26 (2010) xiii–xiv
doi:10.1016/j.ccc.2009.10.005
0749-0704/09/$ – see front matter © 2010 Elsevier Inc. All rights reserved.

criticalcare.theclinics.com

We would like to thank our authors, for their outstanding contributions, and the staff of Elsevier, for their editorial support and patience. Finally, we dedicate this issue to our families—Maria T. DeSancho, MD, MSc, and children Steven Michael and Monica Cristina Pastores; and Judith Halpern and children Lauren and Michael Halpern—for providing the love and support to enable us to work and complete this project.

Stephen M. Pastores, MD, FACP, FCCP, FCCM
Department of Clinical Anesthesiology
Weill Medical College of Cornell University
New York, NY, USA

Critical Care Medicine Fellowship and Research Programs
Department of Anesthesiology and Critical Care Medicine
Memorial Sloan-Kettering Cancer Center
1275 York Avenue, C-1179, New York, NY 10065, USA

Neil A. Halpern, MD, FACP, FCCP, FCCM
Weill Medical College of Cornell University
New York, NY, USA

Critical Care Medicine Service
Department of Anesthesiology and Critical Care Medicine
Memorial Sloan-Kettering Cancer Center
1275 York Avenue, C-1179, New York, NY 10065, USA

E-mail addresses:
pastores@mskcc.org (S.M. Pastores)
halpernn@mskcc.org (N.A. Halpern)

Admission Criteria and Prognostication in Patients with Cancer Admitted to the Intensive Care Unit

Brenda K. Shelton, MS, RN, CCRN, AOCN

KEYWORDS

- Admission • Cancer • Critical care • Critical illness
- Intensive care • Mortality • Oncology • Outcome

Critical care of patients with cancer has progressed despite many challenges in recent decades. In the early 1980s, a cancer diagnosis was considered a contraindication for admission to an intensive care unit (ICU).[1] The advent of successful antineoplastic therapies, improved supportive care, and consumer demand initially validated the benefits of critical care for these patients. A desire to pursue more aggressive therapies in search of enhanced patient outcomes also led to practice changes within the critical care environment in the 1990s.[2] This article provides an overview of these historical perspectives and the current state of the science regarding admission to ICUs, care of patients who have cancer in the ICU, and prognostication for critical illness among patients with cancer.

HISTORICAL PERSPECTIVES OF CANCER AND CRITICAL CARE

ICUs developed in the 1960s and flourished in the 1970s with the implementation of resuscitation standards for acute life-threatening dysrhythmias and perfection of trauma management skills associated with the Vietnam War. Initial critical care was provided for cardiac, surgical, and trauma patients although many patients with chronic medical disorders such as chronic obstructive pulmonary disease and chronic renal failure required the technologies available only in an ICU setting. The first antineoplastic therapies to provide potential for long-term disease-free survival were surgical interventions aimed at removing tumors at an early stage. Late in the 1970s

The Sidney Kimmel Comprehensive Cancer Center at Johns Hopkins, 401 North Broadway, Weinberg Building #1370, Baltimore, MD 21231, USA
E-mail address: sheltbr@jhmi.edu

Crit Care Clin 26 (2010) 1–20
doi:10.1016/j.ccc.2009.10.003
0749-0704/09/$ – see front matter © 2010 Elsevier Inc. All rights reserved.

criticalcare.theclinics.com

medical antineoplastic therapy first realized its major successes with Hodgkin disease and testicular cancer, both of which occur frequently in young adults. Childhood leukemia treatment exceeded these success rates, mandating a revision in ICU admission policies for children. Experience with oncologic therapies such as blood and bone marrow transplantation that produced extreme myelosuppression and organ dysfunction led some academic medical centers to dedicate intensive care beds to provide specialized care to these patients.[3]

Despite advances in antineoplastic therapy and supportive care treatments that provided a growing number of patients who have cancer with an opportunity to become "cancer survivors," the lack of accessibility to intensive care resources persisted. Intensive care clinicians perceived that responses to cancer therapy were poor, and the ability of patients to survive physical insults such as critical illness were deemed appropriate reasons to limit care.[2–4] As oncologic success stories became commonplace, consumers demanded equal treatment, and prognostic variables became better defined, as did acceptance of critical care for these patients.[5] A suggestion to assist clinicians in reversing their biases is described in an article by Le-Cuyer and colleagues[6] and mirrored by an editorial[7] stating that a change of view is needed of patients who have cancer to "see them as people living with a chronic illness that may have minimal impact on their day-to-day lives." The literature suggests that studies published within the last decade report improved outcomes for patients with cancer as opposed to those before 1999,[2,5,8] with some investigators defining intensive care admission after 1996 as an independent predictor for a more positive outcome.[7,9] These improvements in outcomes have been attributed to improved patient triage, enhanced management of oncologic emergencies, perfection of critical care interventions for common acute ICU conditions such as severe sepsis and acute respiratory distress syndrome, and advances in hematology/oncology.[5,8] Patients with cancer are often admitted to ICUs and several variables are used to determine best practices in their management.

Professional society guidelines for intensive care admission, discharge, and triage are available and can be used as a guide for evaluation of patients.[10] Based on a comprehensive review of the literature describing critical care of patients with cancer, this article further defines reasons for appropriate admission to the ICU that are unique to oncologic patients. Clinicians should evaluate and interpret suggested admission criteria based on their institutional capacity, particularly the sophistication of general care available, and patient acuity that requires ICU admission for high levels of nursing care rather than the need for specific intensivist skills. Some patients with cancer have high acuity and the need for increased frequency of assessment and physical interventions may necessitate critical care admission, but not because of clear critical illness.

Approximately 62% of patients with cancer are considered "survivors," as shown by an expected survival beyond 5 years.[5,11] This information paired with the data that show 1 in 10 patients with cancer will require expertise provided by intensive care clinicians demonstrates that selective critical care is reasonable and morally necessary.[12–14]

ICU ADMISSION AND RESTRICTION POLICIES AND PATIENTS WITH CANCER

More than 28% of all health care expenditures occur in the last 6 months of life, and appropriate allocation of scarce critical care beds is an essential component of managing limited resources and controlling health care costs.[14] One method to ensure objective decision-making when triaging patients for ICU admission is to use predetermined admission or restriction criteria developed for adult and pediatric patients by the Society of Critical Care Medicine.[10,15] These guidelines offer options of admission criteria using 1 of 3 models: a prioritization model (eg, highest priority with greatest potential benefit), a diagnosis model (eg, specific medical diagnoses or clinical conditions), or an objective parameters model (eg, specific clinical symptoms such as third-degree heart block or hemoglobin less than 7 mg/dL).[10] The priority model of this document specifically states "priority 4 are those patients who are generally not appropriate for ICU admission.... For example: metastatic cancer unresponsive to chemotherapy and/or radiation therapy (unless the patient is on a specific treatment protocol)."[10] The context of this example may continue to encourage decision-making based on prediction of outcome, a concept that continues to elude definition. If using the prioritization model for creation of admission criteria, the principle of justice would dictate that ICUs use a valid and reliable mortality prediction model for determination of admission. One study defines metastatic cancer as 1 of only 2 variables statistically significant for refusal for ICU admission despite the presence of general guidelines that did not define specific diagnoses.[16]

The operationalization of these recommendations or a similar institution-based document has been inconsistent among ICU clinicians. Published studies assessing the application of recommendations demonstrate that ICU clinicians do not necessarily use these guidelines in daily practice.[17–19] As many as 75% of clinicians do not adhere to their own admission guidelines and 79% do not have restriction guidelines.[19] Within the framework of these recommendations, several investigators have attempted to define objective criteria for triaging patients with cancer for ICU admission. Groeger and Aurora[3] define broad categories of admission criteria: (1) postoperative care, (2) management of medical emergencies related to cancer or its treatment, and (3) monitoring during intensive oncologic treatments. They further state that 3 principles guiding decisions will lead to the best use of critical care resources. First, the clinician should determine whether the status of the critical care complication and the disease suggest a high likelihood of meaningful survival as defined by the patient and physician. Second, is the patient's autonomy or prior expressed wishes being respected? Lastly, the principle of distributive justice should be employed when there are limited ICU resources. These principles were mirrored in a study of Israeli intensive care physicians.[20] The Australian Classification System outlines stages of cancer based on the goals of care and recommends that ICU care should be delivered only if the goals of care are clearly beneficial to quality and quantity of life. These classifications are (1) newly diagnosed, (2) cure is possible, (3) probable control of disease, (4) treatment failure indicates probable supportive care objective, and (5) palliative symptom control. When using this system, critical care is always provided to class 1 and 2 patients, is evaluated on a case-by-case basis for class 3 and 4 patients, and is considered contraindicated for class 5 patients.[21]

COMMON CAUSES OF CRITICAL ILLNESS

Critical illness in patients with cancer can vary as widely as the different tumor types themselves. The critical care literature examining outcomes and reasons for critical illness in patients who have cancer concurs that the best outcomes are realized when careful patient selection for ICU care is employed.[3] Consensus dictates that the best candidates for use of critical care resources among patients with cancer are patients at presentation for their initial cancer diagnosis, when there are clearly promising treatment options for their cancer and critical illness, or when crises occur in patients who do not have active malignancy.[8,22,23] Critical illness, however, arises in many patients in whom clear indications are not present, and each patient should be considered in the context of current malignant disease, status of comorbid health conditions, and ability to survive the critical illness and the time it takes to return to pre-illness level of functioning.[3,22,24] Understanding specific situations that may precipitate critical illness is valuable for planning best care. When there are insufficient data to predict prognosis of a patient confidently, it is reasonable to initiate critical care intervention with reassessment of the patient's status after 3 to 7 days.[3,8,22] This range of time may be necessary to obtain key diagnostic data, or to assess initial responses to interventions. Patients with cancer who prove to have irreversible complications or who do not quickly improve with perceived definitive therapy are less likely to survive the critical illness. No improvement in the patient's critical illness during this "therapeutic trial of critical care interventions" may result in cessation of mechanical support, a decision not to escalate care, or a definitive discussion with a health care proxy regarding additional interventions deemed unhelpful for achieving the goal of comfort. Unique critical care applications in patients with cancer include postoperative care, special considerations of solid tumors and hematologic malignancies, and situations in which the crisis is unrelated to the tumor or its therapy.

When considering all patients with cancer who require ICU care, the most common reasons for ICU admission are: (1) respiratory failure, (2) postanesthetic recovery, (3) infection and sepsis, (4) bleeding, and (5) oncologic emergencies.[3,25] Respiratory failure is the most common reason for ICU admission for all groups of patients with cancer, but the implications vary depending on the reason for respiratory compromise.[2,3,17,24–29] Studies suggest that postoperative support and a positive response to noninvasive ventilation are patient characteristics that indicate a better prognosis.[9,25,27] Some subpopulations have specific common critical illnesses that must always be considered in planning for ICU use and necessary nurse training or resource allocation. For instance, although acute intracranial events such as increased intracranial pressure, hemorrhage, or status epilepticus are uncommon with many cancers, their management must be within the scope of the local ICU if the oncologists are treating patients with brain tumors. Patients with hematologic malignancies also require advanced blood component support, pheresis capabilities, and continuous renal replacement therapy (CRRT) to manage the complications common to their disease. Unique causes of critical illness and potentially valid reasons for admission to an ICU are now described according to the neoplastic diagnosis or treatment modality.

Postoperative Care

One of the most common uses of critical care is for postoperative patients with complex or large tumor resection. Although many patients who have cancer require surgery, those most likely to require postoperative critical care support include brain tumors, esophagogastric cancer, head and neck cancer, hepatic cancer or metastases to the liver, lung cancer, ovarian cancer, pancreatic cancer, and urologic malignancies.[30] Surgical critical care units provide immediate stabilization and recovery after prolonged surgical procedures, monitor for multisystem complications such as bleeding, dysrhythmias, fluid and electrolyte imbalance, glycemic events, hypotension, or ischemic organ failure. Use of critical care in these patients has assisted surgeons to develop more advanced and aggressive procedures that have positively influenced survival. ICU survival in this patient population exceeds 80%, and long-term survival is common.[3,17,25,31] Surgical interventions for supportive care such as semipermanent central line insertions, or palliative interventions such as stent placement are also important for care of patients with cancer who occasionally require intensive care resources.[3] At the forefront for all decisions concerning surgical intervention and ICU care is the concern of immediate survival benefit. The next variable to contribute to decision-making is the status of the underlying cancer and likelihood that the surgical procedure will provide enhanced quality and quantity of life.

Patients with Solid Tumor Malignancies

Patients with solid tumor malignancies also require critical care support when they present initially or with recurrent bulky disease that erodes vessels and tissues, or compresses body organs, causing hemorrhage or organ failure. These patients frequently undergo surgical resection, debulking, or reconstructive surgical procedures. Patients with solid tumors are also more likely to receive palliative surgical interventions such as stenting, embolization, catheter or shunt placement, or diverting procedures. The unique critical care needs of these patients vary based on the location, initial size, stage of disease, and growth rate of the tumor, but principles of care are consistent. In all patients, possible and probable complications can be anticipated and advanced planning about the extent of supportive interventions to be offered should be discussed with patients and their health care decision-makers.

When known, the tumor growth rate may be 1 of the most significant variables to predict critical illness. Tumors with rapid proliferation rates are quick to metastasize and create life-threatening complications but are also the most immediately responsive to antineoplastic therapy. For example, patients presenting with advanced stage small cell lung cancer are at risk for immediate severe, life-threatening complications such as airway obstruction, superior vena cava obstruction, pericardial effusions, or pleural effusions, but may have rapid and dramatic dissipation of symptoms soon after chemotherapy.

Tumor location, size, and stage of disease are the next considerations. Initially, complications should be anticipated related to the location of the primary tumor and what will occur when it shrinks with therapy or when it continues to grow before therapy has adequate time to work or despite treatment. When planned transfer to the ICU has been determined appropriate, predicting likely complications based on the primary tumor location and penetration of nearby organs could facilitate early involvement of intensivists as consultants. Their consultation and awareness of the patient's clinical disease and goals of care can enhance a rapid and more successful transfer of service if needed. For example, a tumor of the esophagus that has extension into the tracheal wall could shrink with therapy, but leave a tracheoesophageal fistula that would require immediate surgery. Another example is a patient with head and neck cancer that is impinging on the carotid artery and could have tumor erosion into the carotid or nearby vessels with massive bleeding. In both cases, the specific emergency and its approximate timing may be predictable, with definable early signs or symptoms, and proactive discussions could help determine the critical care course of care.

The next consideration for patients with solid tumors involves the actual or potential high-risk sites of metastases and crises that may arise. Because the risk of brain metastases is high in patients with small cell lung cancer, clinicians should be constantly vigilant for mental status changes or signs and symptoms of possible seizure activity. Recognition of the metastatic pattern of each tumor type is helpful in planning critical care interventions.

The disease trajectory in patients with solid tumors may vary, enabling many patients with metastatic but slow-growing disease to live long and productive lives despite having metastatic cancer. High functional performance before critical illness has been shown to influence outcomes positively.[17] Functional activity or performance status scoring such as the Karnofsky Performance Scale Index, Functional

Assessment of Cancer Therapy (FACT), or Memorial Symptom Assessment Scale (MSAS) can be useful for identifying patients who will either fare well or do poorly with critical care interventions.[32] As with other malignancies, the need for mechanical ventilation among patients with solid tumors remains an important poor prognostic predictor for mortality.[17,33]

Patients with Hematologic Malignancies

Patients with hematologic malignancies present with different critical care issues from those with solid tumor malignancies. First, the nature of these malignancies is diffuse at diagnosis, producing general body responses to widespread malignancy such as capillary permeability syndrome, clotting, and catabolism that consequently trigger complications such as respiratory distress, hypotension, disseminated intravascular coagulation, renal insufficiency, and hepatic dysfunction.[3,13,34] All treatments for these malignancies include the whole body and total marrow destruction, which leads to severe complications of myelosuppression such as bleeding and sepsis.[34,35] In addition, these tumors are more likely to have rapid proliferation rates that result in excessive cell turnover before and during therapy. The consequences may include critical illnesses such as leukostasis, tumor lysis syndrome, or disseminated intravascular coagulation. These patients frequently present with multisystem dysfunction and respiratory failure, often the result of serious infection. Because many patients experience prolonged marrow suppression, and receive frequent and prolonged antibiotic treatment, it is common for them to have infections with resistant organisms, opportunistic and unusual microbial disease, and refractory infectious complications. Recovery from critical illness in these patients most often directly correlates with their establishment of disease remission and white blood cell recovery. Several studies validate that implementation of mechanical ventilation also predicts for poorer outcome.[28,36–39] Progress has been made in the last decade and recent literature reports patients with hematologic malignancies surviving an ICU episode requiring mechanical ventilation on average of 22% to 42% of the time compared with less than 20% survival in the 1980s and 1990s.[36,39,40] Proposed reasons for this finding reflect the same advances in cancer care that have enhanced outcomes in other patient populations. The length of time a patient's white blood cells are depressed may lead to a more prolonged ICU course while awaiting evidence of bone marrow recovery and resolution of complications.[34,36]

Patients Undergoing Hematopoietic Stem Cell Transplantation

Critical care admission has also been provided based on use of specific therapies. For many years the trajectory of hematopoietic stem cell transplantation (HSCT) required severely myelosuppressive, high-dose chemotherapy, or radiation followed by infusion of a foreign antigenic material (another person's bone marrow or concentrated hematopoietic stem cells). The aim of this intensive therapy is total irradication of cancer. The serious complication rate for these patients who were receiving a potentially curative treatment exceeded 20% to 40%, requiring frequent admission to the ICU.[3,12,34–36,38,41] The rationale for delivering this high level of support has been the hope for cure in these individuals. It was believed that allogeneic transplant patients experienced more frequent and higher severity of critical illness,[36–38,40] but this assumption has not proven true in many studies.[34,36,39,40,42,43] Common reasons for ICU admission for patients with hematopoietic stem cell therapies have included respiratory distress, severe bleeding, sepsis, rejection disorders such as graft-versus-host disease (GVHD), and chemotherapy toxicities such as hepatic venoocclusive disease or renal failure.[29,37,39,44–46] The need for mechanical ventilation and presence of GVHD have been markers for greater severity of illness and have been consistently predictive for poorer outcomes in transplant patients.[36,37,39,40,45–47] One study also affirmed that patients requiring mechanical ventilation with concomitant hepatic and renal dysfunction had the highest mortality.[47] Alveolar hemorrhage as the source of respiratory failure also holds a potential for poorer outcome.[29] One British study spanning 10 years of a large number of patients reported vasopressor use as predictive for lower survival, although this has not proven statistically significant in other studies.[44] For those patients who do immediately survive mechanical ventilation, 6-month survival is considerably better than in many other patients who have cancer, varying from 27% to 88%.[38,46,47]

In the past 2 decades, hematopoietic stem cell treatments have evolved into a more predictable and less toxic therapy, and now many of these same patients experience less myelosuppression, and receive better antirejection therapies, closer genetically matched cellular therapies, and advanced supportive measures.[39] These patients have realized a dramatic decrease in need for critical care support from a high of 44% in the 1980s[27,35,41] to 8% to 20% today.[39,40,44] In a meta-analysis of pediatric HSCT patients,[40] the investigators caution that straightforward interpretation of these advances in outcomes may be premature because of study limitations such as transplant criteria, biases of single center data, reduction in use of invasive mechanical ventilation, or selection bias for critical care intervention that may have changed. Several investigators have reported that ICU survival for HSCT patients has also improved from approximately 20%[34] to 37.8% to 48.3%,[37,39,44] attributable to improved cell-processing techniques, enhanced antirejection regimens, and better supportive care. Long-term survival (6–12 months) of these patients was once as low as 3%,[34] but now averages 21.6% to 32.5%.[39,44]

Other Reasons for Critical Care Support for Patients with Cancer

Other cancer-therapy driven critical care needs have been documented with administration of specific toxic chemotherapy, biotherapy, or radiotherapy treatments. Most antineoplastic therapies are associated with a risk of hypersensitivity.[48] Moderate to severe hypersensitivity reactions have been identified in approximately 2% to 43% of patients receiving therapy.[49] This variability is in part caused by adjustment of treatment regimens, and institution of antianaphylaxis premedications once serious reactions have been identified.[49,50] Intensive vital signs, cardiac monitoring, or life-support after hypersensitivity reactions may be required by some patients. Administration of high-dose interleukin 2 to patients with renal cell cancer or melanoma has required critical care support in many patients, but is still administered because of toxicity reversibility and potential for cure in a small number of patients.[12]

The final indications for use of critical care in patients with cancer are those general medical-surgical problems that arise during the course of antineoplastic therapy. Even when patients present for antineoplastic treatment with a good performance status, there is a high incidence of complications related to underlying medical disorders, such as hyperglycemia with diabetes, or respiratory distress in patients with chronic obstructive pulmonary disease. Cancer therapies may also exacerbate underlying conditions such as coronary artery disease or ulcerative colitis. In many cases, these complications are viewed as reversible given the stable status of the disease at the time the patient began treatment. For conditions in which a clear medical treatment is available that will stabilize the medical complication, aggressive support is usually offered.[51] It may become apparent through the process of aggressive care that these same medical disorders make it impossible for the patient to receive optimal antineo-plastic therapy.

GENERAL PREDICTORS FOR OUTCOME

The research literature that defines outcomes for critical care of patients who have cancer spans close to 3 decades. Some studies stratified patients with cancer as a subgroup, and others studied only patients with cancer. The most consistent finding and predictor of outcome was the status of the malignancy. In newly diagnosed patients in whom there was an effective therapy option, the patients fared better than when the malignancy was persistent despite receiving treatment. Clinicians continue to debate the merit of offering aggressive antineoplastic therapy while the patient is critically ill, although studies support the administration of therapy, showing that it can be safely and successfully performed and provide immediate relief of certain tumor-related critical care crises.[22,51–53] Most patients in these studies, however, had rapidly proliferative hematologic malignancies, making it difficult to generalize these findings to patients with solid tumor malignancies.[51] The authors' experience shows that patients with solid tumor masses causing the critical illness tolerate antineoplastic therapy and their critical illness resolves when and if their tumor shrinks. Those patients who have the best prognosis are those whose malignancy is in remission or quiescent at the time of the critical illness.[3,51] There is considerable vari-ability in findings when comparing early literature (before 1996) and studies published after that time. ICU mortality for patients with cancer before 1996 ranged from 44% to 98%,[26,54–63] but today it ranges from 23% to 57%.[9,25,28] Six-month survival has also improved from 2%–14% to 33%–66%.[25,64] A summary of the literature since 1979 has yielded a consistent number of prognostic indicators for short- and long-term survival from critical illness; these are summarized in **Box 1**. The literature spans a long period, and more recent oncologic advances have influenced outcomes in certain patient populations. For example, advances in cell processing and antirejection treatments have altered the critical illness profile for many HSCT patients. The advent of small molecule tyrosine kinase inhibitors has also improved long-term disease-free status for many chronic leukemia patients who would have previously converted to high-risk acute leukemia. Interventional radiologic procedures have enhanced nonsurgical management of obstructive processes in solid tumors, reducing the need for aggres-sive surgery and ICU care. The advent of effective noninvasive ventilation techniques has also reduced the need for mechanical ventilation and is suggested to be

---

Box 1
Prognostic predictors for improved survival of critical illness by patients with cancer

Postoperative support and monitoring is the only indication for critical care

Quiescent cancer or malignancy in remission

Good performance status at onset of critical illness

Critical illness for less than 7 days

Immune suppression lasting for less than 7 to 10 days

Absence of fungal infection

Absence of comorbidities

Reason for ICU care found to be correctable or amenable to treatment

independently associated with improved survival even after adjustment for matching variables.[9,65]

Early studies of critical care outcomes in patients with cancer describe lower survival rates in patients requiring vasopressors, mechanical ventilation, with prolonged neutropenia, or with septic shock.[4,41,58,62,66] Older age was evaluated as a potential poor prognostic variable in most studies, but did not prove significant, reinforcing that age alone should not be used in planning care for critically ill patients with cancer.[67] These variables do not show the same significance in more recent studies. Survival from mechanical ventilation has improved from 20% in the 1980s [4,26,63] to approximately 32% in studies since 1999.[8,9,64] The cause of the respiratory failure requiring mechanical ventilation is perhaps the most significant contribution to the variability of outcomes for these patients.[3,30] Mechanical ventilation postoperatively has the greatest success rate for extubation, discharge from the hospital, and general outcomes. Patients in whom there is an unclear cause for respiratory failure are least likely to survive mechanical ventilation and ICU stay.[24] Specific predictors for low survival after mechanical ventilation include unknown cause, alveolar hemorrhage, multiorgan failure, refractory malignant disease, and prior performance status.[29,38,42,47,58,60] Prolonged mechanical ventilation in the absence of multiorgan failure is not associated with higher mortality.

Neutropenia is no longer predictive of mortality, although prolonged neutropenia still confers an increased risk for severe and refractory infections.[28,53] More recent studies of critical illness in patients with cancer report outcomes similar to those of other chronic medical patients.[64,66] According to 1 investigator,[68] approximately 15% of patients with cancer require a protracted ICU stay exceeding 21 days, yet their survival to discharge is not so grim as expected (about 18% are alive at discharge). The implication is that length of ICU care may not necessarily be prognostic for poor outcomes, and additional variables must be considered in determining futility for this patient population.[68]

Renal failure in all ICU patients implies a risk of mortality between 40% and 90%, but stable statistics despite advances in renal replacement therapies suggest that the population of patients may be older and surviving other complications to develop renal impairment later.[3] Recent studies since the use of CRRT became common are sparse but suggest improved outcomes in select patients who are not experiencing multiorgan failure.[69–71] Early use of dialysis may predict better outcomes also.[71,72] The presence of active malignancy continues to be an independent predictor of higher mortality in patients with renal failure and cancer.[3] Anecdotal experience and case reports with CRRT suggests reduced mechanical ventilation, decreased use of vasopressors, and improved short-term outcomes in patients experiencing tumor lysis syndrome or hepatorenal failure, in whom survival may be 60% to 75%.[3,69,73,74] The cause of renal impairment is an important variable in determining the overall prognosis associated with mortality in critically ill patients with cancer, with metabolic derangements having more promising outcomes than patients with primary renal disease and multiorgan failure.[3,69]

Several studies have specifically addressed the short- and long-term benefit of cardiopulmonary resuscitation (CPR) in patients with cancer. In most studies of CPR in general care the diagnosis of cancer is described as an independent predictor of poor outcome.[3,62,65,70,72] In most studies, immediate 24-hour survival from resuscitation matches statistics of other critically ill patients at about 38%, but the survival to discharge is lower than the 14% reported for other medical patients.[3,68,72] More recent studies of CPR in patients with cancer demonstrates improved survival to discharge, but a longer rehabilitation and lower 6-month survival rate than with other patient populations.[25] Pediatric resuscitation yields a lower survival rate for all patients, and those with cancer rarely survived to be discharged from the hospital.[62,65] An additional variable that contributes to poorer outcomes in these patients is a lower performance status before the resuscitation.[3,68] In 1 report, patients who were critically ill, then had a cardiac arrest, had a poorer outcome than those patients who experienced a sudden and unexpected arrest.[70] Patients with sudden cardiac arrest had dysrhythmias, sudden metabolic alterations, and cardiac complications; whereas those who suffered cardiopulmonary arrest after becoming critically ill were more likely to suffer from chronic and progressive organ failure.[70] Health care providers should develop a relationship with patients with cancer that enables them to clarify patients' wishes before an acute event, and continually to evaluate and communicate changing goals of care that may influence the patients' decisions regarding resuscitation.

BARRIERS TO PREDICTING OUTCOME IN PATIENTS WHO HAVE CANCER

Before analysis of severity of illness or prognostic scoring systems and their application in critical illness among patients who have cancer, it is essential to consider the potential variables that may interfere with their accuracy. First, all scoring systems are used with patients after they present with critical illness and are hence flawed for use in any capacity as a preadmission screening tool.[10] Potential confounding variables of the prognostication systems when applied to patients with cancer include short-term treatment-related organ compromise associated with cancer treatment, potential influence of chronic immune suppression, unpredictable tumor responses to treatment, the impact of reversible oncologic emergencies on initial acuity measures, and the lack of sensitivity of these same measures in patients whose malignancy is initially understaged. Organ compromise is common after initiation of many anticancer therapies, but the effects are usually time limited. Individual responses to organ toxicity are difficult to predict, as they may be altered by the patient's underlying cancer, previous organ insults, degree of immune compromise, and previous general health. Patients' responses to interventions for sepsis and coagulopathy are influenced by long-term persistent exposures to antigens and development of antimicrobial resistance, factors not easily incorporated into acuity scoring systems. Even in patients newly diagnosed with cancer, who are perceived to have the greatest successful outcome in critical illness, there are ill-defined factors that make 1 person's tumor shrink considerably, whereas in the same time frame, another person's tumor quadruples in size and effect. In these patients, the presence of high acuity scores is less reflective of their prognostic outcome of critical care than of the tumor response to treatment.[75] The converse is true with oncologic emergencies such as tumor lysis syndrome or disseminated intravascular coagulation, which may be a positive reflection of tumor destruction even although acuity is increased in the short term. Many tumor effects and treatment plans are short term, with only a small poorly identifiable window of time to treat the cancer successfully. Thus, tumor- and treatment-related variables influencing acuity scoring may not be truly reflective of mortality, but instead a mirror of the combined effects of tumor growth, destruction, or treatment adverse effects.[17] In some cases, the initial staging incorrectly identifies all existing tumors, influencing individual responses and leading to initially low acuity scores with a resurgence of symptoms as advanced or metastatic disease becomes symptomatic. More often, cancer has a rapid progression of symptoms with unclear variables influencing any 1 individual's chance of fully responding to treatment without lasting adverse effects on organ function.

Several specific studies regarding outcomes of sepsis in patients with cancer have been performed. The prevalence of research interest in this patient population has been attributed to the frequency of this adverse effect of cancer or its treatment, and the necessity for admission to the ICU. It is estimated that 2% to 10% of patients experience an episode of sepsis or septic shock during cancer therapy.[66,67] Because there are unpredictable variables such as organism-specific virulence, the host's level of immunosuppression, and antibiotic resistance, studies have shown that there are few easily identifiable predictors of outcomes.[76] Although this is also true of the general ICU patient, the variables that seem to influence outcome are more often cancer specific rather than infection related in critical illness caused by sepsis.[65,77]

PROGNOSTIC SCORING SYSTEMS AND APPLICATION TO CRITICALLY ILL PATIENTS WHO HAVE CANCER

Prognostic scoring systems for predicting general ICU patients' outcomes and oncology-specific patients' outcomes have been studied extensively, but primarily using a retrospective design, and not yet showing the patient specificity that would be required to use them for individual patient advisement.[71] Despite extensive effort to create the ideal objective tool for critical care outcome prediction, studies continue to show that expert clinicians are better able to use available scoring system data combined with their own knowledge to better predict specific patient outcomes.[19,25,75] Despite this, there remains diversity in predicted cause of critical illness and mortality and postmortem findings.[77] The misdiagnosis of cardiac conditions and opportunistic infections suggests that perhaps improved diagnostic techniques and more accurate diagnosis may yield altered outcomes in these patients. Initial prognostication scoring systems in ICUs implemented in the 1980s include the Acute Physiology and Chronic Health Evaluation (APACHE-I, II, III), and its shortened version called the Simplified Acute Physiology Score (SAPS-II).[43,71,78,79]

The APACHE-III summarizes patient data to produce a severity-of-illness score that is usually performed at admission to the ICU, and 24 to 48 hours later. The degree of organ failure is entered into an equation to predict mortality. In medical-surgical patients and patients with cancer, this has been identified as inadequate to predict individual patient outcomes, but instead is more useful for planning staffing, describing case mix index, or for ICU performance benchmarking. Attempts have been made to modify the APACHE to account for oncologic variables such as reversible hematologic, gastrointestinal, or hepatic failure caused by therapy toxicities. This instrument is called the Intensive Care Mortality Model (ICMM) and provides cancer-specific factors to best identify the unique prognostic risks.[3,71] This model was further developed and tested at 72 hours after admission to the ICU with better discrimination for survivors versus nonsurvivors.[80,81] The ICMM scale used information yielded from the APACHE studies as a baseline, and built on an earlier study of this model,[82] and defines 72 hours as a more sensitive predictive time for assessment of patients with cancer who are critically ill.[66,78,80] SAPS-II uses similar data to the APACHE scoring system, but with fewer data points. The Therapeutic Index Scoring System (TISS-28 or TISS-76) measure severity of illness based on technologies required to provide care. Studies of APACHE scoring in oncology patients overpredicted critical illness, whereas TISS often underpredicted degree of critical illness because of lower use of invasive monitoring and aggressive diagnostic interventions in some patients with cancer.[3] In a systematic review of prognostic models studied in critically ill patients with cancer, use of these models clarified that general prognostic models were adequate for identification of the very sick and very well patients, but tended to

Table 1
Prognostic scoring systems for predicting mortality in patients with cancer

Scoring System	Description	Investigators
APACHE I	Scoring of medical diagnoses, comorbidities, and diagnostic test findings to predict ICU mortality. Performed on day of admission and 48 hours after admission, so not discriminating for patients who are not the "sickest" at the time of admission.	Johnson, Gordon, Fitzgerald, 1986[59]
APACHE II	Refinement of initial criteria with adjustment of normal value ranges and weightings.	Afessa, Tefferi, Dunn, et al, 2003[43] Benoit, Depuydt, Vanderwoude, et al, 2005[52] Ho, 2007[95] Owczuk, Wujtewicz, Sawicka, et al, 2004[96] Sculier, Paesmans, Markiewicz, et al, 2000[97] Schellongowski, Benesch, Lang et al, 2004[81] Soares, Fontes, Dantas, et al, 2004[83] Thakkar, Fu, Sweetenham, et al, 2008[98]
APACHE III	Statistical evaluation methods refined from previous APACHE versions.	Afessa, Tefferi, Dunn, et al, 2003[43] Staudinger, Stoiser, Mullner, et al, 2000[25] Soares, Fontes, Dantas, et al, 2004[83]
SAPS II	Shortened version of APACHE using the variables most significantly predictive for mortality; tended to underestimate mortality in some populations, including patients with cancer	Adda, Coquet, Dramon, et al, 2008[99] Benoit, Vanderwoude, Decruyenaere, et al, 2003[100] Berghmans, Paesmans, Sculier, 2004[101] Guiguet, Blot, Escudier, et al, 1998[78] Kroschinsky, Weise, Illmer, et al, 2002[102] La Gall, Neumann, Hemery, et al, 2005[79] Owczuk, Wujtewicz, Sawicka, et al, 2004[96] Rabbat, Chaoui, Montani et al, 2005[103] Sculier, Paesmans, Markiewicz, et al, 2000[97] Schellongowski, Benesch, Lang et al, 2004[81] Soares, Fontes, Dantas, et al, 2004[83] Timsit, Fosse, Troche, et al, 2001[91]

SAPS III	Refinement of terms and normal values for enhanced prediction of mortality.	Pene, Aubron, Azoulay, et al, 2006[39] Santolaya, Alvarez, Aviles, et al, 2008[93] Soares & Salluh, 2006[86]
ICMM	MPM II was used as a basis to identify common ICU prognostic criteria and enhancement with oncology specific variables for improved mortality prediction in patients with cancer.	Berghmans, Paesmans, Sculier, 2004[101] Groeger, Lemeshaw, Price, et al, 1998[82] Groeger, Glassman, Nierman, et al, 2003[80] Santolaya, Alvarez, Aviles, et al, 2008[93] Soares, Fontes, Dantas, et al, 2004[83]
MPM I	Diagnostic predictions made based on reason for ICU admission, and abnormal diagnostic test results, but without inclusion of primary diagnosis	Groeger, Lemeshaw, Price, et al, 1998[82] Soares, Fontes, Dantas, et al, 2004[83]
MPM II	Attempts to refine sensitivity to identify thresholds of frequency in the case mix of specific diagnoses beyond which the model is not predictive	Groeger, Lemeshaw, Price, et al, 1998[82] Santolaya, Alvarez, Aviles, et al, 2008[93] Soares, Fontes, Dantas, et al, 2004[83]
MPM III	Application of model in broader case mix of recent critically ill patients to validate predictive value; this model was consistent in most groups, but performed less consistently in the medical critical illness group, which comprised approximately 50% of the group	Higgins, Kramer, Nathanson, et al, 2009[87] Nathanson, Higgins, Kramer, et al, 2009[88]
SOFA	Organ failure assessment throughout the ICU hospitalization among septic patients, but name changed from "sepsis-related" to "sequential" once determined it could be applied in other critically ill patients; a single score assigned for each of 6 organ systems based on physiologic (eg, hypotension) and resource needs (eg, need for vasopressors for blood pressure support)	Ho, 2007[95] Minne, Abu-Hanna, de Jonge, 2008[77] Owczuk, Wujtewicz, Sawicka, et al, 2004[96] Peres, Melot, Lopes Ferreira, et al, 2002[84] Santolaya, Alvarez, Aviles, et al, 2008[93] Silfvast, Pettila, Ihalainen, et al, 2003[94] Timsit, Fosse, Troche, et al, 2002[85]
LOD	A system of physiologic and biologic variables collected at the time and intermittently throughout ICU hospitalization with regression analysis of organ dysfunction parameters	Metnitz, Lang, Valentin, et al, 2001[76] Pene, Aubron, Azoulay, et al, 2006[39] Santolaya, Alvarez, Aviles, et al, 2008[93] Timsit, Fosse, Troche, et al, 2001[91]
MODS	Organ failure scoring system with a unique definition of cardiovascular failure compared with SOFA; failure is calculated based on a mathematical formula combining physiologic variables and resource intensity.	Peres, Melot, Lopes Ferreira, et al, 2002[84] Santolaya, Alvarez, Aviles, et al, 2008[93]

underestimate the risk of mortality for patients with cancer. The oncology-specific ICMM model developed by Groeger and colleagues[71,80,82,83] showed better discrimination for oncology-specific prognostic variables and assisted in identification of high-risk patient groups, but the SAPS-II performed best overall across all studies.[71,76–80,82,84–86,97] Use of a modified ICMM at 72 hours after ICU admission provided enhanced discrimination since many patients with cancer do not exhibit their highest acuity at the time of admission like other ICU patients.[80] The Mortality Prediction Model (MPM) II showed sensitivity for mortality prediction when ICU patients were homogeneous in nature, but recent revisions and development of the MPM-III has been tested and validated on a wider range of patients.[87,88] On retrospective data from 2004 and 2005, the severity adjustment model MPM-III calibrates and discriminates across a broad population.[87,88] The application of the MPM-III scoring system in patients with cancer has not been tested. One published risk profile scoring system with a small patient series incorporated cancer- and treatment-related factors, comorbid health conditions, and general health and performance status to create a low, moderate, or high risk for critical illness category.[89] This clinical tool was not further developed or statistically validated.

Because of poor performance of these instruments in patients with sepsis, more recent researchers have attempted to incorporate the prognostic implications of organ failure into predictive models such as the Logistic Organ Failure (LOD), Sequential Organ Failure (SOFA) Score and Multiple Organ Dysfunction Score (MODS).[66,76,84,85,90,91] These scores have been compared with earlier models in an attempt to improve discrimination for predicting specific patients' outcomes. Calculation of organ dysfunction by these models has been successful in categorizing extremes in illness, but remains nonspecific in predicting patient outcomes.[75,77,79] However, they provide meaningful data for clinicians to use in conjunction with their expert judgment to counsel patients and families regarding the severity of their illness and possible outcomes.[76,90,91] Several studies have used these scales on a daily basis rather than on the first day of critical illness, so that trends can be identified.[68,85] This practice is especially important in patients with cancer, who are unlikely to experience their highest level of acuity on admission to the ICU like trauma or surgical ICU patients.[85,89] Even these more sophisticated scoring systems are flawed, and only the SOFA has the desirable sensitivity to predict outcome in patients with shock,[84] sepsis,[92,93] and hematologic malignancy.[76,94] A summary of all the prognostic scoring systems used for assessment of ICU severity of illness in patients with cancer is provided in **Table 1**.

SUMMARY AND RECOMMENDATIONS

There used to be a difference between patients with and without cancer using ICU resources and specific patient outcomes. In the ICU environment, patients with cancer constitute similar frequency of ICU admissions to other medical illnesses, which reflects a distribution of care similar to that seen with inpatient admissions and suggests that opinion biases regarding the appropriate use of critical care in patients with cancer has dissipated. Improved understanding of the interventions performed in select patients that will yield best outcomes has led to equalization of prognosis between patients with cancer and other medical ICU patients. The ICU is frequently used to support patients with cancer after surgery, those presenting with oncologic emergencies, acute treatment-related complications, immune compromise and serious infection, and when medical-surgical disorders become exacerbated. The most predictive influencers of outcome, such as status of the malignancy, degree of organ failure, and perceived reversibility of the crisis, should be considered when determining the appropriateness of critical care use.[5,14,23] Newly diagnosed patients in whom effective therapy has yet to be given or take effect and those with quiescent or disease remission remain the best candidates to receive critical care for any unexpected crisis. No clear scoring system has yet been developed that can prospectively predict survival or response to critical care interventions for patients with cancer. Without statistical guidance, the gold standard for decision-making regarding implementation of critical care for patients with cancer remains collaborative and proactive multidisciplinary planning, including oncology specialists, intensive care clinicians, and patients or their health care proxies.

REFERENCES

1. Shelton BK. Critical care of cancer patients: past, present and future. Semin Oncol Nurs 1994;10(3):146–55.
2. Azoulay E, Recher C, Alberti C, et al. Changing use of intensive care for hematological patients: the example of multiple myeloma. Intensive Care Med 1999; 25(12):1395–401.
3. Groeger JS, Aurora RN. Intensive care, mechanical ventilation, dialysis, and cardiopulmonary resuscitation. Implications for the patient with cancer. Crit Care Clin 2001;17(3):991–7.
4. Carlon GC. Admitting cancer patients to the intensive care unit. Crit Care Clin 1988;4(1):183–91.
5. Brenner H. Long-term survival rates for cancer patients achieved by the end of the 20th century: a period analysis. Lancet 2002;360(9340):1131–5.
6. LeCuyer L, Chevret S, Thiery G, et al. The ICU trial: a new admission policy for cancer patients requiring mechanical ventilation. Crit Care Med 2007;35: 808–14.
7. Raoof ND, Groeger JS. You never know–one of your patients with cancer might surprise you. Crit Care Med 2007;35(3):965–6.
8. Markou N, Demopoulou E, Myrianthefs P. The critically ill patient with cancer–indications for Intensive Care Unit admission and outcomes. J BUON 2008; 13(4):469–78.
9. Azoulay E, Alberti C, Bornstain C, et al. Improved survival in cancer patients requiring mechanical ventilatory support: impact of non-invasive mechanical ventilatory support. Crit Care Med 2001;29:519–25.
10. Guidelines for intensive care admission, discharge and triage. Task Force of the American College of Critical Care Medicine, Society of Intensive Care Medicine. Crit Care Med 1999;27:633–8.
11. Ganz PA, Casillas J, Hahn EE. Ensuring quality care for cancer survivors: implementing the survivorship care plan. Semin Oncol Nurs 2008;24(3):208–17.
12. Alkire K, Shelton BK. Creating critical care oncology beds. Semin Oncol Nurs 1994;10(3):208–21.
13. Shelton BK, Baker L, Stecker S. Critical care of the patient with hematologic malignancy. AACN Clin Issues 1996;7(1):65–78.
14. Seshamani M, Gray A. Time to death and health expenditure: an improved model for the impact of demographic change on health care costs. Age Ageing 2004;33(6):556–61.
15. Guidelines for developing admission and discharge policies for the pediatric intensive care unit. Pediatric Section Task Force on Admission and Discharge Criteria, Society of Critical Care Medicine in conjunction with the American

College of Critical Care Medicine and the Committee on Hospital Care of the American Academy of Pediatrics. Crit Care Med 1999;27(4):843–5.

16. Garrouste-Orgeas M, Montuclard L, Timsit JF, et al. Predictors of intensive care unit refusal in French intensive care units: a multiple-center study. Crit Care Med 2005;33:750–5.
17. Anzoulay E, Moreau D, Alberti C, et al. Predictors of short-term mortality in critically ill patients with solid malignancies. Intensive Care Med 2000;26:1817–23.
18. Azoulay E, Pochard F, Chevret S, et al. Compliance with triage to intensive care recommendations. Crit Care Med 2001;29(11):2132–6.
19. Walter KL, Siegler M, Hall JB. How decisions are made to admit patients to medical intensive care units (MICUs): a survey of MICU directors at academic medical centers across the United States. Crit Care Med 2008;36(2):414–20.
20. Elinav S, Soudry E, Levin PD, et al. Intensive care physicians' attitudes concerning distribution of intensive care resources. A comparison of Israeli, North American and European cohorts. Intensive Care Med 2004;30(6):1140–3.
21. Haines IE, Zalcberg J, Buchanan JD. Not-for-resuscitation orders in cancer patients–principles of decision-making. Med J Aust 1990;153:225–9.
22. Azoulay E, Afessa B. The intensive care support of patients with malignancy: do everything that can be done. Intensive Care Med 2006;32:3–5.
23. Shelton BK. Critical care of patients with cancer. Am J Nurs 2000;100(4):24AA–24BB.
24. Azoulay E, Thiery G, Chevret S, et al. The prognosis of acute respiratory failure in critically ill cancer patients. Medicine 2004;83(6):360–70.
25. Staudinger T, Stoiser B, Maxllner M, et al. Outcome and prognostic factors in critically ill cancer patients admitted to the intensive care unit. Crit Care Med 2000;28(5):1322–8.
26. Estopa R, Kastanos N, Rives A, et al. Acute respiratory failure in severe hematologic disorders. Crit Care Med 1984;12:26–8.
27. Pastores SM. Acute respiratory failure in critically ill patients with cancer. Diagnosis and management. Crit Care Clin 2001;17(3):623–46.
28. Kress JP, Christenson J, Pohlman AS, et al. Outcomes of critically ill cancer patients in a university hospital setting. Am J Respir Crit Care Med 1999;160(6):1957–61.
29. Afessa B, Tefferi A, Litzow MR, et al. Outcome of diffuse alveolar hemorrhage in hematopoietic stem cell transplant recipients. Am J Respir Crit Care Med 2002;166(10):1364–8.
30. Groeger JS, White P Jr, Nierman DM, et al. Outcome for cancer patients requiring mechanical ventilation. J Clin Oncol 1999;17(3):991–7.
31. Leath CA 3rd, Kendrick JE 4th, Numnum TM, et al. Outcomes of gynecologic oncology patients admitted to the intensive care unit following surgery: a university teaching hospital experience. Int J Gynecol Cancer 2006;16:1766–9.
32. McDowelll I In: Measuring health: a guide to rating scales and questionnaires, vol. 3. London: Oxford University Press; 2006.
33. Boussat S, El'rini T, Dubiez A, et al. Predictive factors of death in primary lung cancer patients on admission to the intensive care unit. Intensive Care Med 2000;26:1811–6.
34. Faber-Langendoen K, Caplan AL, McGlave PB. Survival of adult bone marrow transplant patients receiving mechanical ventilation: a case for restricted use. Bone Marrow Transplant 1993;12(5):501–7.
35. Paz HL, Garland A, Weinar M, et al. Effect of clinical outcomes data on intensive care utilization by bone marrow transplant patients. Crit Care Med 1998;26:66–70.

36. Paz HL, Crilley P, Weinar M, et al. Outcome of patients requiring medical ICU admission following bone marrow transplantation. Chest 1993;104(2):527–31.

37. Price KJ, Thall PF, Kish SK, et al. Prognostic indicators for blood and marrow transplant patients admitted to an intensive care unit. Am J Respir Crit Care Med 1998;158:876–84.

38. Khassawneh BY, White P Jr, Anaissie EJ, et al. Outcome from mechanical ventilation after autologous peripheral blood stem cell transplantation. Chest 2002; 121(1):185–8.

39. Pene F, Aubron C, Azoulay E, et al. Outcome of critically ill allogeneic hematopoietic stem-cell transplantation recipients: a reappraisal of indications for organ failure. J Clin Oncol 2006;24(4):643–9.

40. van Gestel JPJ, Bollen CW, van der Tweel I, et al. Intensive care unit mortality trends in children after hematopoietic stem cell transplantation: a meta-regression analysis. Crit Care Med 2008;36(10):2898–904.

41. Torrecilla C, Cortes JL, Chamorro C, et al. Prognostic assessment of the acute complications of bone marrow transplantation requiring intensive therapy. Intensive Care Med 1988;14(4):393–8.

42. Shorr AF, Moores LK, Edenfield WJ, et al. Mechanical ventilation in hematopoietic stem cell transplantation: can we effectively predict outcomes? Chest 1999; 116(4):1012–8.

43. Afessa B, Tefferi A, Dunn WF, et al. Intensive care unit support and acute physiology and chronic health evaluation III performance in hematopoietic stem cell transplant recipients. Crit Care Med 2003;31(6):1715–21.

44. Kew AK, Couban S, Patrick W, et al. Outcome of hematopoietic stem cell transplant recipients admitted to the intensive care unit. Bone Marrow Transplant 2006;12:301–5.

45. Huaringa AJ, Leyva FJ, Giralt SA, et al. Outcome of bone marrow transplantation patients requiring mechanical ventilation. Crit Care Med 2000;28(4):1232–4.

46. Soubani AO, Kseibi E, Bander JJ, et al. Outcome and prognostic factors of hematopoietic stem cell transplantation recipients admitted to a medical ICU. Chest 2004;126(5):1604–11.

47. Bach PB, Schrag D, Nierman DM, et al. Identification of poor prognostic features among patients requiring mechanical ventilation after hematopoietic stem cell transplantation. Blood 2001;98(12):3234–40.

48. Van Gerpen R. Chemotherapy and biotherapy-induced hypersensitivity reactions. J Infus Nurs 2009;32(3):157–65.

49. Gobel B. Hypersensitivity reactions to biological drugs. Semin Oncol Nurs 2005; 23(3):191–200.

50. Viale PH. Management of hypersensitivity reactions: a nursing perspective. Oncology (Williston Park) 2009;23(2 Suppl 1):26–30.

51. Tanvetyanon T. Consideration before administering cytotoxic chemotherapy to the critically ill. Crit Care Med 2005;33(11):2689–91.

52. Benoit DD, Depuydt PO, Vanderwoude KH, et al. Outcome in severely ill patients with hematological malignancies who received intravenous chemotherapy in the intensive care unit. Intensive Care Med 2005;32(1):93–9.

53. Darmon M, Thiery G, Ciroldi M, et al. Intensive care in patients with newly diagnosed malignancies and a need for cancer chemotherapy. Crit Care Med 2005; 33(11):2689–91.

54. Turnbull AD, Graziano C, Baron R, et al. The inverse relationship between cost and survival in the critically ill cancer patient. Crit Care Med 1979;7: 20–3.

55. Snow RM, Miller WC, Rice DL, et al. Respiratory failure in cancer patients. JAMA 1979;241:2039–42.
56. Hauser MJ, Tabak J, Baier H. Survival of patients with cancer in a medical critical care unit. Arch Intern Med 1982;142:527–9.
57. Schuster DP, Marion JM. Precedents for meaningful recovery during treatment in a medical intensive care unit. Outcomes for patients with hematologic malignancy. Am J Med 1983;75(3):402–8.
58. Cox SC, Norwood SH, Duncan CA. Acute respiratory failure: mortality associated with underlying disease. Crit Care Med 1985;13:1005–8.
59. Johnson MH, Gordon PW, Fitzgerald FT. Stratification of prognosis in granulocytopenic patients with hematologic malignancies using the APACHE-II severity of illness score. Crit Care Med 1986;14(8):693–7.
60. Ewer MS, Ali MK, Atta MS. Outcome of lung cancer patients requiring mechanical ventilation for pulmonary failure. JAMA 1986;256:3364–6.
61. Lloyd-Thomas AR, Wright I, Lister TA, et al. Prognosis of patients receiving intensive care for life-threatening complications of hematologic malignancy. Br Med J 1988;296:1025–9.
62. Butt W, Barker G, Walker C, et al. Outcome of children with hematologic malignancy who are admitted to an intensive care unit. Crit Care Med 1988;16:761–4.
63. Peters SG, Meadows JA, Gracey DR. Outcome of respiratory failure in hematologic malignancy. Chest 1988;94:99–102.
64. Moran JL, Soloman PJ, Williams PJ. Assessment of outcome over a 10-year period of patients admitted to a multidisciplinary adult intensive care unit with haematological and solid tumors. Anaesth Intensive Care 2005;33(1):26–35.
65. Slonim AD, Patel KM, Ruttimann UE, et al. Cardiopulmonary resuscitation in pediatric intensive care units. Crit Care Med 1997;25(12):1951–5.
66. Larche J, Azoulay E, Fieux F, et al. Improved survival of critically ill cancer patients with septic shock. Intensive Care Med 2003;29(10):1688–95.
67. Chalfin DB, Carlon GC. Age and utilization of intensive care unit resources of critically ill cancer patients. Crit Care Med 1990;18(7):694–8.
68. Wallace SK, Ewer MS, Price KJ, et al. Outcome and cost implications of cardiopulmonary resuscitation in the medical intensive care unit of a comprehensive cancer center. Support Care Cancer 2002;10(5):425–9.
69. Berghmans T, Meert AP, Markiewicz E, et al. Continuous venovenous haemofiltration in cancer patients with renal failure: a single-centre experience. Support Care Cancer 2004;12(5):306–11.
70. Ewer MS, Kish SK, Martin CG, et al. Characteristics of cardiac arrest in cancer patients as a predictor of survival after cardiopulmonary resuscitation. Cancer 2001;92(7):1905–12.
71. den Boer S, de Keizer NF, de Jonge E. Performance of prognostic models in critically ill cancer patients–a review. Crit Care 2005;9(4):R458–63.
72. Vitelli CE, Cooper K, Rogatkp A, et al. Cardiopulmonary resuscitation and the patient with cancer. J Clin Oncol 1991;9(1):111–5.
73. Agha-Razii M, Amyot SL, Pichette V, et al. Continuous veno-venous hemodiafiltration for the treatment of spontaneous tumor lysis syndrome complicated by acute renal failure and severe hyperuricemia. Clin Nephrol 2000;54(1):59–63.
74. DiCarlo JV, Alexander SR, Agarwal R, et al. Continuous veno-venous hemofiltration may improve survival from acute respiratory distress syndrome after bone marrow transplantation or chemotherapy. J Pediatr Hematol Oncol 2003;25(10):801–5.

75. Sinuff T, Adhikari NK, Cook DJ, et al. Mortality predictions in the intensive care unit: comparing physicians with scoring systems. Crit Care Med 2006;34(3):878–85.
76. Metnitz PG, Lang T, Valentin A, et al. Evaluation of the logistic organ dysfunction system for the assessment of organ dysfunction and mortality in critically ill patients. Intensive Care Med 2001;27:992–8.
77. Minne L, Abu-Hanna A, de Jonge E. Evaluation of SOFA-based models for predicting mortality in the ICU: a systematic review. Crit Care 2008;12: R161–74.
78. Guiguet M, Blot F, Escudier B, et al. Severity-of-illness scores for neutropenic cancer patients in an intensive care unit: which is the best predictor? Do multiple assessment times improve the predictive value? Crit Care Med 1998;26(3): 488–93.
79. Le Gall JR, Neumann A, Hemery F, et al. Mortality prediction using SAPS II: an update for French intensive care units. Crit Care 2005;9:R645–52.
80. Groeger JS, Glassman J, Nierman DM, et al. Probability of mortality of critically ill cancer patients at 72 h of intensive care unit (ICU) management. Support Care Cancer 2003;11:686–95.
81. Schellongowski P, Benesch M, Lang T, et al. Comparison of three severity scores for critically ill cancer patients. Intensive Care Med 2004;30:430–6.
82. Groeger JS, Lemeshow S, Price K, et al. Multicenter outcome study of cancer patients admitted to the intensive care unit: a probability of mortality model. J Clin Oncol 1998;16:761–70.
83. Soares M, Fontes F, Dantas J, et al. Performance of six severity of illness scores in cancer patients requiring admission to the intensive care unit: a prospective observational study. Crit Care Med 2004;8:R194–203.
84. Peres BD, Melot C, Lopes Ferreira F, et al. The Multiple Organ Dysfunction Score (MODS) versus the Sequential Organ Failure Assessment (SOFA) score in outcome prediction. Intensive Care Med 2002;28(11):1619–24.
85. Timsit JF, Fosse JP, Troche G, et al. Calibration and discrimination by daily logistic organ dysfunction scoring comparatively with daily sequential organ failure assessment scoring for predicting hospital mortality in critically ill patients. Crit Care Med 2002;30(9):2003–13.
86. Soares M, Salluh JI. Validation of the SAPS 3 admission prognostic model in patients with cancer in need of intensive care. Intensive Care Med 2006;32: 1839–44.
87. Higgins TL, Kramer AA, Nathanson BH, et al. Prospective validation of the intensive care unit admission Mortality Probability Model (MPM$_0$-III). Crit Care Med 2009;37(5):1619–23.
88. Nathanson BH, Higgins TL, Kramer AA, et al. Subgroup mortality probability models: are they necessary for specialized intensive care units? Crit Care Med 2009;37(8):2375–86.
89. Shelton BK. Preventing crises in the patient with cancer. Oncol Nurs Forum 2000;27(6):905–13.
90. Moreno R, Matos R. Outcome predictions in intensive care. Solving the paradox. Intensive Care Med 2001;27:962–4.
91. Timsit JF, Fosse JP, Troche G, et al. Accuracy of a composite score using daily SAPS II and LOD scores for predicting hospital mortality in ICU patients hospitalized for more than 72 h. Intensive Care Med 2001;27(6):1012–21.
92. Arabi Y, Al Shirawi N, Memish Z, et al. Assessment of six mortality prediction models in patients admitted with severe sepsis and septic shock to the intensive care unit: a prospective cohort study. Crit Care 2003;7:R116–22.

93. Santolaya ME, Alvarez AM, Aviles CL, et al. Predictors of severe sepsis not clinically apparent during the first twenty-four hours of hospitalization in children with cancer, neutropenia, and fever: a prospective, multicenter trial. Pediatr Infect Dis J 2008;27(6):538–43.

94. Silfvast T, Pettila V, Ihalainen A, et al. Multiple organ failure and outcome of critically ill patients with haematological malignancy. Acta Anaesthesiol Scand 2003;47(3):301–6.

95. Ho KM. Combining sequential organ failure assessment (SOFA) score with acute physiologic and chronic health evaluation (APACHE) II score to predict hospital mortality of critically ill patients. Anaesth Intensive Care 2007;35(4):515–21.

96. Owczuk R, Wujtewicz MA, Sawicka W, et al. Patients with haematological malignancies requiring invasive mechanical ventilation: differences between survivors and non-survivors in intensive care unit. Support Care Cancer 2004;13(5):332–8.

97. Sculier JP, Paesmans M, Markiewicz E, et al. Scoring systems in cancer patients admitted for an acute complication in a medical intensive care unit. Crit Care Med 2000;28(8):2786–92.

98. Thakkar SG, Fu AZ, Sweetenham JW, et al. Survival and predictors of outcome in patients with acute leukemia admitted to the intensive care unit. Cancer 2008;112(10):2233–40.

99. Adda M, Coquet I, Darmon M, et al. Predictors of noninvasive ventilation in patients with hematologic malignancy and acute respiratory failure. Crit Care Med 2008;36(10):2766–72.

100. Benoit DD, Vanderwoude RH, Decruyenaere JM, et al. Outcome and early prognostic indicators in patients with a hematologic malignancy admitted to the intensive care unit with a life-threatening complication. Crit Care Med 2003;31(1):104–12.

101. Berghmans T, Paesmans M, Sculier JP. Is a specific oncological scoring system better at predicting the prognosis of cancer patients admitted for an acute medical complication in an intensive care unit than general gravity scores? Support Care Cancer 2004;12(4):234–9.

102. Kroschinsky F, Weise M, Illmer T, et al. Outcome and prognostic features of intensive care unit treatment in patients with hematological malignancies. Intensive Care Med 2002;28(9):1294–300.

103. Rabbat A, Chaoui D, Montani D, et al. Prognosis of patients with acute myeloid leukaemia admitted to intensive care. Br J Haematol 2005;129(3):350–7.

Acute Respiratory Failure in the Patient with Cancer: Diagnostic and Management Strategies

Stephen M. Pastores, MD, FACP, FCCP, FCCM*, Louis P. Voigt, MD, FCCP

KEYWORDS

- Respiratory failure • Cancer • Diagnosis • Management
- Mechanical ventilation • Intensive care
- Critical care • Outcome

Acute respiratory failure (ARF) is the commonest cause for admission to the intensive care unit (ICU) in patients with cancer and is usually associated with a poor outcome, especially in those patients who require mechanical ventilation (MV) for severe acute lung injury (ALI).[1–15] Among patients with hematologic and solid malignancies, the incidence of ARF has ranged from 10% to 50%,[3,15] with an overall mortality of 50%, rising to 75% in those who require MV.[3,4,14–17] Among hematopoietic stem cell transplant (HSCT) recipients requiring MV and ICU admission, the incidence of ARF ranges from 42% to 88% with an overall survival rate of approximately only 15% in those receiving MV.[18–27] The epidemiology, prognostic risk factors, and outcomes of adult cancer patients and among HSCT recipients who develop ARF requiring MV are discussed in greater detail in separate articles in this issue of the *Clinics*.

In recent years, several studies have reported an increase in survival rates in cancer patients requiring MV for ARF.[3,4,28] Investigators have attributed these higher survival rates to recent advances in oncology and critical care in conjunction with more appropriate selection of cancer patients for ICU admission. This article focuses on the major causes of ARF in adult patients with cancer and discusses recent advances in

Conflict of Interest: None.
Financial Support: None.
Department of Anesthesiology and Critical Care Medicine, Memorial Sloan-Kettering Cancer Center, 1275 York Avenue C1179, New York, NY 10065, USA
* Corresponding author.
E-mail address: pastores@mskcc.org (S.M. Pastores).

the diagnostic and management approaches of these disorders in the critical care setting.

CAUSES OF ARF IN PATIENTS WITH CANCER

The myriad causes of ARF in critically ill patients with cancer are listed in **Table 1**. The most frequent causes include pulmonary infections (pneumonia), cardiogenic and noncardiogenic pulmonary edema (ALI/acute respiratory distress syndrome [ARDS]), antineoplastic therapy (chemotherapy, radiation therapy)-induced lung injury, cancer-related medical disorders (such as venous thromboembolism [VTE] and diffuse alveolar hemorrhage [DAH]), direct involvement of the respiratory system by malignancy (eg, airway obstruction), and progression of underlying disease.[4,29,30] Respiratory failure may also occur postoperatively because of atelectasis, pneumonia, pulmonary edema, and development of bronchopleural fistula, particularly in patients undergoing thoracic cancer surgery such as intrapericardial or extrapleural pneumonectomy and esophagectomy.[31–33] Direct involvement of the respiratory system by malignancy resulting in upper or lower airway obstruction and its management is discussed in a separate article on oncologic emergencies in this issue.

PNEUMONIA

Pulmonary infections are the most common cause of ARF in patients with cancer, especially in those with significant comorbidities (eg, chronic obstructive pulmonary disease, cardiac failure), underlying hematologic malignancies, and in those receiving chemotherapy.[34–36] Several factors increase the risk of infection in these patients, including defects in humoral or cell-mediated immunity, neutropenia, use of corticosteroids, frequent exposure to antibiotics, and prolonged hospitalization.

The major organisms causing pneumonia in patients with cancer and impaired humoral (B-cell) immunity such as those with acute and chronic lymphocytic leukemia and multiple myeloma are *Streptococcus pneumoniae* and *Haemophilus influenzae*. In contrast, in patients with cancer and impaired cell-mediated (T-cell) immunity such as those with Hodgkin disease and those receiving high-dose corticosteroids, the predominant organisms are *Pneumocystis jiroveci* (pneumocystis pneumonia [PCP]), mycobacteria, *Cryptococcus* and other pathogenic fungi, *Legionella pneumophila*, and herpes virus (especially cytomegalovirus [CMV]). In patients with chemotherapy-induced neutropenia, pneumonia is usually caused by *Staphylococcus aureus*, *Streptococcus pneumoniae*, gram-negative enteric bacilli (*Pseudomonas aeruginosa* and *Klebsiella pneumoniae*), and opportunistic fungi (especially *Aspergillus*).[37] Among patients with obstructive lung cancer and those who are neutropenic, exposed to broad-spectrum antibiotics and require prolonged MV, *Stenotrophomonas maltophilia* has become an increasing concern given the high rate of antimicrobial resistance and mortality associated with this infection.[38,39]

Patients with cancer who develop bacterial pneumonia tend to have atypical clinical presentations. Although fever is common, cough and sputum production are not. The initial chest radiograph may be normal or demonstrate diffuse interstitial infiltrates; the classic lobar consolidation that is observed in patients who do not have cancer with bacterial pneumonia is often missing.

Bacterial pneumonia may also result from aspiration of pharyngeal or gastric contents in patients who have cancer, especially those with head and neck or esophageal cancers and those who have difficulty clearing their secretions, have dysfunction of the upper airway from laryngeal nerve involvement, or require a tracheostomy. Oncologic patients are usually malnourished, debilitated, and often on prolonged bed rest,

Table 1
Causes of ARF in patients who have cancer

Central Nervous System and Neuromuscular Disorders	Chest Wall and Pleural Disorders	Vascular Disorders	Airway Disorders	Parenchymal Disorders

Drug intoxications
• Narcotics
• Sedatives
• Neuroleptics
Encephalopathies
• Infections
• Metabolic
• Derangements
• Seizures
Intracranial tumors
• Primary
• Metastatic
Neuropathies/myopathies
• Nerve palsies
• Paraneoplastic Syndromes
  - Eaton-Lambert syndrome
  - Myasthenia gravis
  - Guillain-Barré syndrome
	Pleural disorders
	• Malignant pleural effusions
	• Pleural tumors (primary or metastatic)
	• Tension pneumothorax
	Chest wall disorders
	• Chest wall tumors (primary or metastatic)
	• Rib fractures
		Pulmonary thromboembolism
		• VTE
		• Tumor embolism
		• Pulmonary venooc-clusive disease
			Malignant airway obstruction
			• Endobronchial metastases
			• External airway compression
			• Primary tumors of periglottic area
			Others
			• Tracheoesophageal fistula
			• Bronchiolitis obliterans
				Pneumonitis
				• Infections
				• Chemotherapy
				• Radiation therapy
				• Aspiration
				ALI/ARDS
				• Infection
				• Chemotherapy
				• Radiation
				• Transfusion
				Unique complications of HSCT recipients
				• Periengraftment respiratory distress syndrome
				• DAH
				• Idiopathic pneumonia syndrome
				Miscellaneous
				• Lymphangitic carcinomatosis
				• Pulmonary leukostasis
				• Bronchiolitis obliterans organizing pneumonia

are receiving enteral feedings in the supine position, have central nervous system metastases, or require large amounts of narcotic agents for pain control, all of which predispose them to a higher risk of aspiration.[29]

Fungal pneumonia typically occurs in the setting of prolonged neutropenia, treatment with corticosteroids and broad-spectrum antibiotics, and underlying leukemia or lymphoma. *Aspergillus* pneumonia can be a fulminant disease, manifesting with chest pain, dyspnea, and hemoptysis. The chest radiograph may show patchy bronchopneumonia, multiple nodular densities, and peripheral, wedged-shaped infiltrates, and a characteristic halo or air-crescent sign may be seen on computed tomography (CT) scans. Persistently febrile neutropenic patients with pulmonary infiltrates who have *Aspergillus* spp recovered from a respiratory culture (sputum or bronchoalveolar lavage [BAL]) have a high probability of invasive pulmonary aspergillosis and require antifungal therapy.

Identifying the exact cause of pneumonia in patients with cancer with pulmonary infiltrates often requires fiberoptic bronchoscopy with BAL or lung biopsy, as sputum is seldom produced.[37] The overall diagnostic yield of BAL in neutropenic and nonneutropenic nontransplant patients with suspected pneumonia is 49% and 63%, respectively, and only 38% in neutropenic transplant recipients.[40] In neutropenic patients with hematologic malignancies and pulmonary infiltrates, protected specimen brush and protected BAL did not yield better diagnostic results compared with BAL.[41] Other investigators have shown that surgical lung biopsy in patients with hematologic malignancies may provide a specific diagnosis and lead to a significant change in therapy.[42,43]

Pneumocystis jiroveci (formerly known as *Pneumocystis carinii*) pneumonia (PCP) continues to occur frequently in patients with cancer with the use of more intensive treatment regimens and new anticancer and immunomodulating agents.[44] Mortality from PCP is high among patients with lymphoproliferative malignancies and solid tumors receiving long-term corticosteroids.[45,46] The usual presentation is of a subacute, febrile, severe bilateral pneumonia with radiographic evidence of bilateral ground-glass pattern of interstitial infiltrates.[47] The diagnosis of PCP is usually obtained by detection of *P jiroveci* by conventional staining methods (direct and indirect fluorescence antibody and toluidine blue O, Grocott-Gomori silver stain, or Giemsa stains) in samples of induced sputum, BAL fluid, or lung biopsies. Although induced sputum has a high yield for diagnosing PCP in patients infected with the human immunodeficiency virus, its diagnostic sensitivity in patients with cancer is low. *P jiroveci* polymerase chain reaction (PCR) on induced sputum has recently been shown to have excellent sensitivity and negative predictive value and may obviate bronchoscopy in some patients.[48] Trimethoprim-sulfamethoxazole or intravenous (IV) pentamidine with adjunctive corticosteroid therapy to suppress lung inflammation in patients with severe PCP remains the preferred treatment. Atovaquone may be used in patients with mild or moderate PCP who are unable to tolerate trimethoprim-sulfamethoxazole.

CMV, respiratory syncytial virus (RSV), influenza viruses A and B, parainfluenza virus, human adenoviruses, human parainfluenza viruses 1 to 3, human enteroviruses, human rhinoviruses, and the recently discovered human metapneumoviruses are all important causes of pneumonias in patients who have cancer. CMV pneumonia is a particularly serious infection, especially in solid organ and HSCT recipients.[49–52] Fever, nonproductive cough, and dyspnea are common presenting symptoms. Radiographic patterns in CMV pneumonia include lobar consolidation, focal parenchymal haziness, and bilateral reticulonodular infiltrates.[53] CT may reveal ground-glass opacification, bronchial wall thickening, reticular opacities, and nodules. The diagnosis of CMV pneumonia is usually obtained from viral shell vial culture and conventional culture of BAL samples. Pneumonias caused by RSV and influenzae viruses are often encountered during the fall and winter months. In addition to routine fluorescent anti-body testing, PCR testing of respiratory secretions is specific and reliable.[54] Thera-peutic modalities for these viral infections are limited to a few agents (eg, ganciclovir or foscarnet for CMV pneumonia, aerosolized ribavirin for RSV pneumonia) used alone or in combination with IV immunoglobulin (IVIg).

ALI AND ARDS

ALI is a clinical syndrome characterized by the acute onset of severe hypoxemia (as defined by a ratio of the partial pressure of arterial oxygen to the fraction of inspired oxygen [P_{AO_2}/F_{IO_2}] <300) and the presence of bilateral alveolar or interstitial infiltrates in the absence of congestive heart failure.[55] ARDS is a more severe form of lung injury defined by a P_{AO_2}/F_{IO_2} ratio less than 200. Atypical presentation of ARDS with unilateral infiltrates on chest radiograph is noteworthy, particularly in patients with bullous emphysema or in those who have undergone lung resection.

Recent screening studies of patients with ARDS indicate an annual incidence of 13 to 24 cases per 100,000 of the general population.[56–58] In patients with cancer, the exact incidence is unknown but those with sepsis, aspiration of gastric contents, multiple transfusions of blood products, and pneumonia are at high risk for developing ARDS.[59] ALI/ARDS remains the most serious pulmonary complication in patients undergoing lung resection for lung cancer.[60–62] In patients undergoing HSCT, ARDS may also occur from engraftment syndrome or idiopathic pneumonia syndrome.

Pathologically, ALI/ARDS is characterized by diffuse alveolar damage associated with increased permeability of the alveolar-capillary membrane.[63] The hallmark lesion is widespread destruction of the alveolar epithelium and flooding of the alveolar spaces with proteinaceous exudates containing large numbers of neutrophils. In some patients, ARDS resolves after the acute phase, but in many others it generally progresses to the fibrosing alveolitis phase, with persistent hypoxemia, increased alveolar dead space, worsening of lung compliance, and development of severe pulmonary hypertension and right heart failure. Gradual resolution of hypoxemia and improvement in lung compliance characterize the recovery phase.

Although clinical and experimental studies have provided circumstantial evidence of the occurrence of neutrophil-mediated injury in ARDS,[64] neutropenic patients with cancer can develop ARDS, although the neutropenia does not seem to worsen their outcomes.[65] In addition, among neutropenic patients who received granulocyte colony-stimulating factor to increase the number of circulating neutrophils, the incidence or severity of ALI did not increase.[66]

Treatment of ARDS is directed at the underlying cause, if known, and supportive care with MV and prevention and treatment of infections, gastrointestinal hemorrhage and VTE, hemodynamic management, and nutritional support. The ARDS Network studies[67–72] demonstrated that survival of patients with ALI/ARDS can be significantly increased by adhering to pressure- and volume-limited ventilation strategy (targeting tidal volumes of 6 mL/kg of predicted body weight and limiting plateau airway pressures to 30 cm of water or <) and by a conservative strategy of fluid management. In a study of 61 patients with ALI or ARDS, Talmor and colleagues[73] reported that a ventilator strategy using esophageal pressures to estimate the transpulmonary pressure significantly improved oxygenation and compliance in these patients. However, further trials are necessary to confirm the feasibility and clinical benefit of this strategy.

Although an earlier randomized trial suggested benefit with the use of moderate dose methylprednisolone treatment (2 mg/kg/d) for unresolving ARDS,[74] an ARDS Network multicenter randomized controlled trial[75] failed to show benefit in late-phase

ARDS and was associated with a higher rate of neuromuscular weakness. Furthermore, the investigators suggested that corticosteroids may be harmful when initiated more than 2 weeks after the onset of ARDS. However, in a follow-up study, Hough and colleagues[76] did not find a significant association between methylprednisolone treatment and neuromyopathy among 128 survivors of persistent ARDS in the ARDS Network trial. Several investigators have argued that prolonged corticosteroid treatment ($\geq$7 days) substantially and significantly improves meaningful patient-centered outcome variables, and has a distinct survival benefit when initiated before day 14 of ARDS.[77] Other pharmacologic agents such as prostaglandin E, prostacyclin, ketoconazole, lisofylline, procysteine, aerosolized surfactant, and inhaled nitric oxide have also not been shown to have any survival benefit in adult patients with ARDS.

During the past decade, the mortality in ARDS has been observed to decrease to approximately 40%.[78] Investigators have attributed this decline to more effective therapies for sepsis, protective ventilation strategies, increased use of noninvasive positive pressure ventilation (NIPPV), and overall improvements in standard supportive therapy.[79] Adverse risk factors predictive of death at the onset of ARDS include sepsis, chronic liver disease, advanced age, and nonpulmonary organ dysfunction. In most patients who survive the episode of ARDS, pulmonary function usually returns to normal within 6 to 12 months. Patients with severe disease and those requiring prolonged ventilatory support may develop persistent abnormalities in pulmonary function, manifested by mild restriction, airway obstruction, gas exchange abnormalities with exercise, or decreases in the diffusing capacity for carbon monoxide and disabling muscle weakness and neuropsychiatric deficiencies.[80–83] Recent studies have shown the beneficial impact of daily interruption of sedation and spontaneous breathing trials (wake up and breathe protocol) and of early mobilization of mechanically ventilated patients and placed renewed enthusiasm in pursuing a comprehensive multifaceted strategy to curtail long-term complications from ARDS.[84–86]

ANTINEOPLASTIC AGENT-INDUCED LUNG INJURY

Pulmonary toxicity from antineoplastic agents is an important cause of respiratory failure in patients who have cancer. The various clinical syndromes associated with antineoplastic-induced lung injury include acute interstitial pneumonitis, ALI/ARDS, capillary leak syndrome, organizing pneumonia, hypersensitivity reaction, bronchospasm, and DAH. A listing of the most common chemotherapeutic and immunosuppressive agents associated with pulmonary toxicity can be found at http://www.pneumotox.com. A review of the pulmonary complications of novel antineoplastic agents has also been published recently.[87]

Nonproductive cough, exertional dyspnea, and low-grade fever are usually present and gradually develop for several weeks during treatment with the chemotherapeutic agent but also may occur as late as several months after completion of treatment. Bilateral inspiratory crackles at the lung bases may be heard on chest auscultation, reduced lung volumes and diffusing capacity are present on pulmonary function testing, and diffuse or patchy ground-glass opacities or consolidations are seen on chest radiograph and chest CT. Other common nonspecific laboratory findings include leukocytosis, increased erythrocyte sedimentation rate, and increased levels of C-reactive protein and serum Krebs von den Lungen-6 (KL-6) levels.[88] In patients who have previously received radiation to the chest, radiation recall pneumonitis may occur. This syndrome is manifested by fever, cough, dyspnea, and hypoxemia in association with radiographic findings of pulmonary infiltrates in the same field as in the previous radiation therapy. Antineoplastic agents that have been associated with radiation recall pneumonitis include doxorubicin, etoposide, paclitaxel, gemcitabine, and trastuzumab.[87]

Diagnostic evaluation requires integration of the history, physical findings, physiologic and imaging studies, and results of bronchoscopy with BAL, which is often necessary to rule out opportunistic infection, alveolar hemorrhage, or tumor progression or recurrence. In most cases, antineoplastic agent-induced lung injury is a diagnosis of exclusion. Definitive diagnosis usually is made with the findings of atypia of alveolar lining cells, interstitial inflammation, and fibrosis observed on lung specimens obtained by transbronchial or open-lung biopsy in conjunction with the history.

General principles of management include cessation of the implicated antineoplastic agent, avoiding high levels of supplemental oxygen (in bleomycin or mitomycin), and treatment with systemic corticosteroids (methylprednisolone 240 mg IV daily in divided doses in less severe cases to 1 g daily in patients with respiratory failure).[89]

VTE

VTE, manifested as either deep venous thrombosis (DVT) or pulmonary embolism (PE), remains an important and major cause of morbidity and mortality in patients with cancer.[90,91] When adjusted for disease prevalence, the malignancies most strongly associated with thrombotic complications are those of the pancreas, ovary, and brain.[92] Several factors or conditions increase the risk for DVT and PE in patients with cancer, including intrinsic tumor procoagulant activity, antineoplastic drugs (such as platinum compounds, angiogenesis inhibitors, and growth factors), selective estrogen receptor modulators (tamoxifen, raloxifene), surgery, immobilization, and indwelling central venous catheters.[93]

Similar to patients who do not have cancer, patients with cancer who develop PE may present with shortness of breath, pleuritic chest pain, palpitations, dysrhythmias, unexplained hypoxemia, and pleural effusion. CT is currently the diagnostic imaging modality of choice in patients with suspected PE.[94,95] The Prospective Investigation of Pulmonary Embolism Diagnosis II (PIOPED II), which used only multirow detector CT, reported sensitivity and specificity rates of 83% and 96%, respectively.[96] Lower extremity venous ultrasonography demonstrating DVT may support a clinical diagnosis of PE when other imaging modalities are nondiagnostic. Although the measurement of D-dimer levels may assist in guiding the need for diagnostic imaging in patients with low probability for PE, a negative D-dimer test result does not reliably exclude DVT in patients with cancer because the negative predictive value of the test is significantly lower than in patients without cancer.[97] A diagnostic algorithm with a dichotomized version of the Wells clinical decision rule, D-dimer testing, and CT has recently been shown to be useful in guiding therapeutic decisions in almost 98% of patients with clinically suspected PE.[98]

Anticoagulation therapy for PE in patients who have cancer can be challenging because these patients are at higher risk of recurrent VTE than are patients who do not have cancer with thrombosis and also have a greater risk for anticoagulant-associated bleeding complications while receiving therapy to prevent recurrent VTE.[99] Additional treatment considerations include how to manage anticoagulant therapy around the time of invasive procedures; whether to initiate anticoagulation in a patient with a short life-expectancy, or when to discontinue such therapy; and when to use thrombolytic agents or insert inferior vena cava (IVC) filters.[100] These concerns mandate that anticoagulant therapy in patients with cancer be individualized and based on overall therapeutic and palliative goals of care. Unfractionated heparin

(UFH) and low molecular weight heparins (LMWHs) are safe and efficacious in treating cancer patients with PE.[99,101] Current practice is to administer IV heparin using a weight-based regimen (loading dose of 80 IU/kg IV followed by a continuous infusion of 18 IU/kg/h), aiming for an activated partial thromboplastin time of at least 1.5 to 2 times control values. Bleeding and heparin-induced thrombocytopenia with thrombosis (HITT) are major complications of UFH therapy. For patients with HITT, heparin must be discontinued and a nonheparin alternative anticoagulant (eg, lepirudin or argatroban) should be used.[102] LMWHs have several advantages compared with UFH, including ease of administration, greater bioavailability, more predictable pharmacokinetics, avoidance of routine laboratory monitoring of anticoagulant effect, and potential for outpatient use, resulting in cost savings and better quality of life for the patient who has cancer. The safety and efficacy of LMWHs for the treatment of PE have been demonstrated in several clinical trials.[103,104] However, these PE trials enrolled only a limited number of patients with cancer. In addition to their anticoagulant effects, UFH and LMWHs may have an antineoplastic effect through inhibition of angiogenesis, which may confer a survival benefit to cancer patients with VTE.

Thrombolytic therapy with tissue-type plasminogen activator or streptokinase is indicated for patients with PE presenting with hemodynamic instability, such as hypotension and right ventricular failure, or who have evidence of a thrombus in the right atrium or ventricle.[105,106] Despite their ability to cause rapid lysis of pulmonary emboli and immediate hemodynamic improvement, thrombolytic agents have not been shown to improve survival in hemodynamically unstable patients with PE and may cause major bleeding in up to 20% of patients. Patients with brain tumors or metastases have a higher risk for intracranial bleeding with thrombolytic agents.

IVC filters have been used for almost 3 decades to prevent or treat PE in high-risk patients with contraindications or lack of response to anticoagulant therapy. More recently, retrievable IVC filters have been increasingly used. However, the indications for placement of IVC filters in patients with cancer have not been well defined. Several investigators have cautioned against the use of IVC filters in patients with cancer because of the high rate of filter-related complications (eg, leg swelling), the poor overall outcome or questionable benefit in patients with end-stage malignancy, and the lack of benefit in patients with brain cancer.[107] It is the authors' practice to continue anticoagulation in cancer patients with an IVC filter for durations appropriate for their thrombotic disorder unless contraindications exist given their high risk for ongoing thrombotic complications. Although IVC filters when used concurrently with anticoagulant therapy prevent PE in high-risk patients initially, no improvement in immediate or long-term mortality has been demonstrated and many patients develop recurrent DVT caused by thrombosis at the filter site.[108,109]

DAH

Alveolar hemorrhage is a frequent cause of respiratory failure in thrombocytopenic patients (platelet counts <50,000/mm^3) with acute or chronic leukemias or multiple myeloma. The incidence of DAH in recipients of hematopoietic stem cell transplantation ranges from 2% to 12%.[110,111] Pretransplant intensive chemotherapy, including conditioning regimen, total body irradiation, thoracic irradiation, and old age, are known risk factors for DAH.[110] The pathogenesis of DAH in HSCT recipients is believed to involve lung tissue injury, inflammation, and cytokine release (tumor necrosis factor-α [TNF-α], interleukin 12 [IL-12]). Progressive dyspnea, cough, and fever are common; hemoptysis is present in less than one-third of cases. Chest radiograph shows diffuse interstitial and alveolar infiltrates, primarily central, and involving predominantly lower and middle lung zones. The diagnosis is confirmed with the demonstration of progressively bloodier BAL fluid during bronchoscopy and the presence of greater than 20% hemosiderin-laden macrophages in BAL fluid.[110] Alveolar hemorrhage may coexist with various conditions, but invasive aspergillosis and disseminated CMV infection are the most fatal. Treatment is generally supportive with corticosteroids, platelet transfusions, and mechanical ventilator support to treat ARF.[110–112] Systemic and intrapulmonary administration of recombinant factor VIIa (rFVIIa) has been successfully used in several cases.[113,114] Patients with hematologic malignancy and HSCT recipients who develop respiratory failure caused by DAH usually have a dismal outcome, with mortality exceeding 50% in most series.[115]

TRANSFUSION-RELATED ACUTE LUNG INJURY (TRALI)

Patients with cancer, particularly those with hematologic malignancies and patients undergoing major cancer surgery, frequently require transfusion of fresh frozen plasma, platelets, and packed red blood cells, and thus are susceptible to TRALI. This syndrome usually takes the form of noncardiogenic pulmonary edema and is commonly associated with fever, hypotension, severe hypoxemia, pulmonary hypertension, and bilateral lung infiltrates with normal left ventricular function.[116] Similarly, neutropenic patients with cancer are particularly prone to develop respiratory failure during granulocyte transfusions. The mechanism of lung injury related to blood transfusion seems to involve several factors, including passive transfer of antibodies in the donor plasma directed against histocompatibility antigens or granulocyte-specific antigens in the recipient and complement activation.[117,118] Other risk factors are blood products from alloimmunized female donors, which also carry a higher mortality from TRALI. Alternatively, transfusion of donor serum with normal serum IgA concentrations into a recipient lacking in serum IgA but with anti-IgA antibodies may precipitate the development of ALI. The finding of granulocyte, leukoagglutinating, or lymphocytotoxic antibodies in serum from either the donor or the recipient may support the diagnosis. Treatment of TRALI is primarily supportive and often includes ventilatory support.[118] Most cases resolve within a few days although persistent infiltrates and hypoxemia may occur for more than a week in as many as 20% of patients.

RADIATION-INDUCED LUNG INJURY

Radiation-induced lung injury is generally limited to the irradiated lung volume and results in several histopathologic changes, including enlargement and atypia of type II pneumocytes, alveolar wall edema, infiltration of the interstitium by monocytes and fibroblasts, aggregation of alveolar macrophages, and dense collagen fibrosis.[119] Significant lung injury from radiation therapy is dependent on the volume of lung irradiated, the total dose, and the dose per fraction used. Although radiation lung injury can occur with doses of a few hundred cGy, lung damage is nearly universal with doses in excess of 6000 cGy, but may be attenuated by administering radiation in multiple, small fractions. Animal and human studies have demonstrated that the detrimental effects of radiation therapy on the lung are exacerbated by concomitant chemotherapy, repeat courses of radiation therapy, and steroid withdrawal. Radiation-induced lung injury is manifested by an early acute phase (radiation pneumonitis) and a late phase of pulmonary fibrosis. In both syndromes, radiation-induced local inflammatory cytokine production (eg, TNF-α, IL-1, IL-6) and activation of cell adhesion molecules (E-selectin, P-selectin, and ICAM-1) and fibrotic cytokines (transforming growth factor-β, basic fibroblast growth factor, platelet-derived growth factor, and vascular endothelial growth factor) are believed to be the major mechanisms involved in radiation-induced lung injury.[120] Radiation pneumonitis occurs 1 to 3 months after completion of the radiotherapy course and is manifested by the insidious onset of dyspnea, cough, and fever and the presence of interstitial or alveolar infiltrates within the irradiated field on chest radiograph. Although radiation pneumonitis generally is self-limited in its course, severe respiratory failure can occur and may require systemic corticosteroids initially at high doses and then tapered slowly following the clinical response.[121] On the other hand, radiation fibrosis usually occurs 6 to 12 months after irradiation, is irreversible, and the use of corticosteroids may be harmful.

PARANEOPLASTIC SYNDROMES

Approximately 30% of patients with thymomas develop myasthenia gravis and often the respiratory failure worsens around the time of thymectomy. The diagnosis is confirmed with the finding of improvement in muscle strength after the administration of IV edrophonium (Tensilon) and evidence of decremental response of the muscle action potential to repetitive nerve testing on electromyogram (EMG) studies. Supportive measures, in addition to cholinesterase inhibitors such as pyridostigmine and thymectomy, include plasmapheresis, corticosteroids, immunosuppressive therapy, and IVIg.[29]

Lambert-Eaton myasthenic syndrome, an uncommon disorder of neuromuscular junction transmission manifested primarily by muscle weakness, has been strongly associated with small cell lung cancer.[122] The syndrome is caused by decreased release of acetylcholine from the presynaptic nerve terminals resulting from antibodies directed against the voltage-gated calcium channel (VGCC), which interferes with the normal calcium flux required for the release of acetylcholine.[123] The most common clinical presentation is slowly progressive proximal muscle weakness; respiratory failure may occur late in the course of the disease. The diagnosis is usually made based on clinical manifestations and confirmed by the presence of antibodies directed against VGCCs and by electrodiagnostic studies. A high titer P/Q-type VGCC antibody is strongly suggestive. The diagnosis is confirmed by a reproducible postexercise increase in compound muscle action potential amplitude of at least 100% compared with preexercise baseline value. Management is directed at treatment of the underlying malignancy, use of symptomatic therapies that increase the amount of acetylcholine available at the postsynaptic membrane including guanine, aminopyridines such as 3,4-diaminopyridine, and cholinesterase inhibitors, plasma exchange, IVIg, corticosteroids, azathioprine, mycophenolate, and cyclosporine.[124]

Guillain-Barré syndrome (acute sensorimotor neuropathy) has been associated with Hodgkin lymphoma and following treatment with chemotherapeutic agents including vincristine, oxaliplatin, and sunitinib. The clinical features include progressive symmetric muscle weakness accompanied by absent or decreased deep tendon reflexes. Lumbar puncture reveals an elevated cerebrospinal fluid protein with a normal white blood cell count (albuminocytologic dissociation). EMG shows evidence of acute motor and sensory axonal neuropathy. Treatment usually involves plasma exchange and IVIg. The mechanisms underlying the development of ARF in these patients include upper airway compromise caused by weakness of the facial, oropharyngeal, and laryngeal muscles, which interferes with swallowing and secretion clearance, and inspiratory and expiratory respiratory muscle weakness leading to inadequate lung expansion, atelectasis, and increased risk of aspiration and pneumonia.[125] The decision to intubate these patients should be made early guided by regular assessment for clinical signs of respiratory muscle fatigue and objective monitoring of vital capacity and maximum inspiratory and expiratory pressures, to avoid emergency intubation and cardiorespiratory arrest.

MANAGEMENT PRINCIPLES FOR ARF IN THE CRITICAL CARE SETTING

The key management principles for cancer patients who develop ARF include a comprehensive diagnostic work-up including fiberoptic bronchoscopy to identify the cause of the respiratory failure; appropriate and timely use of antimicrobial therapy in those with infectious disorders; and respiratory support including early use of NIPPV rather than invasive MV. The reader is referred to a flow-chart outlining the recommendations for selecting the initial ventilatory strategy in cancer patients with hypoxemic ARF in the article by Soares and colleagues in this issue of the *Clinics*.

Presently, NIPPV can be delivered through a nasal or face mask using a conventional mechanical ventilator or a NIPPV machine. The advantages of NIPPV compared with invasive MV include avoidance of intubation-related trauma, enhanced patient comfort, and reduced need for sedation. In the past decade, the use of NIPPV has increased and several studies have reported its benefits among patients with cancer who develop ARF.[16,17,126] Hilbert and colleagues[16] randomized 52 immunosuppressed patients (one-third had undergone HSCT) with pulmonary infiltrates and early hypoxemic respiratory failure (P_{AO_2}/F_{IO_2} <200) to NIPPV or standard treatment with supplemental oxygen and no ventilatory support. Periods of noninvasive ventilation delivered through a face mask were alternated every 3 hours with periods of spontaneous breathing with supplemental oxygen. Patients in the noninvasive ventilation study arm experienced greater improvements in oxygenation and hospital survival (50% vs 19%) and were less likely to require endotracheal intubation (46% vs 77%). NIPPV may also be a reasonable option in patients with cancer who have refused endotracheal intubation (or have a Do Not Intubate order) but still request aggressive supportive care and in those patients with disabling dyspnea.[127] Most studies indicate that the success of NIPPV is dependent mainly on its early use and the experience of the staff.

Patients who have cancer with severe hypoxemic ARF and those with renal replacement therapy, vasopressor need, or fulfilling the criteria of ARDS, are more likely to fail NIPPV and should be considered for invasive MV. The use of high positive end-expiratory pressure, alveolar recruitment maneuvers, and prone positioning may be attempted as rescue therapy in patients with severe hypoxemia, but these techniques have not been shown to improve survival for patients with ARDS.[128] Similarly, newer modes and methods of MV including high frequency oscillatory ventilation, inverse ratio ventilation, and airway pressure release ventilation may be considered in difficult cases.

PROGNOSIS AND OUTCOME DATA

Although MV remains an important life-support modality for many patients who have cancer with ARF, these patients generally have survival rates less than 20%.[1–15] In recent years, however, there has been optimism about improved survival rates in mechanically ventilated patients with cancer.[7,17]

In addition to general ICU mortality prediction models (eg, Acute Physiology and Chronic Health Evaluation [APACHE] II and III, Mortality Probability Models, Simplified Acute Physiology Score [SAPS] II and III),[129] prediction models that estimate the probability of death after ICU admission for patients with cancer with respiratory failure have been developed. In a prospective, multicenter study of 782 adult patients with cancer receiving ventilator support for respiratory failure, Groeger and colleagues[14] reported an overall survival rate of 24%. Independent adverse prognostic factors were need for intubation for more than 24 hours after developing ARF, diagnosis of leukemia, progression or recurrence of cancer, bone marrow transplantation, presence of disseminated intravascular coagulation, cardiac arrhythmias, and need for vasopressor therapy. Staudinger and colleagues[2] reported a 53% survival rate in 121 of 414 critically ill cancer patients with ARF who were admitted to the ICU. Of the 121 patients, 54 patients had underlying leukemia, 31 had lymphoma, 26 had a solid tumor, and 10 were bone marrow transplant patients. However, only 13% of the patients who survived ICU were still alive after 1 year. Azoulay and colleagues[3] conducted a prospective 5-year observational study of 203 cancer patients with ARF in a medical ICU in a teaching hospital in Paris, France. Fifty-eight percent of the patients had ARF caused by infectious pneumonia, 9% had noninfectious pneumonia, 12% had congestive heart failure, and no identifiable cause was observed in 21%. ICU and hospital mortality rates were 44.8% and 47.8%, respectively. NIPPV was used in 39% of the patients and conventional MV in 56%, with mortality of 48.1% and 75.4%, respectively. Mortality was 100% in the 19 noncardiac patients in whom conventional MV was started after 72 hours. Factors associated with increased mortality were documented invasive aspergillosis, no definite diagnosis, use of vasopressors, first-line conventional MV, conventional MV after NIPPV failure, and late NIPPV. Hospital mortality was lower in patients with cardiac pulmonary edema.

Patients who have cancer and their family members or surrogates need to make informed decisions regarding the use of MV and other life-sustaining treatments in the ICU. The severity of acute organ failures, poor performance status, cancer status, older age, and HSCT are the major determinants of mortality in cancer patients requiring mechanical ventilatory support.[4,7,10,14,27] It is incumbent on physicians to recommend or assist all patients with cancer to complete advance directives stating their desires about withholding or withdrawing advanced life support such as MV in the event of respiratory failure.[29] Increased family satisfaction with end-of-life decision-making has been shown to be associated with the withdrawal of life support, and chart documentation of physician recommendations to withdraw life support, discussions of patients' wishes, and discussions of families' spiritual needs.[130–133] Wright and colleagues[134] showed that end-of-life discussions were associated with less aggressive medical care near death and earlier hospice referrals. In contrast, aggressive care was associated with worse patient quality of life and worse bereavement adjustment. Other investigators have reported that ethics and palliative care consultations greatly benefit end-of-life discussions with family members of patients dying in the ICU.[135,136]

SUMMARY

The diagnosis and management of ARF in patients with cancer poses special challenges to the intensivist. The clinical presentation of ARF in patients with cancer may be less specific than in patients without cancer. Depending on the type of cancer, the degree of immunosuppression, underlying comorbidities, and the modality of cancer treatment, progression or spread of underlying cancer, and disease- or therapy-associated complications are the most common causes of ARF in these patients. Despite significant advances in antineoplastic therapies and supportive management in the ICU, the mortality of cancer patients with ARF requiring MV remains high. The keys to achieving an optimal outcome include timely diagnosis and treatment of reversible causes of respiratory failure, including earlier use of noninvasive ventilation and judicious ventilator and fluid management in patients with ALI. Close collaboration between oncologists and intensivists will ensure the establishment of clear goals and direction of treatment of every patient with cancer who requires MV for ARF.

REFERENCES

1. Hauser MJ, Tabak J, Baier H. Survival of patients with cancer in a medical critical care unit. Arch Intern Med 1982;142:527–9.
2. Staudinger T, Stoiser B, Mullner M, et al. Outcome and prognostic factors in critically ill cancer patients admitted to the intensive care unit. Crit Care Med 2000;28:1322–8.
3. Azoulay E, Thiery G, Chevret S, et al. The prognosis of acute respiratory failure in critically ill cancer patients. Medicine (Baltimore) 2004;83:360–70.
4. Soares M, Salluh JI, Spector N, et al. Characteristics and outcomes of cancer patients requiring mechanical ventilatory support for >24 hrs. Crit Care Med 2005;33:520–6.
5. Peters SG, Meadows JA 3rd, Gracey DR. Outcome of respiratory failure in hematologic malignancy. Chest 1988;94:99–102.
6. Reichner CA, Thompson JA, O'Brien S, et al. Outcome and code status of lung cancer patients admitted to the medical ICU. Chest 2006;130:719–23.
7. Benoit DD, Vandewoude KH, Decruyenaere JM, et al. Outcome and early prognostic indicators in patients with a hematologic malignancy admitted to the intensive care unit for a life-threatening complication. Crit Care Med 2003; 31(1):104–12.
8. Snow RM, Miller WC, Rice DL, et al. Respiratory failure in cancer patients. JAMA 1979;241(19):2039–42.
9. Darmon M, Thiery G, Ciroldi M, et al. Intensive care in patients with newly diagnosed malignancies and a need for cancer chemotherapy. Crit Care Med 2005; 33(11):2488–93.
10. Ewer M, Ali MK, Atta MS, et al. Outcome of lung cancer patients requiring mechanical ventilation for pulmonary failure. JAMA 1986;256(24):3364–6.
11. Lloyd-Thomas AR, Wright I, Lister TA, et al. Prognosis of patients receiving intensive care for life-threatening medical complications of haematological malignancy. Br Med J (Clin Res Ed) 1988;296(6628):1025–9.
12. Schuster DP, Marion JM. Precedents for meaningful recovery during treatment in a medical intensive care unit. Outcome in patients with hematologic malignancy. Am J Med 1983;75(3):402–8.
13. Estopa R, Torres Marti A, Kastanos N, et al. Acute respiratory failure in severe hematologic disorders. Crit Care Med 1984;12(1):26–8.
14. Groeger JS, White P Jr, Nierman DM, et al. Outcome for cancer patients requiring mechanical ventilation. J Clin Oncol 1999;17(3):991–7.
15. Chaoui D, Legrand O, Roche N, et al. Incidence and prognostic value of respiratory events in acute leukemia. Leukemia 2004;18(4):670–5.
16. Hilbert G, Gruson D, Vargas F, et al. Noninvasive ventilation in immunosuppressed patients with pulmonary infiltrates, fever, and acute respiratory failure. N Engl J Med 2001;344(7):481–7.
17. Azoulay E, Alberti C, Bornstain C, et al. Improved survival in cancer patients requiring mechanical ventilatory support: impact of noninvasive mechanical ventilatory support. Crit Care Med 2001;29(3):519–25.

18. Rubenfeld GD, Crawford SW. Withdrawing life support from mechanically ventilated recipients of bone marrow transplants: a case for evidence-based guidelines. Ann Intern Med 1996;125(8):625–33.
19. Huaringa AJ, Leyva FJ, Giralt SA, et al. Outcome of bone marrow transplantation patients requiring mechanical ventilation. Crit Care Med 2000;28(4):1014–7.
20. Afessa B, Tefferi A, Hoagland HC, et al. Outcome of recipients of bone marrow transplants who require intensive-care unit support. Mayo Clin Proc 1992;67(2):117–22.
21. Faber-Langendoen K, Caplan AL, McGlave PB. Survival of adult bone marrow transplant patients receiving mechanical ventilation: a case for restricted use. Bone Marrow Transplant 1993;12(5):501–7.
22. Paz HL, Crilley P, Weinar M, et al. Outcome of patients requiring medical ICU admission following bone marrow transplantation. Chest 1993;104(2):527–31.
23. Denardo SJ, Oye RK, Bellamy PE. Efficacy of intensive care for bone marrow transplant patients with respiratory failure. Crit Care Med 1989;17(1):4–6.
24. Scott PH, Morgan TJ, Durrant S, et al. Survival following mechanical ventilation of recipients of bone marrow transplants and peripheral blood stem cell transplants. Anaesth Intensive Care 2002;30(3):289–94.
25. Price KJ, Thall PF, Kish SK, et al. Prognostic indicators for blood and marrow transplant patients admitted to an intensive care unit. Am J Respir Crit Care Med 1998;158(3):876–84.
26. Jackson SR, Tweeddale MG, Barnett MJ, et al. Admission of bone marrow transplant recipients to the intensive care unit: outcome, survival and prognostic factors. Bone Marrow Transplant 1998;21(7):697–704.
27. Bach PB, Schrag D, Nierman DM, et al. Identification of poor prognostic features among patients requiring mechanical ventilation after hematopoietic stem cell transplantation. Blood 2001;98(12):3234–40.
28. Peigne V, Rusinová K, Karlin L, et al. Continued survival gains in recent years among critically ill myeloma patients. Intensive Care Med 2009;35(3):512–8.
29. Pastores SM. Acute respiratory failure in critically ill patients with cancer. Diagnosis and management [review]. Crit Care Clin 2001;17(3):623–46.
30. Azoulay E, Schlemmer B. Diagnostic strategy in cancer patients with acute respiratory failure [review]. Intensive Care Med 2006;32(6):808–22.
31. Ginsberg RJ, Hill LD, Eagan RT, et al. Modern thirty-day operative mortality for surgical resections in lung cancer. J Thorac Cardiovasc Surg 1983;86:654–8.
32. Licker M, Fauconnet P, Villiger Y, et al. Acute lung injury and outcomes after thoracic surgery [review]. Curr Opin Anaesthesiol 2009;22(1):61–7.
33. Murthy SC, Rozas MS, Adelstein DJ, et al. Induction chemoradiotherapy increases pleural and pericardial complications after esophagectomy for cancer. J Thorac Oncol 2009;4:395–403.
34. Stover DE, Kaner RJ. Pulmonary complications in cancer patients [review]. CA Cancer J Clin 1996;46(5):303–20.
35. Collin BA, Ramphal R. Pneumonia in the compromised host including cancer patients and transplant patients. Infect Dis Clin North Am 1998;12(3):781–805.
36. Alberts WM. Pulmonary complications of cancer treatment. Curr Opin Oncol 1997;9(2):161.
37. Vento S, Cainelli F, Temesgen Z. Lung infections after cancer chemotherapy [review]. Lancet Oncol 2008;9(10):982–92.
38. Safdar A, Rolston KV. Stenotrophomonas maltophilia: changing spectrum of a serious bacterial pathogen in patients with cancer [review]. Clin Infect Dis 2007;45(12):1602–9.

39. Paez JI, Costa SF. Risk factors associated with mortality of infections caused by *Stenotrophomonas maltophilia*: a systematic review [review]. J Hosp Infect 2008;70(2):101–8.
40. Gruson D, Hilbert G, Valentino R, et al. Utility of fiberoptic bronchoscopy in neutropenic patients admitted to the intensive care unit with pulmonary infiltrates. Crit Care Med 2000;28:2224–30.
41. Boersma WG, Erjavec Z, van der Werf TS, et al. Bronchoscopic diagnosis of pulmonary infiltrates in granulocytopenic patients with hematologic malignancies: BAL versus PSB and PBAL. Respir Med 2007;101(2):317–25.
42. Zihlif M, Khanchandani G, Ahmed HP, et al. Surgical lung biopsy in patients with hematological malignancy or hematopoietic stem cell transplantation and unexplained pulmonary infiltrates: improved outcome with specific diagnosis. Am J Hematol 2005;78(2):94–9.
43. White DA, Wong PW, Downey R. The utility of open lung biopsy in patients with hematologic malignancies. Am J Respir Crit Care Med 2000;161:723–9.
44. Thomas CF Jr, Limper AH. Pneumocystis pneumonia. N Engl J Med 2004;350: 2487–98.
45. Roblot F, Imbert S, Godet C, et al. Risk factors analysis for *Pneumocystis jiroveci* pneumonia (PCP) in patients with haematological malignancies and pneumonia. Scand J Infect Dis 2004;36:848–54.
46. Rai KR, Freter CE, Mercier RJ, et al. Alemtuzumab in previously treated chronic lymphocytic leukemia patients who also had received fludarabine. J Clin Oncol 2002;20:3891–7.
47. Bollee G, Sarfati C, Thiery G, et al. Clinical picture of *Pneumocystis jiroveci* pneumonia in cancer patients. Chest 2007;132:1305–10.
48. Azoulay E, Bergeron A, Chevret S, et al. Polymerase chain reaction for diagnosing pneumocystis pneumonia in non-HIV immunocompromised patients with pulmonary infiltrates. Chest 2009;135:655–61.
49. Martino R, Porras RP, Rabella N, et al. Prospective study of the incidence, clinical features, and outcome of symptomatic upper and lower respiratory tract infections by respiratory viruses in adult recipients of hematopoietic stem cell transplants for hematologic malignancies. Biol Blood Marrow Transplant 2005;11:781–96.
50. Nichols WG, Corey L, Gooley T, et al. Parainfluenza virus infections after hematopoietic stem cell transplantation: risk factors, response to antiviral therapy, and effect on transplant outcome. Blood 2001;98:573–8.
51. Chemaly RF, Ghosh S, Bodey GP, et al. Respiratory viral infections in adults with hematologic malignancies and human stem cell transplantation recipients: a retrospective study at a major cancer center. Medicine (Baltimore) 2006;85:278–87.
52. Peck AJ, Englund JA, Kuypers J, et al. Respiratory virus infection among hematopoietic cell transplant recipients: evidence for asymptomatic parainfluenza virus infection. Blood 2007;110:1681–8.
53. Shorr AF, Susla GM, O'Grady NP. Pulmonary infiltrates in the non-HIV-infected immunocompromised patient: etiologies, diagnostic strategies, and outcomes [review]. Chest 2004;125(1):260–71.
54. van Elden LJ, van Kraaij MG, Nijhuis M, et al. Polymerase chain reaction is more sensitive than viral culture and antigen testing for the detection of respiratory viruses in adults with hematological cancer and pneumonia. Clin Infect Dis 2002;34:177–83.
55. Bernard GR, Artigas A, Brigham KL, et al. The American-European Consensus Conference on ARDS. Definitions, mechanisms, relevant outcomes, and clinical trial coordination. Am J Respir Crit Care Med 1994;149:818–24.

56. Luhr OR, Antonsen K, Karlsson M, et al. Incidence and mortality after acute respiratory failure and acute respiratory distress syndrome in Sweden, Denmark, and Iceland. The ARF Study Group. Am J Respir Crit Care Med 1999;159:1849–61.
57. Wind J, Versteegt J, Twisk J, et al. Epidemiology of acute lung injury and acute respiratory distress syndrome in The Netherlands: a survey. Respir Med 2007; 101:2091–8.
58. Rubenfeld GD, Caldwell E, Peabody E, et al. Incidence and outcomes of acute lung injury. N Engl J Med 2005;353(16):1685–93.
59. Rubenfeld GD, Herridge MS. Epidemiology and outcomes of acute lung injury [review]. Chest 2007;131(2):554–62.
60. Jeon K, Yoon JW, Suh GY, et al. Risk factors for post-pneumonectomy acute lung injury/acute respiratory distress syndrome in primary lung cancer patients. Anaesth Intensive Care 2009;37(1):14–9.
61. Kutlu CA, Williams EA, Evans TW, et al. Acute lung injury and acute respiratory distress syndrome after pulmonary resection. Ann Thorac Surg 2000;69(2): 376–80.
62. Dulu A, Pastores SM, Park B, et al. Prevalence and mortality of acute lung injury and ARDS after lung resection. Chest 2006;130(1):73–8.
63. Ware LB, Matthay MA. The acute respiratory distress syndrome. N Engl J Med 2000;342:1334–49.
64. Laufe MD, Simon RH, Flint A, et al. Adult respiratory distress syndrome in neutropenic patients. Am J Med 1986;80(6):1022–6.
65. Kress JP, Christenson J, Pohlman AS, et al. Outcomes of critically ill cancer patients in a university hospital setting. Am J Respir Crit Care Med 1999;160: 1957–61.
66. Nelson S, Belknap SM, Carlson RW, et al. A randomized controlled trial of filgrastim as an adjunct to antibiotics for treatment of hospitalized patients with community-acquired pneumonia. CAP Study Group. J Infect Dis 1998;178(4): 1075–80.
67. Wheeler AP, Bernard GR, Thompson BT, et al. Pulmonary-artery versus central venous catheter to guide treatment of acute lung injury. N Engl J Med 2006; 354:2213–24.
68. Wiedemann HP, Wheeler AP, Bernard GR, et al. Comparison of two fluid-management strategies in acute lung injury. N Engl J Med 2006;354:2564–75.
69. Mercat A, Richard JC, Vielle B, et al. Positive end-expiratory pressure setting in adults with acute lung injury and acute respiratory distress syndrome: a randomized controlled trial. JAMA 2008;299:646–55.
70. Stewart RM, Park PK, Hunt JP, et al. Less is more: improved outcomes in surgical patients with conservative fluid administration and central venous catheter monitoring. J Am Coll Surg 2009;208:725–35.
71. Brower RG, Lanken PN, MacIntyre N, et al. Higher versus lower positive end-expiratory pressures in patients with the acute respiratory distress syndrome. N Engl J Med 2004;351:327–36.
72. Ventilation with lower tidal volumes as compared with traditional tidal volumes for acute lung injury and the acute respiratory distress syndrome. The Acute Respiratory Distress Syndrome Network. N Engl J Med 2000;342:1301–8.
73. Talmor D, Sarge T, Malhotra A, et al. Mechanical ventilation guided by esophageal pressure in acute lung injury. N Engl J Med 2008;359(20):2095–104.
74. Meduri GU, Headley AS, Golden E, et al. Effect of prolonged methylprednisolone therapy in unresolving acute respiratory distress syndrome: a randomized controlled trial. JAMA 1998;280:159–65.

75. Steinberg KP, Hudson LD, Goodman RB, et al. Efficacy and safety of corticosteroids for persistent acute respiratory distress syndrome. N Engl J Med 2006; 354:1671–84.
76. Hough CL, Steinberg KP, Taylor Thompson B, et al. Intensive care unit-acquired neuromyopathy and corticosteroids in survivors of persistent ARDS. Intensive Care Med 2009;35(1):63–8.
77. Meduri GU, Marik PE, Chrousos GP, et al. Steroid treatment in ARDS: a critical appraisal of the ARDS network trial and the recent literature. Intensive Care Med 2008;34(1):61–9.
78. Zambon M, Vincent JL. Mortality rates for patients with acute lung injury/ARDS have decreased over time. Chest 2008;133:1120–7.
79. Erickson SE, Martin GS, Davis JL, et al. Recent trends in acute lung injury mortality: 1996–2005. Crit Care Med 2009;37(5):1574–9.
80. Davidson TA, Caldwell ES, Curtis JR, et al. Reduced quality of life in survivors of acute respiratory distress syndrome compared with critically ill control patients. JAMA 1999;281:354–60.
81. Dowdy DW, Bienvenu OJ, Dinglas VD, et al. Are intensive care factors associated with depressive symptoms 6 months after acute lung injury? Crit Care Med 2009;37(5):1702–7.
82. Hopkins RO, Weaver LK, Collingridge D, et al. Two-year cognitive, emotional, and quality-of-life outcomes in acute respiratory distress syndrome. Am J Respir Crit Care Med 2005;171:340–7.
83. Herridge MS, Cheung AM, Tansey CM, et al. Canadian Critical Care Trials Group. One-year outcomes in survivors of the acute respiratory distress syndrome. N Engl J Med 2003;348(8):683–93.
84. Kress JP, Pohlman AS, O'Connor MF, et al. Daily interruption of sedative infusions in critically ill patients undergoing mechanical ventilation. N Engl J Med 2000;342(20):1471–7.
85. Girard TD, Kress JP, Fuchs BD, et al. Efficacy and safety of a paired sedation and ventilator weaning protocol for mechanically ventilated patients in intensive care (Awakening and Breathing Controlled trial): a randomised controlled trial. Lancet 2008;371(9607):126–34.
86. Schweickert WD, Pohlman MC, Pohlman AS, et al. Early physical and occupational therapy in mechanically ventilated, critically ill patients: a randomised controlled trial. Lancet 2009;373(9678):1874–82.
87. Vahid B, Marik PE. Pulmonary complications of novel antineoplastic agents for solid tumors [review]. Chest 2008;133(2):528–38.
88. Ohnishi H, Yokoyama A, Yasuhara Y, et al. Circulating KL-6 levels in patients with drug induced pneumonitis. Thorax 2003;58(10):872–5.
89. Camus P, Kudoh S, Ebina M. Interstitial lung disease associated with drug therapy [review]. Br J Cancer 2004;91(Suppl 2):S18–23.
90. Sallah S, Wan JY, Nguyen NP. Venous thrombosis in patients with solid tumors: determination of frequency and characteristics. Thromb Haemost 2002;87:575–9.
91. Heit JA, Silverstein MD, Mohr DN, et al. Risk factors for deep vein thrombosis and pulmonary embolism: a population-based case-control study. Arch Intern Med 2000;160:809–15.
92. Lee AY, Levine MN. Venous thromboembolism and cancer: risks and outcomes. Circulation 2003;107(23 Suppl 1):I17–21.
93. DeSancho MT, Rand JH. Bleeding and thrombotic complications in critically ill patients with cancer [review]. Crit Care Clin 2001;17(3):599–622.

94. Stein PD, Woodard PK, Weg JG, et al. PIOPED II investigators. Diagnostic pathways in acute pulmonary embolism: recommendations of the PIOPED II investigators. Am J Med 2006;119(12):1048–55.

95. Anderson DR, Kahn SR, Rodger MA, et al. Computed tomographic pulmonary angiography vs ventilation-perfusion lung scanning in patients with suspected pulmonary embolism: a randomized controlled trial. JAMA 2007;298(23):2743–53.

96. Stein PD, Fowler SE, Goodman LR, et al. PIOPED II Investigators. Multidetector computed tomography for acute pulmonary embolism. N Engl J Med 2006;354(22):2317–27.

97. Lee AY, Julian JA, Levine MN, et al. Clinical utility of a rapid whole-blood D-dimer assay in patients with cancer who present with suspected acute deep venous thrombosis. Ann Intern Med 1999;131(6):417–23.

98. van Belle A, Büller HR, Huisman MV, et al. Christopher Study Investigators. Effectiveness of managing suspected pulmonary embolism using an algorithm combining clinical probability, D-dimer testing, and computed tomography. JAMA 2006;295(2):172–9.

99. Petralia GA, Kakkar AK. Treatment of venous thromboembolism in cancer patients. Semin Thromb Hemost 2007;33(7):707–11.

100. Pastores SM. Management of venous thromboembolism in the intensive care unit. J Crit Care 2009;24(2):185–91.

101. Kearon C, Kahn SR, Agnelli G, et al. American College of Chest Physicians. Antithrombotic therapy for venous thromboembolic disease: American College of Chest Physicians evidence-based clinical practice guidelines (8th Edition). Chest 2008;133(Suppl 6):454S–545S, Erratum in: Chest 2008;134(4):892.

102. Warkentin TE, Greinacher A, Koster A, et al. American College of Chest Physicians. Treatment and prevention of heparin-induced thrombocytopenia: American College of Chest Physicians evidence-based clinical practice guidelines (8th Edition). Chest 2008;133(Suppl 6):340S–80S.

103. Simonneau G, Sors H, Charbonnier B, et al. A comparison of low-molecular-weight heparin with unfractionated heparin for acute pulmonary embolism. The THESEE Study Group. Tinzaparine ou Héparine Standard: Évaluations dans l'Embolie Pulmonaire. N Engl J Med 1997;337(10):663–9.

104. The Columbus Investigators. Low-molecular-weight heparin in the treatment of patients with venous thromboembolism. N Engl J Med 1997;337(10):657–62.

105. Carlbom DJ, Davidson BL. Pulmonary embolism in the critically ill. Chest 2007;132(1):313–24.

106. Konstantinides S. Clinical practice. Acute pulmonary embolism. N Engl J Med 2008;359(26):2804–13.

107. Schunn C, Schunn GB, Hobbs G, et al. Inferior vena cava filter placement in late-stage cancer. Vasc Endovascular Surg 2006;40(4):287–94.

108. Decousus H, Leizorovicz A, Parent F, et al. A clinical trial of vena caval filters in the prevention of pulmonary embolism in patients with proximal deep-vein thrombosis. Prévention du Risque d'Embolie Pulmonaire par Interruption Cave Study Group. N Engl J Med 1998;338(7):409–15.

109. Streiff MB. Vena caval filters: a review for intensive care specialists. J Intensive Care Med 2003;18(2):59–79.

110. Afessa B, Tefferi A, Litzow MR, et al. Diffuse alveolar hemorrhage in hematopoietic stem cell recipients. Am J Respir Crit Care Med 2002;166:641–5.

111. Lewis ID, DeFor T, Weisdorf DJ. Increasing incidence of diffuse alveolar hemorrhage following allogeneic bone marrow transplantation: cryptic etiology and uncertain therapy. Bone Marrow Transplant 2000;26:539–43.

112. Metcalf JP, Rennard SI, Reed EC, et al. Corticosteroids as adjunctive therapy for diffuse alveolar hemorrhage associated with bone marrow transplantation: University of Nebraska Medical Center Bone Marrow Transplant Group. Am J Med 1994;96:327–34.

113. Pastores SM, Papadopoulos E, Voigt L, et al. Diffuse alveolar hemorrhage after allogeneic hematopoietic stem-cell transplantation: treatment with recombinant factor VIIa. Chest 2003;124(6):2400–3.

114. Heslet L, Nielsen JD, Levi M, et al. Successful pulmonary administration of activated recombinant factor VII in diffuse alveolar hemorrhage. Crit Care 2006;10(6):R177.

115. Kotloff RM, Ahya VN, Crawford SW. Pulmonary complications of solid organ and hematopoietic stem cell transplantation. Am J Respir Crit Care Med 2004; 170(1):22–48.

116. Jawa RS, Anillo S, Kulaylat MN. Transfusion-related acute lung injury [review]. J Intensive Care Med 2008;23(2):109–21.

117. Triulzi DJ. Transfusion-related acute lung injury: current concepts for the clinician. Anesth Analg 2009;108(3):770–6.

118. Gajic O, Moore SB. Transfusion-related acute lung injury [review]. Mayo Clin Proc 2005;80(6):766–70.

119. Marks LB, Yu X, Vujaskovic Z, et al. Radiation-induced lung injury [review]. Semin Radiat Oncol 2003;13(3):333–45.

120. Provatopoulou X, Athanasiou E, Gounaris A. Predictive markers of radiation pneumonitis. Anticancer Res 2008;28(4C):2421–32.

121. Ghafoori P, Marks LB, Vujaskovic Z, et al. Radiation-induced lung injury. Assessment, management, and prevention. Oncology (Williston Park) 2008;22(1): 37–47 [discussion: 52–3].

122. Titulaer MJ, Wirtz PW, Willems LN, et al. Screening for small-cell lung cancer: a follow-up study of patients with Lambert-Eaton myasthenic syndrome. J Clin Oncol 2008;26:4276.

123. Lang B, Pinto A, Giovannini F, et al. Pathogenic autoantibodies in the Lambert-Eaton myasthenic syndrome. Ann N Y Acad Sci 2003;998:187.

124. Maddison P, Newsom-Davis J. Treatment for Lambert-Eaton myasthenic syndrome [review]. Cochrane Database Syst Rev 2005;(2):CD003279.

125. Mehta S. Neuromuscular disease causing acute respiratory failure. Respir Care 2006;51(9):1016–21.

126. Soares M, Salluh JI, Azoulay E. Noninvasive ventilation in patients with malignancies and hypoxemic acute respiratory failure: a still pending question. J Crit Care 2009 [Epub ahead of print].

127. Marik PE. Noninvasive positive-pressure ventilation in patients with malignancy [review]. Am J Hosp Palliat Care 2007;24(5):417–21.

128. Girard TD, Bernard GR. Mechanical ventilation in ARDS: a state-of-the-art review [review]. Chest 2007;131(3):921–9.

129. Soares M, Salluh JI. Validation of the SAPS 3 admission prognostic model in patients with cancer in need of intensive care. Intensive Care Med 2006; 32(11):1839–44.

130. Curtis JR, White DB. Practical guidance for evidence-based ICU family conferences [review]. Chest 2008;134(4):835–43.

131. Lautrette A, Darmon M, Megarbane B, et al. A communication strategy and brochure for relatives of patients dying in the ICU. N Engl J Med 2007;356(5): 469–78. [Erratum in: N Engl J Med 2007 Jul 12;357(2):203].

132. Lilly CM, De Meo DL, Sonna LA, et al. An intensive communication intervention for the critically ill. Am J Med 2000;109(6):469–75.

133. Gries CJ, Curtis JR, Wall RJ, et al. Family member satisfaction with end-of-life decision making in the ICU. Chest 2008;133(3):704–12.

134. Wright AA, Zhang B, Ray A, et al. Associations between end-of-life discussions, patient mental health, medical care near death, and caregiver bereavement adjustment. JAMA 2008;300(14):1665–73.

135. Schneiderman LJ, Gilmer T, Teetzel HD, et al. Effect of ethics consultations on nonbeneficial life-sustaining treatments in the intensive care setting: a randomized controlled trial. JAMA 2003;290(9):1166–72.

136. Campbell ML, Guzman JA. Impact of a proactive approach to improve end-of-life care in a medical ICU. Chest 2003;123(1):266–71.

Mechanical Ventilation in Cancer Patients: Clinical Characteristics and Outcomes

Márcio Soares, MD, PhD[a],*, Pieter O. Depuydt, MD, PhD[b], Jorge I.F. Salluh, MD, PhD[a]

KEYWORDS

- Cancer • Mechanical ventilation • Acute respiratory failure
- Noninvasive ventilation • Outcome

Acute respiratory failure (ARF) with the need for mechanical ventilation (MV) is a severe and frequent complication, and a leading reason for admission to the intensive care unit (ICU) in patients with malignancies. For decades, ARF developing in these patients was considered to be a consequence of refractory pulmonary disorders invariably associated with very high mortality. Nevertheless, over the past several years, this clinical scenario has changed significantly as improved survival rates have been reported from different specialized centers. Investigators attribute the increased survival to advances in oncology, hematology, and critical care (including ventilatory strategies) coupled with a more appropriate selection of patients for ICU admission.

This article reviews the epidemiology and outcomes of adult patients with malignancies requiring ventilatory support, focusing mainly on the studies published over the last decade. Studies on patients with do-not-intubate orders treated with noninvasive positive pressure ventilation (NIPPV) as the upper limit of respiratory support, and on patients requiring ventilatory support for a short period during postoperative care following scheduled surgeries were not considered. In addition, data on ARF developing in allogeneic bone marrow transplant (BMT) recipients were not included, as this subgroup of patients has significant peculiarities as well as still a dismal outcome.

Conflicts of interest: none.

Financial support: Dr Soares is supported in part by an individual research grant from CNPq - Conselho Nacional de Desenvolvimento Científico e Tecnológico (Brazil).

[a] Intensive Care Unit, Instituto Nacional de Câncer, Praça Cruz Vermelha, 23–10 andar, 20230-130, Rio de Janeiro, RJ, Brazil

[b] Department of Intensive Care Medicine, Ghent University Hospital, De Pintelaan 185 9000 Gent, Belgium

* Corresponding author.

E-mail address: marciosoaresms@yahoo.com.br (M. Soares).

EPIDEMIOLOGY

Information on the incidence of ARF and need for ventilatory support in patients with malignancies is still limited, but it seems to vary largely depending on the studied population. Approximately 5% of patients with solid tumors will experience ARF during the course of their disease,[1,2] but the incidence may be higher in patients with lung and head and neck cancers. In hematology patients, the incidence is variable, running from 4% to almost half of the population.[1-5] In the study of Azoulay and colleagues,[1] the incidence of ARF ranged from 6% in patients with Hodgkin disease to 12% in patients with acute and chronic myelogenous leukemias. The incidence of ARF in recipients of autologous BMT similarly is estimated at between 6% and 11%, which is lower than the incidence reported in patients who had undergone allogeneic BMT.[6,7]

ARF requiring MV is a leading reason for ICU admission, and many patients will need MV support while in the ICU. Studies in unselected patients with malignancies admitted to ICUs demonstrated that MV was provided in 44% to 69% of these patients.[8-15] In general, the frequency of ARF was similar in patients with solid tumors (54%–72%)[13,14,16] or hematological malignancies (43%–88%).[14,17-21] In the Sepsis Occurrence in Acutely III Patients (SOAP) study, 473 (15%) of 3147 patients admitted to 198 European ICUs over a 2-week period had a diagnosis of malignancy, 64% of whom received MV.[14] The frequency and duration of MV use in cancer patients were similar to those observed in noncancer patients. However, almost 70% were surgical patients. In addition, 64% to 89% of neutropenic patients[22,23] and 85% to 90% of septic shock patients[24,25] receive MV while in the ICU.

REASONS FOR MECHANICAL VENTILATION

Besides infectious complications and decompensation of concurrent respiratory and cardiovascular diseases, the main reasons for MV in cancer patients include direct involvement of the respiratory system by malignancy, cancer-related medical disorders, and respiratory distress associated with anticancer therapies.[2,26] Outcomes vary largely regarding the underlying reason for MV. For instance, patients with respiratory failure secondary to cardiogenic pulmonary edema are more likely to survive,[1] whereas patients with pulmonary involvement due to the malignancy are more prone to die.[27] In addition, the lack of a definite diagnosis of ARF leading to MV is independently associated with high mortality rates.[1,2,28] This issue is very important, especially if one considers that a significant number of these cases is related to potentially treatable disorders. Pastores and colleagues[29] recently demonstrated that the antemortem diagnoses were frequently discordant from autopsy results in critically ill cancer patients, occurring in 26% of the patients. Among the major missed diagnoses were pulmonary infections including *Pneumocystis jirovecii* pneumonia, *Legionella* infections, invasive aspergillosis, candida, and viral (cytomegalovirus, herpes simplex virus) pneumonia. Therefore, extensive diagnostic workup and aggressive empiric treatments should be employed for patients with a high degree of immunosuppression and severe ARF needing MV.

Severe infections are a major life-threatening condition in cancer patients, especially for those with severe comorbidities, with hematologic malignancies, or those undergoing chemotherapy.[15,24,30] Despite the high mortality rate, bacterial infections seem to be associated with better outcomes when compared with opportunistic infections in patients with severe sepsis and ARF, and when compared with noninfectious causes of ARF other than cardiogenic pulmonary edema.[1,2,17,31-34]

Direct involvement of the respiratory tract is usually due to neck or mediastinal bulky neoplastic disease leading to tracheal compression or invasion, but also may be related to disseminated parenchymal disease or lymphangitis. This severe medical condition usually leads to ARF and, unless when caused by highly chemotherapy-responsive tumors, carries a grim prognosis. Direct neoplastic involvement is considered the main reason for MV in 8% to 11% of cases.[1,27] Soares and colleagues,[27] in a prospective cohort study evaluating 463 cancer patients requiring ventilatory support, observed that compression or invasion of major or distal airways was independently associated with increased hospital mortality. This increased risk for death holds true especially for patients with lung cancer requiring ICU admission.[35]

Cancer-related medical conditions, such as paraneoplastic syndromes, thrombophilia, immunosuppression, requirement for blood product transfusion, and nonrespiratory organ invasion or perforation, are risk factors for ARF through development of venous thromboembolic disease, severe sepsis, transfusion-related acute lung injury, or fluid overload. In a large cohort study, pulmonary embolism was a major cause of ARF, occurring in 7% of MV patients.[27] Venous thromboembolism has been associated with a 6- to 8-fold increase in mortality in cancer patients.[36]

Finally, drug-related pulmonary toxicity is a major concern for clinicians caring for cancer patients. Antineoplastic agent-induced pulmonary toxicity should be a diagnosis of exclusion, and other causes of respiratory failure including bacterial or opportunistic pneumonia, cardiogenic pulmonary edema, and alveolar hemorrhage should be excluded. Although the incidence of pulmonary toxic effects from chemotherapy is low, several side effects such as bronchospasm, hypersensitivity reactions, lung fibrosis, and pulmonary hemorrhage have been reported. The increasing use of chemotherapy and the introduction of novel agents with widened indications pose a challenge for the near future.[37,38] Preexisting lung disease such as chronic obstructive pulmonary disease (COPD), previous radiation therapy, diffuse pulmonary metastasis, and pulmonary fibrosis have been associated with pulmonary toxicity. In addition, a high inspired oxygen fraction may trigger bleomycin pneumonitis.[37,39]

OUTCOME EVALUATION AND PROGNOSTIC FACTORS
Short-Term Outcomes

ARF with the need for ventilatory support is usually associated with high mortality and morbidity. Until the 1990s, the outcome for these patients was considered very poor, with several studies reporting mortality rates greater than 80%.[40–45] Fortunately, studies from the past decade have documented improved survival rates in patients with diverse malignancies requiring MV. Nonetheless, the need for invasive MV remains a major outcome predictor in critically ill patients with malignancies, and still carries a relatively high mortality.[8–11,13,14,16,18,20,21,23,25,28,46,47]

The results of the main studies in patients with malignancies requiring ventilatory support published over the past decade are depicted in **Table 1**. Mortality varies according to multidimensional variables including patient-related characteristics in terms of underlying diagnosis and comorbidities, severity of acute illness, level of ICU support, and ICU policies (eg, criteria used to implement end-of-life care, to admit and discharge patients from the ICU). Overall hospital mortality rates ranged from 55% to 83%, with an average of 66%. Most of the studies were single centered and performed at specialized institutions. In general, mortality rates were lower in patients receiving NIPPV (37%–75%)[1,27,32,34,49,52–54] than in patients who received invasive positive pressure ventilation (IPPV) as the first-line ventilatory strategy (62%–83%).[1,7,9,10,17–21,27,28,32,34,46,48–50,54] In addition, the risk of death was higher

Table 1
Mortality rates and prognostic indicators in different studies published in the last decade (1999–2009) on oncology and hematology patients requiring ventilatory support in the intensive care unit

Authors, Year	Study Design	Patients	First-line IPPV/NIPPV	ST/HM	Hospital Mortality (%)	Independent Prognostic Factors
Groeger et al, 1999[48]	Cohort, prospective, multicenter	782	782/0	305/477	76	Intubation after 24 h, leukemia, progression or recurrence of cancer, allogeneic BMT, cardiac arrhythmias, disseminated intravascular coagulation, vasopressors need were associated with mortality; prior surgery with curative intent was protective
Kress et al, 1999[9]	Cohort, retrospective, single center	153	153/0	—	67	ARDS, hepatic and cardiovascular failures
Azoulay et al, 2001[49]	Cohort, retrospective, single center	237	189/48	50/169	73[a]	SAPS II score was associated with mortality; NIV use was protective.
Khassawneh et al, 2002[7,b]	Cohort, retrospective, single center	78	78/0	7/71	74	Multivariate analyses not performed
Vallot et al, 2003[50]	Cohort, retrospective, single center	168	168/0	104/64	83	Leukopenia
Azoulay et al, 2004[1,c]	Cohort, prospective, single center	148	69/79	—	62	Invasive aspergillosis, lack of definite diagnosis of ARF, vasopressors need, NIV failure (especially after 2 days on NIV), first-line need of MV were associated with mortality; congestive heart failure and successful use of NIV were protective

Study	Type					Comments
Depuydt et al, 2004[32]	Cohort, retrospective, single center	166	140/26	0/166	71	SAPS II score and diagnosis of AML were associated with mortality; female gender, endotracheal intubation <24 h of ICU admission, and bacteremia were protective
Soares et al, 2005[27]	Cohort, prospective, single center	463	444/19	359/104	64	Older age, poor performance status, cancer recurrence/progression, PaO_2/FiO_2 ratio <150, SOFA score and airway/pulmonary invasion or compression by tumor
Azoulay et al, 2008[28,d]	Cohort, prospective, multicenter	110	110/0	NA	69	History of BMT, need for vasopressors or dialysis, intubation during ICU stay were associated with mortality
Lecuyer et al, 2008[51,e]	Cohort, Retrospective. multicenter	1232	967/265	0/1232	55	SAPS II score, need of IPPV, renal replacement therapy and vasopressors, ARDS, shock, and coma were associated with ICU mortality
Adda et al, 2008[52]	Cohort, Retrospective, single center	99	0/99	0/99	62	NIV failure and the number of hours on NIV were associated with mortality, and direct ICU admission and inaugural disease were protective
Depuydt et al, 2009[34,f]	Cohort, retrospective, single center	91	67/24	0/91	78	SOFA and cancer-specific scores were associated with mortality; bacterial infection was protective
Combined	—	3727	3167/560	825/2471	66	—

Abbreviations: AML, acute myeloid leukemia; ARDS, acute respiratory distress syndrome; BMT, bone marrow transplant; HM, hematological malignancies; ICU, intensive care unit; IPPV, invasive positive pressure ventilation; MV, mechanical ventilation; NA, not available; NIPPV, noninvasive positive pressure ventilation; NIV, noninvasive ventilation; SAPS, Simplified Acute Physiology Score; SOFA, Sequential Organ Dysfunction Score; ST, solid tumor.
[a] 30-day mortality; hospital mortality was not reported.
[b] All patients received autologous peripheral stem cell transplant.
[c] 203 patients with ARF were studied, but 55 patients received high-concentration oxygen mask only.
[d] 148 patients with ARF were studied; there was limited information on NIV patients.
[e] 1753 patients with ARF were studied, but 521 patients received high-concentration oxygen mask only.
[f] 137 patients with ARF were studied, but 46 patients received high-concentration oxygen mask only.

in patients who required ventilatory support later in the course of their critical illness compared with those who did so at ICU admission.[1,52,55] Ventilatory support–related aspects are discussed later.

Cancer-Related Characteristics

The diagnosis of "cancer" encompasses a wide range of diseases with diverse clinical and biologic behavior, and the impact of the need for MV on the patients' outcomes in different groups of malignancies (and vice versa) has been a major source of debate. Patients traditionally have been studied and grouped into 2 large categories (ie, solid tumors and hematological malignancies), and studies evaluating specific groups of critically ill cancer patients requiring MV are still scarce. Until recently, patients with hematological malignancies were considered in general to be at higher risk for mortality than patients with solid tumors. However, studies from the past decade have documented similar mortality rates in hematology (48%–85%) and oncology patients (48%–85%) with need for MV.[9,16–21,27,32,48–50] In addition, the effect of the type or group of malignancy on the patients' short-term outcome appeared to be insignificant when adjusted for other relevant outcome predictors in multivariate analyses.[9,27,49] Even specific groups of patients such as those with leukemias, lung, and head and neck cancer, traditionally considered to be at a higher risk of death in cases of ARF, have been reported to experience considerable improvements in survival rates.[35,56–61] In addition, short-term mortality is neither related to the stage at diagnosis nor remission status (partial or complete), but is significantly worse in patients with cancer recurrence or progression.[27,28,48] In contrast, patients who received allogeneic BMT remain a subgroup of cancer patients with disproportionately worse outcome, particularly when severe graft-versus-host disease, or hepatic, renal, or cardiovascular dysfunctions coexist.[28,48,62–70] In contrast, patients treated with autologous BMT have survival rates closer to nontransplanted patients.[7,15,48,65] For example, Khassawneh and colleagues[7] reported that 26% of 78 autologous peripheral BMT patients who received MV were discharged from the hospital and 60% of them were alive at 6 months of follow-up. Finally, whereas the outcomes of neutropenic patients requiring MV were previously considered to be grim,[41,43] recent studies have observed that neither the presence of neutropenia nor recent exposure to chemotherapy were associated with increased risk of death.[27,28,30,49]

Severity of Illness and Acute Organ Dysfunctions

The severity of acute physiologic derangements and organ dysfunctions are the main predictors of short-term mortality.[27,28,32,35,48,49] Patients with cancer frequently require MV in the context of multiple organ failure: for example, between 30% to 90% and 9% to 60% of these patients require concomitant vasopressors or renal replacement therapy, respectively.[1,24,27,32,48–50,55,71] Here, the number of additional failing organs is directly associated with worse prognosis. Organ dysfunction scores such as the Sequential Organ Failure Assessment (SOFA) and Logistic Organ Dysfunction (LOD) scores have been used to quantify the global burden on organ dysfunctions. In addition to baseline values, subsequent changes in these scores over the first few days of ICU admission correlate strongly with mortality.[24,54,55] Thus, the start of additional life-sustaining therapies, such as renal replacement therapy or vasopressors, after several days on MV indicates that the patient's clinical condition may not be responding to ICU care and hence heralds a poor outcome.[55] Furthermore, the presence of organ failure other than ARF is associated with increased risk for NIPPV failure[1,52] and, particularly, acute kidney injury correlates with longer MV duration and weaning from ventilatory support.[72]

Age, Performance Status, and Comorbidities

Aging is associated with the reduction of physiologic capacity and with higher prevalence of chronic diseases, including cancer. Soares and colleagues[47] reported that the frequency of MV use was similar in cancer patients aged 60 years or older and younger patients. The impact of age in critically ill cancer patients is controversial. Although some investigators have reported a relatively worse outcome in elderly patients,[13,23,27] in most studies age was not an independent risk factor for death.[1,9,28,32,34,48–50] However, it is clear that in the elderly cancer patient, selection for candidates for ICU admission in the setting of intercurrent critical illness should be more rigorous.

Patients with cancer often present with severe comorbidities that may have major implications for their outcomes. In these patients, the functional capacity and autonomy is routinely evaluated by the performance status. It has been well documented that a compromised performance status (Karnofsky score <70 or Eastern Cooperative Oncology Group scale of 3–4) before hospital admission and the presence of severe associated comorbid conditions are major determinants of poorer short- and long-term survival in ICU patients with cancer, including those requiring MV.[8,11,27,46,47]

Long-Term Outcomes

There is as yet limited information on medium- and long-term outcomes in patients with cancer who were mechanically ventilated during ICU stay. In a large study of 862 patients with cancer (70% requiring MV), the 6-month mortality was 58%.[47] Massion and colleagues[21] reported that 21 of 84 patients with hematological malignancies (57% of whom were mechanically ventilated) were alive at 6 months' follow-up. Staudinger and colleagues[13] reported 1-year survival rates of 23% in a cohort of 414 patients, 62% of whom were on MV. Finally, Ferrá and colleagues[20] evaluated 100 hematological patients (81 on MV), and found a 2-year survival rate of 15%. However, ideal prognostic evaluation must take into consideration multidimensional aspects other than mortality, including those related to health-related quality of life (HRQOL) and self-perception of quality of care; however, such information is currently lacking. Symptoms of pain, stress, insomnia, depression, and anxiety are frequent in patients who survive critical illnesses, and may compromise functional capacity and limit the ability to work and socialize. Perhaps as a consequence of the "stigma" in carrying a grim prognosis, studies evaluating the outcomes in critically ill patients with cancer have almost exclusively focused on mortality as the outcome of interest. Nelson and colleagues[73] observed the occurrence of painful or distressful experiences in up to 75% of cancer patients admitted to the ICU. Yau and colleagues[74] studied 92 patients with hematological malignancies, and found that most of the survivors perceived their HRQOL as "good" one year after ICU admission. However, additional studies are urgently needed.

The Use of Severity-Of-Illness Scores

Severity-of-illness scores are inaccurate in predicting individual outcome in cancer patients admitted to the ICU. General scores, such as the different versions of the Acute Physiology and Chronic Health Evaluation (APACHE), Simplified Acute Physiology Score (SAPS), and Mortality Probability Models (MPM), usually have a poor performance in critically ill patients with cancer due to inadequate calibration and underestimation of mortality.[8,12,75–77] In 2006, a preliminary validation of the SAPS 3 admission prognostic model was conducted in patients with cancer in need of ICU care,[12] but additional studies are necessary. The limitations of general severity of illness scores have led to the development of a specific score to predict hospital mortality in patients with cancer requiring MV.[48] This model comprises 8 variables obtained at ICU admission: intubation after 24 hours, diagnosis of leukemia, disease progression, or recurrence, allogeneic BMT, prior surgery with curative intent, cardiac arrhythmias, presence of disseminated intravascular coagulation, and need for vasopressors.[48] However, to the authors' knowledge there has been no prospective independent validation of this model outside of the 5 academic tertiary care hospitals where the study was performed.

TRIAGE FOR INTENSIVE CARE UNIT ADMISSION

In the authors' opinion, cancer patients who develop ARF requiring ventilatory support are appropriate candidates for ICU admission. As previously discussed, improvements in survival have been demonstrated in different centers and the knowledge on patients' outcomes has expanded significantly over the past several years. However, the decision to admit a patient with cancer requiring ventilatory support to the ICU remains complex, involving multidimensional domains, and is still a matter of substantial controversy among hemato-oncologists and intensive care physicians. In deciding on ICU admission, besides the availability of hospital/ICU admission guidelines, intensivists take into consideration patient-related characteristics, expected post-ICU outcomes and HRQOL, published evidence, personal experience, and patient's wishes and values. The aforementioned prognostic scores are inaccurate and should not be used for ICU triage,[75,76] and even physicians from the same institution vary significantly regarding admission and treatment decisions.[78] Therefore, the decision-making process must be based on the case-by-case clinical judgment at the bedside. Nevertheless, in an interesting study, Thiéry and colleagues[79] demonstrated that the short-term mortality rates in patients not admitted to the ICU because they were considered "too well" and "too sick" to benefit from intensive care were 21.3% and 74%, respectively. These results clearly suggest that clinical evaluation is imprecise on an individual basis, and that errors of judgment are potentially associated with increased mortality. Adda and colleagues[52] reported that delay from ICU admission to institution of ventilatory support is associated with noninvasive ventilatory failure and worse outcomes.

For all these stated reasons, broadening of ICU admission policies has been advised.[80–83] Investigators from the Saint Louis Hospital in Paris, France have forged the concept of the "ICU trial," which consists of full-code management for a limited period (3–7 days, in general) followed by a reappraisal of the appropriate level of care.[55,80,81] Nevertheless, the length of ICU admission per se should not be used in the clinical decision-making process regarding the continuation of treatment in these patients.[84] There is general agreement that patients with active newly diagnosed malignancies and those in cancer remission presenting with acute complications should receive full ICU management and organ support. In these cases, the benefit from intensive care was demonstrated even when urgent anticancer treatments were required in the ICU by patients with acute complications related to high-grade malignancies.[85,86] One exception may be the patients with ARF secondary to small cell lung carcinoma. Although a fast response to cancer chemotherapy may be expected a priori, results demonstrated that none of the patients admitted with ARF survived their hospital stay.[35] On the other hand, ICU admission may be considered nonbeneficial or inappropriate in patients with a poor performance status and those for whom potentially life-extending treatment is unavailable. In the other cases, a trial of ICU support should be considered paramount to identify high-risk cancer patients who could benefit from early aggressive management of organ failures in the ICU.

INVASIVE AND NONINVASIVE MECHANICAL VENTILATORY SUPPORT IN ACUTE RESPIRATORY FAILURE

Whereas the ultimate outcome of ARF depends on the reversibility of the underlying cause, correction of hypoxemia and oxygen delivery as well as hypercapnic acidosis is pivotal to ensure patient survival while the underlying cause is identified and treated. Positive pressure ventilation can be delivered through endotracheal intubation (ie, IPPV) or through a nasal or facial mask, or a helmet (ie, NIPPV). In contrast to IPPV, NIPPV preserves the integrity of the upper airway functions and defense mechanisms (allowing swallowing, coughing, and vocalization) and decreases the need for sedation.[87] As a consequence, the incidence of ventilator-associated pneumonia is lower in patients exposed to NIPPV than to IPPV.[88] In a setting of hypercapnic ARF failure resulting from COPD, and to a lesser extent in that of cardiogenic pulmonary edema, NIPPV is now accepted as the preferential initial mode of respiratory support,[89] as several randomized controlled trials (RCTs), which compared NIPPV with supplemental oxygen only, have observed a reduction in need for intubation, a reduction of intubation-related complications, a shorter ICU length of stay, and a better survival associated with its use.[90–93] These encouraging results have prompted clinicians to use NIPPV up-front in other categories of patients presenting with ARF, such as patients receiving immunosuppressive therapy or those with underlying hematological or solid malignancy.

NIPPV versus IPPV or Oxygen Therapy in Cancer Patients: The Studies

Data on the use of NIPPV in cancer patients are provided by 2 small RCTs,[94,95] as well as a larger set of observational studies. Both interventional studies randomized immunocompromised patients with hypoxemic ARF (defined as a ratio of PaO_2 to the fraction of inspired oxygen [PaO_2/FiO_2] of <200) to treatment with either NIPPV or with standard supplemental oxygen. Antonelli and colleagues[95] studied 40 solid organ transplant patients; NIPPV averted intubation in 80% (significantly more than in patients treated with supplemental oxygen only), and was associated with reduced ICU, but not hospital mortality. Hilbert and colleagues[94] included a heterogeneous population of immunocompromised patients (56 patients), 30 of whom were hematological (cancer) patients: intubation was avoided in 54%, and both ICU and hospital mortality were significantly lower in the NIPPV-treated compared with the control arm. In both studies, the lower ICU mortality in NIPPV-treated patients was mainly due to the lower rate of fatal complications following intubation. From these trials, it seems that NIPPV effectively restores gas exchange as well as unloads the respiratory pump in an early phase of hypoxic ARF in otherwise stable patients, reducing the need for intubation and its associated complications.

The observational studies include case series of cancer patients subjected to a trial of NIPPV[96,97] as well as studies identifying prognostic indicators in cancer patients with ARF or requiring MV.[1,27,32,34,49,52,59,98] Some of the latter studies compared outcome between NIPPV-exposed (cases) versus no NIPPV-exposed patients (controls).[32,34,49,98] In these studies, control patients consisted of patients initially treated with IPPV[32,49,98] or of patients treated with supplemental oxygen or IPPV.[34] In most reports, the study population included both solid and hematologic cancer patients, but some considered hematologic cancer patients only.[32,34,59,98] NIPPV was applied in a variable proportion of patients, ranging from 4%[27] to 39%,[98] and avoided intubation in a third[32,98] to half of the cases.[49,52] In most, but not all studies,[32,34] the use of NIPPV, as compared with IPPV, was associated with better survival. However, only 3 studies adjusted the association between outcome and the use of NIPPV as (initial) mode of ventilatory support for severity-of-illness: the study of Azoulay and colleagues[1] revealed a protective effect associated with the use of NIPPV, whereas the 2 reports by Depuydt and colleagues[32,34] could not confirm this.

NIPPV or IPPV in Nonpalliative Cancer Patients: Weighing the Evidence

Several factors are to be kept in mind when interpreting the results of studies of ventilatory support in cancer patients; some of these may help to explain the differences between the findings of the interventional and some of the observational studies. First, it should be stressed that the interventional studies were designed to compare respiratory support by NIPPV to supplemental oxygen only, and considered intubation as an end point.[94,95] In contrast, most of the observational studies compared patients treated with NIPPV or IPPV as initial mode of ventilatory support.[32,49] Patients who required immediate intubation, eg, because of septic shock, were excluded in the interventional trials. Inclusion of these sicker patients in the observational studies may have biased the results to the detriment of IPPV patients. For example, in a study in critically ill patients with acute myeloid leukemia, showing a lower mortality in initially NIPPV- as compared with IPPV-treated patients, all patients with initial IPPV were intubated before ICU admission, which suggests a more profound clinical deterioration before institution of MV in the invasively ventilated patients.[98] Second, in the interventional studies, patients were likely to receive NIPPV earlier in the course of their critical illness. In the observational studies, the time lag to ICU referral remains unknown and is probably variable. A longer delay to the start of NIPPV has been shown to be an independent predictor of NIPPV failure,[52] which may explain the high failure rates in the noninterventional trials. Third, the underlying cause of ARF has been shown to be strongly correlated with outcome, and is likely to be an important confounder when assessing the association between outcome and the initial choice of ventilatory support (discussed earlier). Finally, the outcome in patients receiving NIPPV is much worse in the interventional than in the more recent observational studies. In the studies by Antonelli and colleagues[94] and Hilbert and colleagues,[95] ICU mortality rates in patients who ultimately received IPPV were 78% and 87%, respectively. In the more recent observational studies, mortality in invasively ventilated patients ranged from 50% to 70%[1,27,32,34,49]; obviously, these better results reduced the likelihood of finding a significant survival benefit associated with the use of NIPPV compared with IPPV.

NIPPV or IPPV in Nonpalliative Cancer Patients: A Matter of Selection

In the reports published to date, NIPPV failed in roughly half of the cases, despite the compliance with generally established contraindications for NIPPV.[89] More worryingly, NIPPV failure and conversion to IPPV appeared to be associated with very high mortality rates up to greater than 90%[1,32]; in addition, conversion of NIPPV to IPPV itself was an independent predictor of mortality.[1,52] Although this observation may reflect the poor prognosis associated with nonreversible ARF (for which NIPPV is more likely to fail than in rapidly reversible ARF), a causal relationship between adverse outcome and the inappropriate use of NIPPV cannot be ruled out. As discussed earlier, mortality in cancer patients treated with IPPV has decreased to 60% to 70% in the more recent reports (see **Table 1**).[1,27,32,34,49,51] This improvement implies that in nonpalliative cancer patients, IPPV should not be considered as the last resort after every other therapy has failed, but may be a preferable first-line mode of respiratory support in an earlier stage of ARF in some patients. As such, the framework of indications and contraindications for NIPPV applicable for the general population[89] may require modification for the specific population of critically ill cancer patients. Identification of predictors for NIPPV failure in cancer patients such as those provided by Adda and colleagues is therefore important in improving the selection of patients. In a population of 99 cancer patients who received NIPPV, failure of NIPPV was significantly associated with a delay in initiating NIPPV, a diagnosis of acute respiratory distress syndrome (ARDS), and extrapulmonary organ failure, that is, need for vasopressors and for renal replacement therapy. In addition, increasing respiratory rate under NIPPV was an early predictor of NIPPV failure.[52]

Aside from patient characteristics, tolerance of NIPPV, and hence the rate of NIPPV success, may depend on the appropriate choice of the type of ventilator, mode of NIPPV, and patient-ventilator interface. No studies have compared different NIPPV ventilators or ventilatory modes in immunocompromised patients, but data about the choice of interface are provided by one center. In a prospective uncontrolled study in 17 hematological patients with hypoxemic ARF, providing continuous positive airway pressure (CPAP) through a helmet avoided intubation in all patients; in a matched historical control group, CPAP applied through a facial mask failed in half of the cases.[99] However, application of NIPPV with a helmet requires expertise as well as adequate monitoring of the patient, as some investigators reported a substantial risk of ventilatory dysfunction (carbon dioxide rebreathing[100] and rapid hypoxia in case of ventilatory flow disconnection[101]) associated with this type of interface.

Mechanical Ventilatory Support in Cancer Patients: Recommendations

Using the criteria of the Society of Critical Care Medicine (Level 1: convincingly justifiable on scientific evidence, including RCTs; Level 2: reasonably justifiable by available scientific evidence and strongly supported by expert critical care opinion; Level 3: adequate scientific evidence is lacking but widely supported by available data and expert critical care opinion), the following practical recommendations rated by the strength of evidence can be of help in selecting the initial ventilatory strategy in patients with malignancies and hypoxemic ARF (**Fig. 1**,[102]):

(a) Nonpalliative cancer patients who develop hypoxemia (PaO_2/FiO_2 <200) should be considered for a trial of NIPPV at the ICU. Providing supplemental oxygen only in these patients has shown to be inferior to institution of NIPPV (Level 1). Delaying NIPPV in hypoxemic patients has been shown to be predictive for NIPPV failure, which in itself is associated with increased mortality (Level 2).

(b) Some nonpalliative cancer patients with hypoxemic ARF should be considered for IPPV instead of NIPPV: contraindications for NIPPV as identified in the general population should also be respected in cancer patients (Level 1). In addition, patients with renal replacement therapy, vasopressor need, or fulfilling the criteria of ARDS are more likely to fail NIPPV (Level 2). Patients with a potentially rapidly reversible cause of hypoxemic ARF such as cardiogenic pulmonary edema, fluid overload and, to a lesser extent, pneumonia may be better candidates for NIPPV than patients with an unknown cause of ARF. Providing NIPPV to a hypoxemic patient who is likely to fail NIPPV may cause harm (Level 2).

(c) Cancer patients who develop hypercapnia are candidates for a NIPPV trial, based on good clinical results in the noncancer patients with hypercapnic ARF, such as COPD patients (Level 1). However, the same contraindications for NIPPV and

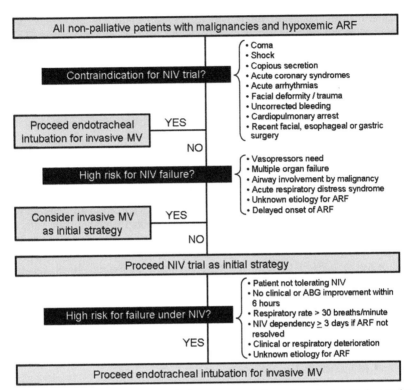

Fig. 1. Flow chart summarizing practical recommendations to select initial ventilatory strategy in patients with malignancies and hypoxemic ARF. ABG, arterial blood gas analysis; ARF, acute respiratory failure; MV, mechanical ventilation; NIV, noninvasive ventilation. (*From* Soares M, Salluh JIF, Azoulay E. Noninvasive ventilation in patients with malignancies and hypoxemic acute respiratory failure: a still pending question. J Crit Care 2009. DOI: 10.1016/j.jcrc.2009.04.001. [Epub ahead of print]; with permission.)

    awareness for risk factors for NIPPV failure as in hypoxemic ARF should be respected (Level 1).

(d) Prolonged NIPPV should be avoided. Late NIPPV failure has been shown to be an independent predictor for mortality (Level 2). Increased respiratory rate while treated with NIPPV is an early predictor of NIPPV failure and should lead the clinician to consider converting NIPPV to IPPV (Level 2). In addition, patient intolerance, failure to improve within 6 hours of NIPPV, prolonged dependency of NIPPV (>3 days), and an unknown cause of ARF are risk factors for NIPPV failure, and should lead to consideration of airway intubation instead (Level 2).

SUMMARY

Survival of patients with malignances admitted to the ICU in need of MV has improved over the last decade. This improvement can be ascribable to advances in patient management in hematology and oncology and in critical care, but certainly also to a better selection of patients for ICU admission. The current scenario of better outcomes coupled with imprecision in patient selection criteria and broadening of ICU admission policies should prompt clinicians to offer initial "full-code" management followed by regular reassessment of the appropriate level of care. Because failure of NIPPV is frequent and associated with increased mortality, caution is needed in recommending NIPPV as the initial mode of ventilatory support in patients with cancer. Early identification of patients in whom NIPPV can be effective is as important as the recognition of early indicators that NIPPV will probably fail. Recommendations were formulated to assist physicians in the selection of the more appropriate initial ventilatory strategy. Finally, close collaboration between intensivists and hemato-oncologists is essential for identification of high-risk patients who can benefit from early aggressive management in the ICU.

REFERENCES

1. Azoulay E, Thiéry G, Chevret S, et al. The prognosis of acute respiratory failure in critically ill cancer patients. Medicine (Baltimore) 2004;83(6):360–70.
2. Azoulay E, Schlemmer B. Diagnostic strategy in cancer patients with acute respiratory failure. Intensive Care Med 2006;32(6):808–22.
3. Azoulay E, Fieux F, Moreau D, et al. Acute monocytic leukemia presenting as acute respiratory failure. Am J Respir Crit Care Med 2003;167(10):1329–33.
4. Chaoui D, Legrand O, Roche N, et al. Incidence and prognostic value of respiratory events in acute leukemia. Leukemia 2004;18(4):670–5.
5. Lim Z, Pagliuca A, Simpson S, et al. Outcomes of patients with haematological malignancies admitted to intensive care unit. A comparative review of allogeneic haematopoietic stem cell transplantation data. Br J Haematol 2007;136(3): 448–50.
6. Shorr AF, Moores LK, Edenfield WJ, et al. Mechanical ventilation in hematopoietic stem cell transplantation: can we effectively predict outcomes? Chest 1999;116(4):1012–8.
7. Khassawneh BY, White P Jr, Anaissie EJ, et al. Outcome from mechanical ventilation after autologous peripheral blood stem cell transplantation. Chest 2002;121(1):185–8.
8. Groeger JS, Lemeshow S, Price K, et al. Multicenter outcome study of cancer patients admitted to the intensive care unit: a probability of mortality model. J Clin Oncol 1998;16(2):761–70.
9. Kress JP, Christenson J, Pohlman AS, et al. Outcomes of critically ill cancer patients in a university hospital setting. Am J Respir Crit Care Med 1999; 160(6):1957–61.
10. Maschmeyer G, Bertschat FL, Moesta KT, et al. Outcome analysis of 189 consecutive cancer patients referred to the intensive care unit as emergencies during a 2-year period. Eur J Cancer 2003;39(6):783–92.
11. Soares M, Salluh JI, Ferreira CG, et al. Impact of two different comorbidity measures on the 6-month mortality of critically ill cancer patients. Intensive Care Med 2005;31(3):408–15.
12. Soares M, Salluh JI. Validation of the SAPS 3 admission prognostic model in patients with cancer in need of intensive care. Intensive Care Med 2006; 32(11):1839–44.
13. Staudinger T, Stoiser B, Müllner M, et al. Outcome and prognostic factors in critically ill cancer patients admitted to the intensive care unit. Crit Care Med 2000;28(5):1322–8.
14. Taccone FS, Artigas AA, Sprung CL, et al. Characteristics and outcomes of cancer patients in European ICUs. Crit Care 2009;13(1):R15.

15. Peigne V, Rusinová K, Karlin L, et al. Continued survival gains in recent years among critically ill myeloma patients. Intensive Care Med 2009;35(3):512–8.
16. Azoulay E, Moreau D, Alberti C, et al. Predictors of short-term mortality in critically ill patients with solid malignancies. Intensive Care Med 2000;26(12):1817–23.
17. Benoit DD, Vandewoude KH, Decruyenaere JM, et al. Outcome and early prognostic indicators in patients with a hematologic malignancy admitted to the intensive care unit for a life-threatening complication. Crit Care Med 2003; 31(1):104–12.
18. Kroschinsky F, Weise M, Illmer T, et al. Outcome and prognostic features of intensive care unit treatment in patients with hematological malignancies. Intensive Care Med 2002;28(9):1294–300.
19. Evison J, Rickenbacher P, Ritz R, et al. Intensive care unit admission in patients with haematological disease: incidence, outcome and prognostic factors. Swiss Med Wkly 2001;131(47–48):681–6.
20. Ferrà C, Marcos P, Misis M, et al. Outcome and prognostic factors in patients with hematologic malignancies admitted to the intensive care unit: a single-center experience. Int J Hematol 2007;85(3):195–202.
21. Massion PB, Dive AM, Doyen C, et al. Prognosis of hematologic malignancies does not predict intensive care unit mortality. Crit Care Med 2002;30(10): 2260–70.
22. Blot F, Guiguet M, Nitenberg G, et al. Prognostic factors for neutropenic patients in an intensive care unit: respective roles of underlying malignancies and acute organ failures. Eur J Cancer 1997;33(7):1031–7.
23. Darmon M, Azoulay E, Alberti C, et al. Impact of neutropenia duration on short-term mortality in neutropenic critically ill cancer patients. Intensive Care Med 2002;28(12):1775–80.
24. Larché J, Azoulay E, Fieux F, et al. Improved survival of critically ill cancer patients with septic shock. Intensive Care Med 2003;29(10):1688–95.
25. Pène F, Percheron S, Lemiale V, et al. Temporal changes in management and outcome of septic shock in patients with malignancies in the intensive care unit. Crit Care Med 2008;36(3):690–6.
26. Pastores SM. Acute respiratory failure in critically ill patients with cancer. Diagnosis and management. Crit Care Clin 2001;17(3):623–46.
27. Soares M, Salluh JI, Spector N, et al. Characteristics and outcomes of cancer patients requiring mechanical ventilatory support for >24 hrs. Crit Care Med 2005;33(3):520–6.
28. Azoulay E, Mokart D, Rabbat A, et al. Diagnostic bronchoscopy in hematology and oncology patients with acute respiratory failure: prospective multicenter data. Crit Care Med 2008;36(1):100–7.
29. Pastores SM, Dulu A, Voigt L, et al. Premortem clinical diagnoses and post-mortem autopsy findings: discrepancies in critically ill cancer patients. Crit Care 2007;11(2):R48.
30. Vandijck DM, Benoit DD, Depuydt PO, et al. Impact of recent intravenous chemotherapy on outcome in severe sepsis and septic shock patients with hematological malignancies. Intensive Care Med 2008;34(5):847–55.
31. Salluh JI, Bozza FA, Pinto TS, et al. Cutaneous periumbilical purpura in disseminated strongyloidiasis in cancer patients: a pathognomonic feature of potentially lethal disease? Braz J Infect Dis 2005;9(5):419–24.
32. Depuydt PO, Benoit DD, Vandewoude KH, et al. Outcome in noninvasively and invasively ventilated hematologic patients with acute respiratory failure. Chest 2004;126(4):1299–306.

33. Benoit DD, Depuydt PO, Peleman RA, et al. Documented and clinically suspected bacterial infection precipitating intensive care unit admission in patients with hematological malignancies: impact on outcome. Intensive Care Med 2005; 31(7):934–42.
34. Depuydt PO, Benoit DD, Roosens CD, et al. The impact of the initial ventilatory strategy on survival in hematological patients with acute hypoxemic respiratory failure. J Crit Care; 2009. DOI:10.1016/j.jcrc.2009.02.016. [Epub ahead of print].
35. Soares M, Darmon M, Salluh JI, et al. Prognosis of lung cancer patients with life-threatening complications. Chest 2007;131(3):840–6.
36. Sørensen HT, Mellemkjaer L, Olsen JH, et al. Prognosis of cancers associated with venous thromboembolism. N Engl J Med 2000;343(25):1846–50.
37. Dimopoulou I, Bamias A, Lyberopoulos P, et al. Pulmonary toxicity from novel antineoplastic agents. Ann Oncol 2006;17(3):372–9.
38. Vahid B, Marik PE. Pulmonary complications of novel antineoplastic agents for solid tumors. Chest 2008;133(2):528–38.
39. Takano T, Ohe Y, Kusumoto M, et al. Risk factors for interstitial lung disease and predictive factors for tumor response in patients with advanced non-small cell lung cancer treated with gefitinib. Lung Cancer 2004;45(1):93–104.
40. Peters SG, Meadows JA 3rd, Gracey DR. Outcome of respiratory failure in hematologic malignancy. Chest 1988;94(1):99–102.
41. Lloyd-Thomas AR, Wright I, Lister TA, et al. Prognosis of patients receiving intensive care for lifethreatening medical complications of haematological malignancy. Br Med J (Clin Res Ed) 1988;296(6628):1025–9.
42. Schuster DP, Marion JM. Precedents for meaningful recovery during treatment in a medical intensive care unit. Outcome in patients with hematologic malignancy. Am J Med 1983;75(3):402–8.
43. Epner DE, White P, Krasnoff M, et al. Outcome of mechanical ventilation for adults with hematologic malignancy. J Investig Med 1996;44(5):254–60.
44. Hauser MJ, Tabak J, Baier H. Survival of patients with cancer in a medical critical care unit. Arch Intern Med 1982;142(3):527–9.
45. Snow RM, Miller WC, Rice DL, et al. Respiratory failure in cancer patients. JAMA 1979;241(19):2039–42.
46. Boussat S, El'rini T, Dubiez A, et al. Predictive factors of death in primary lung cancer patients on admission to the intensive care unit. Intensive Care Med 2000;26(12):1811–6.
47. Soares M, Carvalho MS, Salluh JI, et al. Effect of age on survival of critically ill patients with cancer. Crit Care Med 2006;34(3):715–21.
48. Groeger JS, White P Jr, Nierman DM, et al. Outcome for cancer patients requiring mechanical ventilation. J Clin Oncol 1999;17(3):991–7.
49. Azoulay E, Alberti C, Bornstain C, et al. Improved survival in cancer patients requiring mechanical ventilatory support: impact of noninvasive mechanical ventilatory support. Crit Care Med 2001;29(3):519–25.
50. Vallot F, Paesmans M, Berghmans T, et al. Leucopenia is an independent predictor in cancer patients requiring invasive mechanical ventilation: a prognostic factor analysis in a series of 168 patients. Support Care Cancer 2003;11(4):236–41.
51. Lecuyer L, Chevret S, Guidet B, et al. Case volume and mortality in haematological patients with acute respiratory failure. Eur Respir J 2008;32(3):748–54.
52. Adda M, Coquet I, Darmon M, et al. Predictors of noninvasive ventilation failure in patients with hematologic malignancy and acute respiratory failure. Crit Care Med 2008;36(10):2766–72.

53. Meert AP, Close L, Hardy M, et al. Noninvasive ventilation: application to the cancer patient admitted in the intensive care unit. Support Care Cancer 2003; 11(1):56–9.

54. Lamia B, Hellot MF, Girault C, et al. Changes in severity and organ failure scores as prognostic factors in onco-hematological malignancy patients admitted to the ICU. Intensive Care Med 2006;32(10):1560–8.

55. Lecuyer L, Chevret S, Thiery G, et al. The ICU trial: a new admission policy for cancer patients requiring mechanical ventilation. Crit Care Med 2007;35(3): 808–14.

56. Soares M, Salluh JI, Toscano L, et al. Outcomes and prognostic factors in patients with head and neck cancer and severe acute illnesses. Intensive Care Med 2007;33(11):2009–13.

57. Adam AK, Soubani AO. Outcome and prognostic factors of lung cancer patients admitted to the medical intensive care unit. Eur Respir J 2008;31(1):47–53.

58. Park HY, Suh GY, Jeon K, et al. Outcome and prognostic factors of patients with acute leukemia admitted to the intensive care unit for septic shock. Leuk Lymphoma 2008;49(10):1929–34.

59. Rabbat A, Chaoui D, Montani D, et al. Prognosis of patients with acute myeloid leukaemia admitted to intensive care. Br J Haematol 2005;129(3):350–7.

60. Reichner CA, Thompson JA, O'Brien S, et al. Outcome and code status of lung cancer patients admitted to the medical ICU. Chest 2006;130(3):719–23.

61. Shen HN, Cheng KC, Hou CC, et al. Clinical features and short-term outcome of critically ill patients with head and neck cancer in the medical intensive care unit. Am J Clin Oncol 2009. DOI:10.1097/COC.0b013e3181931236. [Epub ahead of print].

62. Pène F, Aubron C, Azoulay E, et al. Outcome of critically ill allogeneic hemato-poietic stem-cell transplantation recipients: a reappraisal of indications for organ failure supports. J Clin Oncol 2006;24(4):643–9.

63. Huaringa AJ, Leyva FJ, Giralt SA, et al. Outcome of bone marrow transplantation patients requiring mechanical ventilation. Crit Care Med 2000;28(4):1014–7.

64. Jackson SR, Tweeddale MG, Barnett MJ, et al. Admission of bone marrow trans-plant recipients to the intensive care unit: outcome, survival and prognostic factors. Bone Marrow Transplant 1998;21(7):697–704.

65. Afessa B, Tefferi A, Dunn WF, et al. Intensive care unit support and acute phys-iology and Chronic Health Evaluation III performance in hematopoietic stem cell transplant recipients. Crit Care Med 2003;31(6):1715–21.

66. Paz HL, Garland A, Weinar M, et al. Effect of clinical outcomes data on intensive care unit utilization by bone marrow transplant patients. Crit Care Med 1998; 26(1):66–70.

67. Price KJ, Thall PF, Kish SK, et al. Prognostic indicators for blood and marrow transplant patients admitted to an intensive care unit. Am J Respir Crit Care Med 1998;158(3):876–84.

68. Gruson D, Hilbert G, Portel L, et al. Severe respiratory failure requiring ICU admission in bone marrow transplant recipients. Eur Respir J 1999;13(4): 883–7.

69. Ewig S, Torres A, Riquelme R, et al. Pulmonary complications in patients with haematological malignancies treated at a respiratory ICU. Eur Respir J 1998; 12(1):116–22.

70. Bach PB, Schrag D, Nierman DM, et al. Identification of poor prognostic features among patients requiring mechanical ventilation after hematopoietic stem cell transplantation. Blood 2001;98(12):3234–40.

71. Soares M, Salluh JI, Carvalho MS, et al. Prognosis of critically ill patients with cancer and acute renal dysfunction. J Clin Oncol 2006;24(24):4003–10.
72. Vieira JM Jr, Castro I, Curvello-Neto A, et al. Effect of acute kidney injury on weaning from mechanical ventilation in critically ill patients. Crit Care Med 2007;35(1):184–91.
73. Nelson JE, Meier DE, Oei EJ, et al. Self-reported symptom experience of critically ill cancer patients receiving intensive care. Crit Care Med 2001;29(2): 277–82.
74. Yau E, Rohatiner AZ, Lister TA, et al. Long term prognosis and quality of life following intensive care for life-threatening complications of haematological malignancy. Br J Cancer 1991;64(5):938–42.
75. Schellongowski P, Benesch M, Lang T, et al. Comparison of three severity scores for critically ill cancer patients. Intensive Care Med 2004;30(3):430–6.
76. Soares M, Fontes F, Dantas J, et al. Performance of six severity-of-illness scores in cancer patients requiring admission to the intensive care unit: a prospective observational study. Crit Care 2004;8(4):R194–203.
77. den Boer S, de Keizer NF, de Jonge E. Performance of prognostic models in critically ill cancer patients—a review. Crit Care 2005;9(4):R458–63.
78. Barnato AE, Hsu HE, Bryce CL, et al. Using simulation to isolate physician variation in intensive care unit admission decision making for critically ill elders with end-stage cancer: a pilot feasibility study. Crit Care Med 2008;36(12):3156–63.
79. Thiéry G, Azoulay E, Darmon M, et al. Outcome of cancer patients considered for intensive care unit admission: a hospital-wide prospective study. J Clin Oncol 2005;23(19):4406–13.
80. Azoulay E, Afessa B. The intensive care support of patients with malignancy: do everything that can be done. Intensive Care Med 2006;32(1):3–5.
81. Darmon M, Azoulay E. Critical care management of cancer patients: cause for optimism and need for objectivity. Curr Opin Oncol 2009;21(4):318–26.
82. Pène F, Soares M. Can we still refuse ICU admission of patients with hematological malignancies? Intensive Care Med 2008;34(5):790–2.
83. Raoof ND, Groeger JS. You never know—one of your patients with cancer might surprise you. Crit Care Med 2007;35(3):965–6.
84. Soares M, Salluh JI, Torres VB, et al. Short- and long-term outcomes of critically ill patients with cancer and prolonged ICU length of stay. Chest 2008;134(3): 520–6.
85. Benoit DD, Depuydt PO, Vandewoude KH, et al. Outcome in severely ill patients with hematological malignancies who received intravenous chemotherapy in the intensive care unit. Intensive Care Med 2006;32(1):93–9.
86. Darmon M, Thiery G, Ciroldi M, et al. Intensive care in patients with newly diagnosed malignancies and a need for cancer chemotherapy. Crit Care Med 2005; 33(11):2488–93.
87. Rajan T, Hill NS. Noninvasive positive pressure ventilation. In: Fink MP, Abraham E, Vincent JL, et al, editors. Textbook of critical care. 5th edition. Philadelphia: Elsevier Saunders; 2005. p. 519–26.
88. Girou E, Schortgen F, Delclaux C, et al. Association of noninvasive ventilation with nosocomial infections and survival in critically ill patients. JAMA 2000; 284(18):2361–7.
89. British Thoracic Society Standards of Care Committee. Non-invasive ventilation in acute respiratory failure. Thorax 2002;57(3):192–211.
90. Lightowler JV, Wedzicha JA, Elliott MW, et al. Noninvasive positive pressure ventilation to treat respiratory failure resulting from exacerbations of chronic

obstructive pulmonary disease: Cochrane systematic review and meta-analysis. BMJ 2003;326(7382):185.

91. Keenan S, Sinuff T, Cook D, et al. Which patients with acute exacerbation of chronic obstructive pulmonary disease benefit from noninvasive positive pressure ventilation? Ann Intern Med 2003;138(11):861–70.

92. Keenan S, Sinuff T, Cook D, et al. Does noninvasive positive pressure ventilation improve outcome in acute hypoxemic failure? A systematic review. Crit Care Med 2004;32(12):2516–23.

93. Masip J, Roque M, Sanchez B. Noninvasive ventilation in acute cardiogenic pulmonary edema: systematic review and meta-analysis. JAMA 2005;294(24): 3124–30.

94. Hilbert G, Gruson D, Vargas F, et al. Noninvasive ventilation in immunosuppressed patients with pulmonary infiltrates, fever, and acute respiratory failure. N Engl J Med 2001;344(7):481–7.

95. Antonelli M, Conti G, Bufi M, et al. Noninvasive ventilation for treatment of acute respiratory failure in patients undergoing solid organ transplantation: a randomized trial. JAMA 2000;283(2):235–41.

96. Hilbert G, Gruson D, Vargas F, et al. Noninvasive continuous positive airway pressure in neutropenic patients with acute respiratory failure requiring intensive care unit admission. Crit Care Med 2000;28(9):3185–90.

97. Varon J, Walsh GL, Fromm RE. Feasibility of noninvasive mechanical ventilation in the treatment of acute respiratory failure in postoperative cancer patients. J Crit Care 1998;13(2):55–7.

98. Rabitsch W, Staudinger T, Locker G, et al. Respiratory failure after stem cell transplantation: improved outcome with non-invasive ventilation. Leuk Lymphoma 2005;46(8):1151–7.

99. Principi T, Pantanetti S, Catani F, et al. Noninvasive continuous positive airway pressure delivered by helmet in hematological malignancy patients with hypoxemic acute respiratory failure. Intensive Care Med 2004;30(1):147–50.

100. Taccone P, Hess D, Caironi P, et al. Continuous positive airway pressure delivered with a 'helmet': effects on carbon dioxide rebreathing. Crit Care Med 2004;32(10):2090–6.

101. Patroniti N, Saini M, Zanella A, et al. Danger of helmet continuous positive airway pressure during failure of fresh gas source supply. Intensive Care Med 2007; 33(1):153–7.

102. Soares M, Salluh JIF, Azoulay E. Noninvasive ventilation in patients with malignancies and hypoxemic acute respiratory failure: a still pending question. J Crit Care 2009. DOI:10.1016/j.jcrc.2009.04.001. [Epub ahead of print].

Diagnosis and Management of Infectious Complications in Critically Ill Patients with Cancer

Raghukumar Thirumala, MD[a], Madhusudanan Ramaswamy, MD[a],
Sanjay Chawla, MD, FCCP[a,b],*

KEYWORDS

• Infection • Cancer • Critically ill • Immunosuppressed

Patients who have cancer have a greater tendency to acquire infections than the general population. The critically ill cancer patient is at a high risk for infections and its resulting complications. Multiple factors are responsible for this heightened risk of infection. In addition to complex cancer treatments, disruption of physical barriers including mucosal and integumentary systems, neutropenia, cellular and humoral immune dysfunction, splenectomy, presence of indwelling vascular catheters, and local tumor effects contribute to the increased risk of infection. In this population, organisms with low virulence potential are capable of causing significant morbidity and mortality.[1–3] Organisms that cause infections in critically ill patients who have cancer span the entire gamut including bacteria, viruses, fungi, and protozoa.

Sepsis remains a common reason for hospital admission, accounting for approximately 750,000 admissions per year in the United States with a rising incidence.[1,4] Patients who have cancer have a 30% higher risk for death from sepsis, which accounts for approximately 10% of all cancer deaths.[2,4,5] Infection is a major cause of prolonged hospitalization and organ dysfunction in patients who have cancer. The National Institutes of Health estimated the direct medical costs for cancer in 2008 to be $93.2 billion.[6] It is estimated that the annual hospital costs for patients who have cancer with severe sepsis alone is in excess of $3 billion.[5] A total of

[a] Critical Care Medicine Service, Department of Anesthesiology and Critical Care Medicine, Memorial Sloan-Kettering Cancer Center, 1275 York Avenue, C1179, New York, NY 10021, USA
[b] Department of Clinical Anesthesiology, Weill Cornell Medical College, New York, NY, USA
* Corresponding author. Critical Care Medicine Service, Department of Anesthesiology and Critical Care Medicine, Memorial Sloan-Kettering Cancer Center, 1275 York Avenue, C1179, New York, NY 10021.
E-mail address: chawlas@mskcc.org (S. Chawla).

Crit Care Clin 26 (2010) 59–91
doi:10.1016/j.ccc.2009.09.007
0749-0704/09/$ – see front matter © 2010 Elsevier Inc. All rights reserved.

criticalcare.theclinics.com

1,479,350 new cancer cases and 562,340 deaths from cancer are projected to occur in the United States in 2009.[7]

EPIDEMIOLOGY

Patients who have cancer are ten times more likely to acquire sepsis than patients who do not have cancer and account for 2.3% to 25% of severe sepsis and septic shock cases.[2,4,5,8,9] Hematologic cancers (66.4 per 1000) are more likely to develop severe sepsis as compared with solid tumors (7.6 per 1000) and have a higher mortality rate.[5,9] The length of stay and hospital costs for patients who have cancer and severe sepsis was nearly three times that of patients who have cancer but not severe sepsis.

Racial and gender disparities in the incidence of sepsis among patients who have cancer have been noted. Non-white patients who have cancer have consistently higher rates of sepsis. The etiology remains uncertain but factors, such as disparity in access to care and differences in receiving aggressive care, have been suggested. The incidence of sepsis is higher in men relative to women. The source of sepsis is often related to the anatomic site of the primary tumor. It is more common to encounter respiratory infections in patients who have lung cancer and genitourinary infections in patients who have prostate cancer.[2]

CELLULAR HOST DEFENSE DYSFUNCTION
Innate Immunity

The first line of cellular defense of the host is the innate (or natural) immune system, which is in part comprised of phagocytic cells including neutrophils, monocytes, dendritic cells, and tissue macrophages. These cells defend the host from microbial invasion in a nonspecific manner through recognition of pathogen-associated molecular patterns including unique lipopolysaccharides and peptidoglycans, lipoteichoic acids, and mannans. Defense mechanisms include phagocytosis, release of oxidative and nonoxidative mediators, complement activation, and release of cytokines to signal other elements of the immune system. Neutrophils represent the largest proportion of phagocytes, are the primary cell to arrive at the site of infection and have the greatest degree of oxidative burst.

Defects to neutrophils may be either quantitative or qualitative.[10–12] Chemotherapeutic agents, such as melphalan, busulfan, methotrexate, carboplatin, cisplatin, paclitaxel, doxorubicin, cyclophosphamide and etoposide lead to neutropenia by direct bone marrow suppression.[13] Radiation therapy, glucocorticoids, and hyperglycemia can impair neutrophil function and delay neutrophil recovery.[14–16] The three factors that are important in determining the risk of infection associated with neutropenia are the rate of neutrophil decline, degree of neutropenia (absolute neutrophil count [ANC]) and duration of neutropenia.[17–20]

Adaptive Immunity

The adaptive (or acquired) immune system represents a more specialized and targeted component that can be further divided into two separate mechanisms: (1) humoral (B lymphocytes, immunoglobulins and complement system); and (2) cell mediated (T lymphocytes and antigen presenting cells). Additionally, these responses maintain an immunologic memory that is not seen with the innate immune system.[21]

B cells produce immunoglobulins that bind to extracellular foreign antigens including bacterial, viral, and certain fungal pathogens. Immunoglobulins target organisms for phagocytosis by opsonization, activate the complement system, and block pathogen binding to mucosal or target cells.[22] Patients who have B-cell defects, including chronic lymphocytic leukemia (CLL), multiple myeloma, Waldenström macroglobulinemia, and allogeneic hematopoietic stem-cell transplantation (HSCT) recipients are susceptible to overwhelming infections with encapsulated organisms, such as *Streptococcus pneumoniae, Haemophilus influenzae* type b, and *Neisseria meningitidis*.[23–26] Additionally, chemotherapy and radiation can increase the risk for infection.[27] The monoclonal antibody rituximab, used to treat B-cell malignancies, can predispose to infections from encapsulated bacteria and herpes virus up to several months after treatment.[28] Alemtuzumab, a monoclonal antibody used for second line treatment of B-cell CLL and T-cell lymphoma, increases the risk for infection from *Pneumocystis jirovecii* (formerly *Pneumocystis carinii*), fungi and cytomegalovirus (CMV).[29,30]

T-cell receptors, in contrast to immunoglobulins, are displayed on the surface of T cells and enable destruction of intracellular pathogens including viruses, bacteria, fungi, and mycobacteria by recognition of single peptide-major histocompatibility complexes.[31] T cells activate phagocytes, regulate B-cell immunoglobulin production and T-cell mediated cytotoxicity. Malignancies, such as CLL, T-cell leukemia/lymphoma, hairy cell leukemia, Hodgkin's disease and thymoma, and HSCT are associated with impaired T-cell function.[23,32–34] Chemotherapeutic agents, such as fludarabine, cladribine, cyclophosphamide, methotrexate, and corticosteroids can lead to lymphopenia and lymphocyte dysfunction.[35] Patients who have CLL and are treated with fludarabine are at additional risk for various pathogens, including *Listeria monocytogenes, P jirovecii*, CMV, herpes simplex virus (HSV), varicella zoster virus (VZV), and mycobacteria.[35–37] In addition, cyclosporine and tacrolimus, commonly used as immunosuppressants following HSCT, impair T-helper cell function by blocking production of cytokines and other cell-signaling mechanisms. Newer agents, such as temozolomide, cause CD4+ lymphopenia and increase the risk for infections, such as *Pneumocystis* and *Aspergillus* pneumonia.[38,39] **Table 1** lists common pathogens based on the associated immune defect and by organ system involvement.

NEUTROPENIC FEVER

Fever in patients who are neutropenic is an oncologic emergency that necessitates the prompt administration of appropriate antibiotics. Mortality is high when the administration of antibiotics is delayed.[40] Despite improvements in long-term survival, infections remain a common complication of cancer therapy and accounts for the majority of chemotherapy-associated deaths.[41]

Definition

Fever in patients who are neutropenic is defined as a single oral temperature of greater than or equal to 38.3°C (101°F) or a temperature of greater than or equal to 38.0°C (100.4°F) for more than 1 hour. Neutropenia is defined as a neutrophil count of less than 500 cells/mm^3 or a count of less than 1000 cells/mm^3 with a predicted imminent decrease to less than 500 cells/mm^3.[42]

Initial Evaluation

The 2002 Infectious Disease Society of America guidelines stipulate that evaluation of fever in patients who are neutropenic should include a comprehensive history and physical examination with attention for subtle signs and symptoms.[42] Indicators of inflammation may be minimal or absent in patients who are severely neutropenic, especially if accompanied by anemia.[40] Therefore, careful search for sites of infection should include examination of the periodontium, pharynx, perineum and anal

Table 1
System involvement, immune defect, and pathogens commonly associated with critically ill patients who have cancer

Organ Systems		Granulocytopenia	B-cell and Humoral Defects	T-cell Defects
Pulmonary	Bacterial	Staphylococcus aureus Streptococcus pneumoniae Streptococcus pyogenes Klebsiella spp Pseudomonas spp	Streptococcus pneumoniae Haemophilus influenzae	Legionella pneumophila Nocardia asteroides Rhodococcus equi Mycobacterium tuberculosis
	Viral	HSV		CMV Influenza Parainfluenza RSV VZV
	Fungal	Aspergillus spp		Pneumocystis jiroveci Cryptococcus neoformans Histoplasma capsulatum Strongyloides stercoralis
	Parasites			
Gastrointestinal	Bacterial	Escherichia coli Pseudomonas spp Klebsiella spp Clostridium spp CMV	Salmonella spp	Salmonella spp Listeria monocytogenes
	Viral			CMV HSV
	Fungal	Candidia spp		

Central Nervous System	Bacterial	*Staphylococcus aureus* *Streptococcus pneumoniae* *Pseudomonas aeruginosa*	*Streptococcus pneumoniae* *Haemophilus influenzae* *Neisseria meningitidis*	*Aspergillus spp* *Listeria monocytogenes* *Nocardia asteroides* *Mycobacterium tuberculosis*
	Viral	CMV HSV		CMV EBV HHV-6 HSV VZV
	Fungal	*Aspergillus fumigatus* *Candida spp* *Mucoraceae*		*Cryptococcus neoformans*
	Parasites			*Toxoplasma gondii*
Genitourinary	Bacterial	*Escherichia coli* *Pseudomonas aeruginosa*		
	Viral			
	Fungal	*Candida spp*		

region, eye, bone marrow aspiration site, vascular catheter access sites, and perionychium.

Complete blood counts, blood urea nitrogen, creatinine, hepatic panel, and chest radiograph should be obtained in all patients. High-resolution CT (HRCT) will reveal evidence of pneumonia in more than one half of febrile neutropenic patients who have normal findings on chest radiographs.[43] For all patients who have intravascular catheters, a minimum of one set of blood samples should be obtained for culture from each lumen and from a peripheral vein.[44] If a catheter entry site is inflamed or draining, the fluid exuded should be examined by Gram staining and culture for bacteria and fungi. Cultures of urine samples are indicated if signs and symptoms of urinary tract infection (UTI) exist, a urinary catheter is in place, or the findings of urinalysis are abnormal. In a series of febrile neutropenic patients with cancer who had UTIs, only 11% of the subjects who had an ANC of less than 100 cells/mm^3 had pyuria.[40] Cultures of the stool and cerebrospinal fluid (CSF) should be considered as guided by symptoms and physical examination. Aspiration or biopsy of skin lesions suspected of being infected should be performed for cytologic testing, Gram staining, and culture. Levels of C-reactive protein, interleukin (IL)-6, IL-8, and procalcitonin may be affected by bacteremia in febrile neutropenic patients, but the association is not sufficiently consistent to recommend for routine clinical practice.[42]

Risk Assessment

Determining the clinical risk of patients with neutropenic fever is essential to help identify those suitable for outpatient antibiotic therapy and stratify individuals who may benefit from empiric antifungal therapy.[45] Two assessment systems have been developed to risk stratify patients.[46,47] According to the Multinational Association of Supportive Care in Cancer (MASCC) system various factors (absence of hypotension, absence of dehydration, burden of illness, age <60 years) that were associated with a better outcome were assigned an integer weight to develop a risk-index score. A risk-index score greater than or equal to 21 identified low risk patients with a less than 5% risk of complications, but if the risk score is less than or equal to 21 the risk of complications and death is significantly higher. The risk of developing bacteremia and poor outcome after treatment is even greater if the MASCC risk index is less than 15.[47]

Spectrum of Infection

Bacterial infections are the most common causes of infection and at least one half of patients with neutropenic fever with counts less than 100 cells/mm^3 have bacteremia. The organisms causing bacteremia are listed in **Table 2**. Fungi are common causes of secondary infections among patients who received broad-spectrum antibiotics. The primary sites of infection are the gastrointestinal (GI) tract, vascular access devices, and lung.[42]

Bacterial infections

The spectrum of bacterial infections occurring in neutropenic fever has changed over the past three decades.[48] In the 1970s and 1980s enteric Gram-negative bacilli, such as *Escherichia coli*, *Pseudomonas*, and *Enterobacter* species predominated being the etiologic agents in 60% to 70% of cases, whereas Gram-positive organisms, such as *Staphylococcus aureus*, *Staphylococcus epidermidis,* and *Streptococcal* species accounted for 20% to 30% of infections.[49] In the 1990s, Gram-positive infections began to outnumber Gram-negative infections. The reasons for the shift could be attributable to routine use of central venous catheters (CVC), use of quinolone prophylaxis, and

Table 2
Commonly implicated bacterial causes of febrile episodes in neutropenia

Gram Positive Cocci and Bacilli	Gram Negative Cocci and Bacilli	Anaerobic Cocci and Bacilli

Staphylococcus spp
  Coagulase positive
    (Staphylococcus aureus)
  Coagulase negative
    (Staphylococcus epidermidis)
	Escherichia coli
	Klebsiella spp
	
	Pseudomonas aeruginosa
		Bacteroides spp
		Clostridium spp
		
		Fusobacterium spp

Streptococcus spp
  Streptococcus viridans
  Streptococcus pneumoniae
  Streptococcus pyogenes
    (Less common)
	Acinetobacter spp
	Enterobacter spp
	Proteus spp
	Stenotrophomonas
	  maltophilia spp
		Peptococcus and
		Peptostreptococcus spp

Enterococcus faecalis/faecium		
Corynebacterium spp		
Listeria monocytogenes		

increased use of proton pump inhibitors. Anaerobic bacteremia occurs in less than 5% of patients who have febrile neutropenia and has not changed over the past 30 years.[48] Patients who have intra-abdominal infections, neutropenic colitis, perirectal abscesses or periodontal disease are at risk for anaerobic bacteremia.

The emergence of resistant nosocomial isolates has also had an impact on infections in patients who are neutropenic. Particularly, methicillin-resistant *S aureus* (MRSA) and vancomycin-resistant *Enterococci* continued to increase in frequency in the 1990s.[48] This increase has made a significant impact in the choice of therapeutic antimicrobials. Another group of organisms that has been increasingly found as a cause of bacteremia in patients who have cancer and HSCT is *Streptococcus viridans*. The source of infection is the oropharynx in the setting of mucositis and it could manifest as toxic shock syndrome.[50]

Fungal infections

Infections caused by fungal organisms continue to have a significant impact on mortality in patients who have cancer. The most common risk factors for fungal infections include prior use of steroids and antibiotics, advanced age, tissue damage, intensity of chemotherapy, and presence of an indwelling central catheter.[51] *Candida* species remain the most common cause of fungal infection in patients who are neutropenic followed by *Aspergillus* species. Candidemia is most frequently caused by *Candida albicans* followed by *C glabrata*, *C tropicalis* and *C parapsilosis*. The clinical presentation is broad, ranging from catheter-related infections, single-organ candidiasis to disseminated candidiasis.[51]

Aspergillosis is seen in 30% of protracted, severe neutropenia cases and affects the lungs and sinuses.[52] *Aspergillus fumigatus* is the most common species that causes invasive disease. These infections are common in HSCT recipients, patients older than 18 years of age, positive CMV serology, and delayed engraftment.[53] Evidence on chest CT scan of a halo or air crescent sign is felt to be highly indicative of *Aspergillus* infection.[54]

Management

Empiric antibiotic therapy should be administered promptly to all patients who are neutropenic at the onset of fever. In the selection of initial antibiotic regimen, one should consider the type, frequency of occurrence, and antibiotic susceptibility of bacterial isolates recovered from other patients at the same hospital. **Fig. 1** provides a simplified algorithm for empiric antibiotic therapy.

Several studies have shown no striking differences between monotherapy and multidrug combinations for empiric coverage of uncomplicated neutropenic fever.[55] Monotherapy with ceftazidime should be avoided because of resistance through extended spectrum β-lactamases and type 1 β-lactamases.[56] Quinolones or aminoglycosides as monotherapy are not recommended as the initial antibiotic choice.[42]

The single most important determinant of successful discontinuation of antibiotics is the ANC. If the neutrophil count is greater than or equal to 500 cells/mm^3, and if patients are afebrile for greater than or equal to 48 hours, and if no infection is identified after 3 days of treatment, antibiotics may be stopped. On the other hand, if a specific etiology is found, the appropriate antibiotics are continued for a minimum of 7 days. If the ANC remains less than or equal to 500 cells/mm^3, and if patients are afebrile for greater than or equal to 48 hours, the proper antibiotic course is guided by the initial risk assessment of patients and is less well defined.[42]

There is usually no indication for the empiric use of antiviral drugs in the treatment of patients who have febrile neutropenia unless there is clinical or laboratory evidence of viral disease. The routine use of granulocyte transfusion is not usually advocated. Use of colony-stimulating factors can shorten the duration of neutropenia but does not reduce duration of fever, use of antimicrobials, or decrease in infection-related

---

Empiric Antibiotic Therapy of Febrile Neutropenia in the High Risk Patient

Neutrophil count <500 cells/mm^3 and fever (≥38°C)

↓

Monotherapy in uncomplicated cases, with cefepime or a carbapenem*

OR

Dual therapy is indicated in complicated cases or suspicion of resistance, with an antipseudomonal cephalosporin, antipseudomonal extended spectrum β-lactams or carbapenem PLUS aminoglycoside or quinolone*

↓

Fever continues despite 3 days of antibiotics and no clear source, add empiric vancomycin

↓

Fever continues despite 5–7 days of antibiotics and resolution of neutropenia is not imminent, add empiric antifungal therapy with amphotericin B or voriconazole.**

Fig. 1. Simplified algorithm to guide initiation and modifications in antimicrobial coverage for hospitalized patients with neutropenic fever. *Vancomycin should be added to initial coverage in cases with severe mucositis, prior use of quinolone prophylaxis, clinically suspected catheter-related blood stream infections (CRBSI), known colonization with penicillin, and cephalosporin-resistant pneumococci or MRSA, hypotension, or evidence of cardiovascular impairment. **Fluconazole represents an alternative to amphotericin B in patients who have renal insufficiency and in institutions where there are fewer non-albicans *Candida* infections.

mortality rates. Additionally, colony-stimulating factors can lead to splenomegaly and potentially increase the risk for splenic rupture.[57]

RESPIRATORY INFECTIONS

Pneumonia is a common complication seen in patients who have cancer, particularly in those who have neutropenia. Pulmonary infiltrates are seen in 15% to 25% of patients who have profound neutropenia after intensive chemotherapy and are associated with a particularly high risk of mortality.[58] Chemotherapy and immune defects of underlying hematologic disorders increases the risk for infections.[10] Between 25% and 50% of infiltrates are not caused by infection and may be caused by pulmonary edema, drug toxicity, cancer progression, or radiotherapy.[59]

Incidence

In a case series of 104 subjects who had cancer with pulmonary infiltrates, 49% had bacterial infection, 26% had a viral infection, 21% had a fungal infection, and 4% had *P jirovecii* infection.[60] The commonly identified pathogens were *Pseudomonas aeruginosa*, *S aureus*, *Aspergillus* species, CMV and HSV. In a study involving subjects who had leukemia, Gram-negative bacteria caused 70% of infections, polymicrobial infections in 12% of cases, and a fungal etiology was identified in 12%.[61]

Bacterial infection

Bacterial pathogens are the most common cause of respiratory infections complicating cancer chemotherapy. Gram-positive pathogens include *S aureus*, *Streptococcus pyogenes*, *S pneumoniae*, and *Enterococcus faecalis*, whereas *E coli*, *P aeruginosa*, and *Klebsiella* spp are the most common Gram-negative pathogens.

The underlying malignancy and associated immune defects increases the risk for specific types of infections. *S aureus* pneumonia is common in patients who receive prophylactic antibiotics against Gram-negative bacteria, elderly, diabetics, alcohol abuse, and during influenza epidemics. *S viridans* pneumonia is common in patients who have leukemia and who have mucositis after high-dose cytarabine therapy.[62] *S pneumoniae* and *H influenza* are commonly seen in multiple myeloma and CLL, where defects in the immunoglobulin function are observed. *P aeruginosa* and *K pneumoniae* are seen in patients who have neutropenia or leukemia. Diagnosis of bacterial pneumonia is confirmed by performing quantitative cultures of lower respiratory secretions (endotracheal aspirates, bronchoalveolar lavage [BAL], or protected specimen brush samples) to define the presence of pneumonia and the etiologic pathogen. Antibiotic selection should be dictated by the local/institutional microbiology and resistance patterns.

Legionella species are recognized as opportunistic pathogens causing severe pneumonia in immunosuppressed hosts. *L pneumophila* serogroup 1 appears to be more virulent than other serogroups; however, non-pneumophila *Legionella* species are common in hospital potable water systems and can be a cause of infection in hospitalized, immunosuppressed hosts. Most of the affected patients had impairment of cellular immunity, such as lymphopenia, or immune dysfunction caused by systemic use of steroids or antineoplastic agents. The vast majority of the patients in one series had hematologic malignancies.[63] Diagnosis is confirmed by performing legionella direct fluorescent antibody (DFA) on bronchoscopy specimens in patients who had suspected pulmonary infection, whereas urinary legionella antigen detects predominantly *L pneumophila* serogroup 1. Treatment is with a quinolone or azithromycin for 21 days.

Stenotrophomonas maltophilia is commonly seen in patients who have lung cancer, patients on prolonged mechanical ventilation, patients who have neutropenia, those who received broad-spectrum antibiotics, or have leukemia.[64] Infection is not accompanied by an inflammatory process and usually follows colonization of the respiratory tract. Lobar consolidation without pleural effusion is common. Factors associated with high mortality are bacteremia, refractory neutropenia, and delay in appropriate antibiotic treatment. Despite appropriate treatment, more than 50% of patients die of progressive infection or hemorrhage. Trimethoprim-sulfamethoxazole (TMP/SMX) is the treatment of choice. The newer fluoroquinolone, moxifloxacin, is superior to ciprofloxacin because it inhibits many ciprofloxacin resistant strains.[65] Other agents, such as tigecycline, ceftazidime, cefepime, ticarcillin/clavulanate, and piperacillin/tazobactam, have variable activity.[66] Combination therapy allows for synergism, however, its role is unclear and the efficacy needs further evaluation.[66,67]

Nocardia are aerobic, branching Gram-positive bacilli that are also weakly acid-fast that frequently cause necrotizing pneumonia and cavitation in patients who are immunosuppressed.[68] Infection with *Nocardia* species is associated with high mortality. Diagnosis is established by examination of the sputum or pleural fluid, BAL or percutaneous lung aspiration with Gram staining and modified acid-fast staining. TMP/SMX is the first line treatment and is usually given parenterally. The duration of treatment is 1 year or more in patients who are immunosuppressed. Other therapeutic options include amikacin, carbapenems, third generation cephalosporins, and linezolid.

Disseminated tuberculosis (TB) is seen in patients who are immunocompromised, particularly leukemia, and is associated with a high mortality rate.[69] The diagnosis of TB involves detection of mycobacteria in biologic samples. Drug-susceptible TB treatment involves standardized 6 months of anti-TB drug regimens.[70] *Mycobacterium avium* infections are common in children who have leukemia during periods of lymphocytopenia.[71] *Rhodococcus equi* infection should be considered together with *M tuberculosis* and *Nocardia* infections in the differential diagnosis of cavitary or nodular pneumonia in patients who are immunocompromised.[72]

Ventilator associated pneumonia (VAP) is difficult to diagnose in patients who have cancer, who often present with neutropenia and refractory thrombocytopenia. The use of fiberoptic bronchoscopy and the need for bronchial brushing may induce severe bronchial hemorrhage.[73] A blinded plugged telescoping catheter was a reasonably accurate technique for the diagnosis of VAP in patients who have cancer, though less sensitive when compared with fiberoptic protected specimen brush technique.[73]

Viral infections

Common viruses causing respiratory infection include influenza, parainfluenza, respiratory syncytial virus (RSV), CMV, and HSV. RSV accounts for 30% to 49% of all respiratory viruses in patients who are immunocompromised and have hematologic malignancies.[74] In cancer patients, RSV usually presents as an upper respiratory tract illness that can progress to fatal pneumonia in approximately 60% of cases.[75] Patients who have profound myelosuppression, persistent lymphocytopenia, corticosteroid use, and high Acute Physiology and Chronic Health Evaluation (APACHE) scores have the highest risk for progressing to pneumonia and death.[76] In these patients, pneumonia has a mortality rate of 60% to 80%. This rate has decreased considerably, possibly because of earlier diagnosis and more aggressive therapy.[75] Reverse transcriptase polymerase chain reaction (PCR) is more sensitive than antigen testing by DFA. Antigen testing might be helpful for patients who shed the virus at high levels.[77] Aerosolized ribavirin is the treatment of choice and should be administered to high-risk patients who have leukemia. Therapy with the monoclonal antibody, palivizumab (Synagis - MedImmune, LLC, Gaithersburg, MD) has been used as an adjunct to aerosolized ribavirin and has been well tolerated.[78]

CMV infection and pneumonia is most common in patients who have lymphoma or leukemia. The risk of infection is increased by the use of agents, such as cytarabine and fludarabine; treatment with T-cell suppressors, such as steroids and methotrexate; and use of T-cell depleting drugs, such as rituximab and alemtuzumab.[79] The diagnosis of CMV pneumonia involves detection of virus in lung tissue by use of immunohistochemical staining, histopathological assessment, or culture. The diagnostic yield by cytology or immunohistochemical staining from BAL samples is low. However, the yield with viral-shell vial culture and conventional culture of BAL samples is high.[80] The conventional culture is the gold standard for the diagnosis but takes 6 weeks to obtain final results, whereas the rapid viral culture by shell vial method takes 48 hours and has a sensitivity of 68% to 100%.[81] The treatment of choice is ganciclovir or foscarnet.

Reactivation of latent HSV is common in patients who have neutropenia that occurs during induction chemotherapy and in patients who have lymphoma, acute leukemia, as well as during the conditioning phase of HSCT. HSV-1 pneumonitis may follow oral or genital HSV either through contiguous spread from the oropharynx or hematogenous dissemination.[82] Although rare, it should be considered in neutropenic hematologic patients undergoing chemotherapy when they are not responding to antibacterial or antifungal treatment. The radiographic findings show bilateral infiltrates, which are nonspecific. Definitive diagnosis of HSV pneumonia is difficult and is established by culture of BAL fluid or blood or detection of virus in the lung tissue.[83] Treatment is with intravenous (IV) acyclovir.

Infections caused by other viruses, such as influenza and parainfluenza, are also seen. The single most important predictor of mortality in influenza pneumonia is absolute lymphopenia.[74] A specific reverse-transcriptase PCR that detects RNA from influenza A and B and parainfluenza viruses from nasal-wash samples are very sensitive for rapid diagnosis.[84] Infection with enterovirus and adenovirus has also been reported in patients who have lymphoma and leukemia with lower respiratory infections.[85] Human metapneumovirus infection has been reported in 2.7% of respiratory disease in patients who have hematological cancer.[86] Routine diagnostic testing remains a challenge, as the virus requires special cell lines and a long incubation period for growth. There are anecdotal reports on the successful use of ribavirin, but more studies are needed to determine efficacy in randomized trials.[87]

Fungal infections

Aspergillosis is usually acquired by inhalation of *Aspergillus* conidia and the most common manifestation is pneumonia. Invasive pulmonary aspergillosis can occur in patients who are neutropenic and is commonly fatal with mortality as high as 60%.[88] Chest CT usually shows small, round, and dense peripheral lesions that increase in size over time.[89] A halo sign is the first reliable sign of infection during neutropenia and has a high specificity and low sensitivity. On the other hand, nodular cavitated lesions are more frequent in patients who are not neutropenic.[89] *Aspergillus* that is seen on sputum samples might represent colonization and not necessarily indicate infection. Contamination can occur during bronchoscopic sampling or during handling of the samples in the laboratory. Microbiological cultures of *Aspergillus* from BAL are positive in fewer than a third of patients.[90] The gold standard is detection of hyphae by histopathologic or cytopathologic examination of a biopsy sample of lung tissue, either by video-assisted thoracoscopic surgery or transbronchial biopsy. PCR is highly sensitive and specific, and was negative in 1.4% of samples from subjects with histologically confirmed aspergillosis.[91] However, consensus guidelines do not recommend PCR testing in BAL samples or blood samples, but recommend *Aspergillus* antigen detection in such samples.[92] The role of serum galactomannan in the early detection of pulmonary aspergillosis is unclear.[93] Early diagnosis is difficult; however, early recognition and prompt antifungal treatment is key to improved survival. The drug of choice is liposomal amphotericin B 3 mg/kg/d.[94] Clinical response in patients who have confirmed aspergillosis is the same between two preparations of amphotericin B.[95] Voriconazole was found to be more efficacious with fewer side effects when compared with amphotericin B deoxycholate.[96] Posaconazole can be used in refractory cases and is associated with a partial response.[97] Caspofungin led to a partial or complete response as salvage treatment in up to 45% of patients' refractory to other antifungal agents.[98] Despite the theoretical advantages of increasing neutrophils, colony-stimulating factors are ineffective and clinical deterioration might occur during neutrophil recovery.[99]

Fusarium species, a fungus distributed in soil and plants, most commonly affects lungs and skin. Pulmonary manifestations are similar to *Aspergillus*. Treatment is with voriconazole, itraconazole, or amphotericin B. Overall mortality rate is 50% to 80%. Zygomycosis can be difficult to diagnose because blood cultures are negative and bronchial washings rarely yield hyphal forms. High-dose liposomal amphotericin B and radical surgical debridement are the treatment of choice.[100]

P jirovecii pneumonia (PCP) is less common among patients who have cancer, including those who have undergone HSCT when compared with patients who have AIDS.[101] The incidence among patients who had hematologic malignancies was higher than the incidence among patients who had solid tumors, with the majority of episodes of PCP occurring in either leukemia (49%) or lymphoma (45%).[102] Corticosteroids are a major risk factor for PCP, particularly among patients who have solid tumors. Other predisposing factors include intensity of chemotherapy and low CD 4 count. CMV coinfection is common in patients who have PCP.[103] Previous studies have indicated that typical radiographic features of PCP are bilateral interstitial infiltrates, whereas pleural effusions and pneumothorax are rarely observed.[104] The diagnostic yield of BAL cytology is high. TMP/SMX is the standard treatment but might be suboptimal in hematological malignancies.[105] The most common combination therapy was TMP/SMX plus pentamidine and there was a trend toward combination antimicrobial therapy being more commonly used in sicker patients who required mechanical ventilation than in patients who did not.[102] Caspofungin, an echinocandin is active against the cystic form of *P jirovecii* in animal models. In combination with TMP/SMX caspofungin was used in a very small number of subjects. As a result, the role of echinocandins in patients who have cancer and PCP remains uncertain. Optimum duration of treatment is unclear, with 2 weeks being sufficient for most patients who have cancer and treatment with 3 weeks showing better outcome.[102] Prophylaxis with TMP/SMX should be considered in patients who have lymphoblastic leukemia, patients on prednisone greater than or equal to 20 mg for more than 1 month, and in patients who have low CD4 counts.[106]

Parasitic Infection

Strongyloides stercoralis is an intestinal nematode that causes fatal opportunistic infections in immunocompromised hosts, particularly after steroid therapy. Hyperinfections and widespread dissemination of larvae may lead to hemorrhagic pneumonitis (because of larva-induced mucosal injury during larval migration in the hyperinfection syndrome), enteritis, and Gram-negative bacteremia. Diagnosis is made by demonstrating the organisms in stool specimens or by cytology in a sputum specimen. Mortality from disseminated strongyloidiasis approaches 80% and the treatment of choice is oral thiabendazole.[107]

GASTROINTESTINAL INFECTIONS

Normally the GI tract acts as a barrier to the external environment. Disruption of the GI mucosa leads to translocation of enteric pathogens. Risk factors for infection in patients who have cancer include mechanical disruption, such as mucositis, chemotherapy, radiotherapy, immune dysfunction, altered microbial flora, surgery, altered motility, and antimicrobial exposure. GI infections commonly seen in critically ill patients who have cancer include typhlitis, *Clostridium difficile* associated diarrhea (CDAD), and hepatosplenic candidiasis.

Typhlitis

Typhlitis (also reported as neutropenic enterocolitis, necrotizing enterocolitis, neutropenic enteropathy or ileocecal syndrome), occurs most commonly after intensive chemotherapy for acute leukemia, but has also been reported in patients who have untreated hematologic malignancies, neutropenia from other causes, following HSCT and in those receiving immunosuppressive therapy for solid tumors.[108,109] The incidence rate varies from 0.8% to 25% with mortality rates of 50% or higher.[110] The precise pathogenesis is poorly understood but chemotherapy, neutropenia, and immune dysfunction likely lead to mucosal edema, ulceration, necrosis, and focal hemorrhage in the terminal ileum, cecum, and right colon.[108,109] Chemotherapeutic agents, such as cytosine arabinoside (ara-C) and etoposide (VP-16), have been most commonly implicated; however, agents, including vinorelbine, docetaxel, paclitaxel, carboplatin, gemcitabine, 5-fluorouracil, vincristine, doxorubicin, methotrexate, and cyclophosphamide have also been associated.[108,111] Likely pathogens include *Pseudomonas* spp, *E coli*, *Klebsiella* spp, *Clostridium septicum*, *C difficile* and *Candida* spp and CMV.[3,108,109,112] Recurrent bacteremia frequently occurs.[109]

　　Patients who have typhlitis present with fever, right lower quadrant pain with or without rebound tenderness, diarrhea, abdominal distension or less commonly nausea and vomiting, or a palpable mass in the right lower quadrant.[108,109] CT scan or ultrasound are the preferred modalities and demonstrate bowel wall thickening or pneumatosis.[108,113,114] Fever, abdominal pain, and bowel wall thickening greater than 4 mm is consistent with the diagnosis of typhlitis. In patients who have bowel wall thickness greater than 10 mm, mortality is as high as 60%.[110,114,115]

　　Initial management of typhlitis includes strict bowel rest, nasogastric decompression, intravenous fluids, consideration for total parenteral nutrition, broad-spectrum antimicrobial therapy (empirically or based on blood culture results), and surgical consultation. Antimicrobial therapy must provide coverage of enteric Gram-negatives with an extended-spectrum β-lactam/β-lactamase combination, carbapenem, or third or fourth generation cephalosporin plus metronidazole. Metronidazole should be added when *C difficile* is suspected.[108] Empiric antifungal coverage for *Candida* should also be considered.[112] Indications for surgical intervention include acute perforation, toxic megacolon, bowel necrosis, persistent GI bleeding or clinical deterioration. Surgery should be delayed if possible until neutrophil recovery occurs. Although no randomized trials of colony-stimulating factors have been conducted in this condition, their use has been recommended in patients at high risk for complications and poor outcomes associated with neutropenia.[110,116]

Clostridium Difficile Associated Diarrhea

CDAD is a toxin mediated disease that occurs most commonly in the elderly hospitalized patient receiving either antibiotics or chemotherapy and its prevalence is rising.[117,118] In 2005, the identification of the highly virulent strain (BI/NAP1/027) was found to be responsible for the rise in infection rates in North America. It is characterized by fluoroquinolone resistance and is associated with increased toxin production causing a higher mortality rate than other strains.[117,118] Clinically significant strains produce two exotoxins (toxin A and B). Antibiotic exposure to ampicillin, cephalosporins, clindamycin, or fluoroquinolones, bowel surgery, or chemotherapy can disrupt the normal bowel flora and predispose for C difficile colonization.[117–119] Additionally, prolonged hospitalization of more than 4 weeks can increase the rate of acquisition.[119] Patients can present with mild to severe diarrhea, fever, leukocytosis, and abdominal pain. Severe cases will manifest pseudomembranes in the colon, toxic megacolon (which may present without diarrhea), perforation, sepsis, shock, and death.

All hospitalized patients who have cancer who develop diarrhea should be suspected of having CDAD, especially those who have neutropenia.[119] Testing for C difficile-associated glutamate dehydrogenase antigen allows for screening of stool samples, however, a positive result requires toxin testing to confirm the diagnosis.[120] Enzyme immunoassay kits can detect toxin A, toxin B or both and can provide results in 2 to 4 hours, but are less sensitive and kits that do not detect toxin B may miss a small number of strains that only produce this toxin.[121] Detection of the C difficile toxin B in stool samples by cell-culture cytotoxin assay is specific but takes up to 48 hours to yield a result. CT findings include bowel wall thickening greater than 8 mm, wall nodularity and pancolitis.[114] Endoscopy should be performed to identify pseudomembranes in patients where rapid diagnosis is required, if the stool tests are not specific enough, if there is ileus without diarrhea, or if other diagnoses are being considered.[121] Sigmoidoscopy may miss a small number of cases if colonoscopy is not performed. Lower-GI endoscopy should be avoided in the setting of neutropenia.

Treatment of CDAD begins with discontinuation of the offending agent, however, this may not be feasible in patients who are critically ill and results of testing may not be readily available. Because the final diagnosis may be delayed, empiric administration is generally warranted in the ICU setting. Metronidazole (either oral or intravenous) represents the initial drug of choice, whereas oral vancomycin should be used for severe disease.[122] Dual therapy may be of benefit in fulminant disease.[117] A 10- to 14-day course will lead to resolution in greater than 90% of cases, however 5% to 30% of patients may have relapse in 1 to 2 weeks either because of infection by the original organism or reinfection by a new strain. Vancomycin enema can be used when oral administration is not possible and treatment with metronidazole has failed or in severe cases.[122] For patients who have fulminant disease or toxic megacolon without response to treatment or suspicion of perforation, subtotal colectomy with ileostomy may be required. Hemicolectomy should be avoided as reports suggest an increased mortality, which nevertheless is as high as 35% to 80%.[117,121] The use of antidiarrheals or narcotics should be avoided because of the concern of toxin retention and possible development of toxic megacolon.[117,121] Newer agents, such as rifaximin, tolevamer, and difimicin are undergoing clinical investigation.

Hepatosplenic Candidiasis

Hepatosplenic candidiasis, also known as chronic disseminated candidiasis, typically occurs in febrile leukemic patients with neutropenia after receiving chemotherapy. Patients develop fever, right upper quadrant pain, and elevated alkaline phosphatase. Some patients may have hepatomegaly or splenomegaly.[123]

Blood cultures are negative in hepatosplenic candidiasis and diagnosis requires ultrasound, CT, or MRI once neutrophil counts have recovered. CT demonstrates multiple focal lesions, occasionally with peripheral enhancement, but these findings are not pathognomonic. Other disseminated processes, such as miliary tuberculosis, invasive molds, or malignancy, can mimic this process and therefore CT guided biopsy is generally recommended to confirm the diagnosis.[123,124]

Initial management of hepatic candidiasis is with amphotericin B or a liposomal formulation for 1 to 2 weeks followed by fluconazole for several months. Newer antifungal agents, including caspofungin, micafungin, and voriconazole, have been used successfully in small numbers of patients. Treatment should continue for several months until there is radiographic resolution or calcification to prevent relapse.[125]

CENTRAL NERVOUS SYSTEM INFECTIONS

Infections of the central nervous system (CNS) can mimic tumor recurrence or metabolic derangements and clinicians must be vigilant because signs and symptoms may be subtle and nonspecific.[126,127] Symptoms include mild headache, fever, personality changes, delirium, or seizures, but patients who have cancer generally do not have nuchal rigidity or focal deficits and may present only with malaise, especially in the setting of leukopenia.[126,128] Patients who have leukemia, lymphoma, primary CNS tumors, solid tumors undergoing aggressive chemotherapy, and HSCT are most commonly at risk for CNS infections.[126,129] The spectrum of infection includes meningitis, cerebritis, brain abscess, and meningoencephalitis.

Pathogenesis

Pathogens that cause meningitis must cross the blood brain barrier and can lead to cerebral edema, vasculitis with possible infarction, and impaired CSF absorption, all of which may progress to herniation.[126,130] The most common causes of bacterial meningitis in patients who have cancer that have not had neurosurgery are *L monocytogenes*, *S aureus*, and *S pneumoniae*.[126,129] Patients who have *L monocytogenes* present most commonly with fever and a minority have gastroenteritis.[131] Neurosurgical patients are more likely to develop meningitis caused by *S aureus*, *Streptococcus bovis*, and coagulase-negative *Staphylococcus*.[127,128] Occasionally infection caused by Gram-negative organisms, such as *P aeruginosa*, *E coli*, *Klebsiella*, *Enterobacter* and *Proteus* species, can occur.[126]

Patients who have neutrophil defects (quantitative or qualitative), such as acute leukemia or chemotherapy-induced neutropenia may have an acellular CSF in the setting of severe infection.[132] Encapsulated bacteria, such as *S pneumoniae* and *H influenzae*, are the most common pathogens in patients who have B cell and immunoglobulin dysfunction, whereas individuals with T-cell abnormalities are predisposed to developing infections caused by viruses and intracellular bacteria, such as *Listeria monocytogenes*, *Nocardia asteroides*, and *Aspergillus*.

A deficiency in cell-mediated immunity or corticosteroid use predisposes to meningitis caused by *Cryptococcus neoformans*, which can present with fulminant infection or as focal mass lesions.[127] Patients who have neutrophil dysfunction, prolonged neutropenia, those receiving high-dose corticosteroids, chemotherapy, or broad-spectrum antibiotics, or those with CMV infection are at risk for developing *Aspergillus* CNS infection, either by direct extension through paranasal sinuses or hematogenous spread from the lungs.[3,126,127,129] Manifestations include small hemorrhagic infarctions, abscess formation, and mycotic aneurysms.[126,127,133] Less common fungal pathogens include *Candida* and *Mucoraceae* (Mucorales or Zygomycetes). *Candida* meningitis is usually seen in patients who have received a long course of prior antibiotics and have other manifestations of candidiasis.[126,129] *Mucoraceae* is seen in patients who are neutropenic with poor glycemic control, hematologic malignancies, or corticosteroid treatment.[129]

Encephalitis can occur alone, with meningitis, or as a result of meningitis. Signs and symptoms include fever, headache, delirium, focal deficits, and seizures that may be focal or generalized. Presentation may be difficult to distinguish from paraneoplastic syndromes with anti-Hu, or anti-Ma, or Ta antibodies.[129] Pathogens that can lead to encephalitis include Epstein-Barr virus (EBV), VZV, CMV, HSV 1 and 2, and human herpesvirus (HHV) 6, the latter of which is associated with HSCT. VZV can present with an acute, necrotizing encephalitis or a multifocal stroke-like presentation, which can mimic progressive multifocal leukoencephalopathy (PML).[127,129] Reactivation is generally the cause in most cases and patients receiving radiation and corticosteroids are at higher risk. West Nile virus causes meningoencephalitis in patients who have humoral immune defects, such as B-cell dyscrasias and HSCT.[127]

A focal deficit should lead to suspicion of brain abscess caused by bacterial pathogens or *Aspergillus*, *Toxoplasma gondii*, *Mycobacterium tuberculosis*, or *N asteroides*.[129] *Nocardia* can cause infection in hosts with impaired cell-mediated immunity and post-HSCT, with infection generally beginning in the lungs. Manifestations include abscess, mass-like lesions that can mimic metastases, and less commonly meningitis.[126,129] Patients who have Hodgkin's disease and allogeneic HSCT are at higher risk for *T. gondii* infection.[126]

Patients who have undergone craniotomy or recent manipulation of devices, such as an intraventricular shunt or Ommaya reservoir are at risk for infection from organisms, such as *S aureus*, coagulase-negative Staphylococcus, *S epidermidis*, *Propionibacterium acnes*, or *Candida*.[126,129] Development of ventricular shunt or Ommaya reservoir infections usually occurs within 2 months of placement.[134]

Diagnosis

Brain CT or MRI can help to evaluate for metastatic disease or other mass lesions. Platelet counts should be greater than $50,000/mm^3$ to perform lumbar puncture. CSF biochemical patterns are similar to the general population; however, patients who have leukopenia may not have pleocytosis. CSF pleocytosis with lymphocytes is the most common finding in patients who have cancer.[132] Culture of large amounts of CSF (10–20 mL) can confirm a diagnosis if the fluid appears clear and there is a low burden of organisms.[126] India ink examination can rapidly diagnose *C neoformans* infection and CSF serologic testing of cryptococcal antigen is highly sensitive.[127,129] Diagnosis of Aspergillus infection can be difficult and requires a high index of suspicion and recognition of the characteristic clinical presentation in at-risk patients.

Patients who develop encephalitis may have only a CSF lymphocytic pleocytosis with normal protein and glucose levels. Serologic testing and PCR can be useful to confirm a diagnosis of CMV, enteroviruses, EBV, HHV-6, HSV type 1 and 2, and VZV.[127,129] In cases of suspected West Nile virus infection serologic tests, detection of antibodies, and nucleic acid in CSF are diagnostic.[127] Diagnosis of infection of a ventricular shunt or Ommaya reservoir requires positive cultures from the device.[134]

Management

In situations where the suspicion of meningitis is strong and symptoms are acute, treatment must start immediately as progression to death can occur rapidly. Empiric antibiotic therapy is based on the intrinsic immune defect and likely pathogens and local resistance patterns. Initial therapy includes vancomycin and ceftriaxone, whereas ceftazidime is administered for those at risk for *P aeruginosa*. In patients who have T-cell defects, sulfadiazine or TMP/SMZ should be added for coverage of

N asteroides. Ampicillin should be added in suspected cases of *Listeria*.[127,129] Dexamethasone should be administered with the first dose of antibiotics and continued for 4 days in patients suspected to have bacterial meningitis, which has been shown to reduce neurologic sequelae and mortality.[135,136] Infected devices must be removed and externalized drainage used until infection has cleared.

Initial antifungal coverage generally starts with amphotericin B. In addition to systemic therapy, intrathecal amphotericin B by way of an Ommaya reservoir may be helpful in severe infections.[137] In patients who have cryptococcal meningitis, treatment with flucytosine should be added for the first 2 weeks followed by either fluconazole or itraconazole for 8 to 10 weeks as maintenance therapy.[138]

Intravenous acyclovir is used for treatment of EBV, HSV, or VZV encephalitis, whereas ganciclovir is used for CMV infection. In patients who have HSCT and HHV-6 infection, treatment is with foscarnet. Empiric treatment should be started in suspected cases of *T gondii* with sulfadiazine and pyrimethamine. Most patients demonstrate a good response within 10 to 14 days and biopsy should be sought if clinical or radiographic response is not seen with appropriate therapy.[126,127,129]

CATHETER RELATED BLOOD STREAM INFECTIONS

Intravascular catheter-related infections are a major cause of morbidity and mortality in patients who have cancer and are associated with excessive hospital costs. It is estimated that catheter-related blood stream infections (CRBSI) range between 1.0 to 1.9/1,000 catheter days.[139] The four commonest types of intravascular silicone catheters are tunneled catheters (eg, Hickman, Groshong and Broviac [Bard Access Systems, Inc, Salt Lake City, UT]); non-tunneled CVC; implantable ports (eg, PORT-A-CATH [Smiths Group PLC, Smiths Medical, London, England]); and peripherally inserted central catheters.

Pathogenesis

The pathogenesis of non-tunneled CVC infection is often related to the extraluminal colonization of the catheter, which originates from the skin, and less commonly from hematogenous seeding of the catheter tip, or intraluminal colonization of the hub and lumen of the CVC.[140] However, in tunneled CVC or implantable devices contamination of the catheter hub and intraluminal infection are the most common routes of infection. The microorganisms most commonly associated are coagulase-negative Staphylococci, *S aureus*, various species of aerobic Gram-negative bacilli, and *C albicans*. Patients who are neutropenic and receiving chemotherapy and those with mucositis or graft-versus-host disease of the intestine may have a tendency for hematogenous seeding of the catheters with organisms originating from the GI tract. Other factors contributing to the etiology of CRBSI include parenteral nutrition solutions and lipid emulsions, which promote the growth of bacteria and fungi, such as *C parapsilosis* and *Malassezia furfur*.[141]

Diagnosis

Suspicion for CRBSI should be high if patients present with fever or chills and no other source of infection can be identified other than a CVC, especially if blood cultures are positive for *S epidermidis*, *S aureus*, or *Candida* species. Diagnosis relies mostly on isolating the same organism from paired cultures of blood samples taken simultaneously from the CVC and a peripheral vein or the isolation of the same organism from a catheter tip culture and from peripheral blood cultures.

The techniques to diagnose CRBSI, includes quantitative and non-quantitative cultures. The differential time to positivity is a non-quantitative test of simultaneous blood cultures drawn from a CVC and peripheral vein, where the culture from the CVC becomes positive at least 2 hours before the one drawn from the peripheral vein.[142] The other methods of testing include simultaneous quantitative catheter cultures showing fivefold the number of colonies from a blood culture shown from CVC and compared with one drawn from peripheral vein. Finally, if the CVC tip semi-quantitative culture (roll plate) reveals greater than or equal to 15 colony forming units or CVC tip quantitative culture (sonication) reveals greater than or equal to100 CFU, then the diagnosis of CRBSI is favored.[143]

Management

The treatment of CRBSI depends on several factors, such as the underlying severity of disease, risk factors for infection, and the type of organism. Guidelines published by the Infectious Diseases Society of America in 2001 helps in the management of CRBSI.[44] The initial step involves determining whether the catheter is the true source of infection.

In the case of infection caused by coagulase-negative Staphylococci, the long-term CVC may be retained and therapies with systemic antibiotics like nafcillin or vancomycin (in case of methicillin resistance) for 7 to 10 days is usually sufficient.[144]

Infection with S aureus is associated with high rates of complications, such as endocarditis, septic thrombophlebitis, and osteomyelitis. If there are no other access sites, systemic antibiotics with a β-lactam or vancomycin with antibiotic lock therapy for 14 days is recommended. Antibiotic lock therapy involves instilling a highly concentrated antibiotic solution into a catheter lumen and allowing the solution to dwell for a specified time period for the purpose of sterilizing the lumen. In most cases, removal of the catheter is recommended and treatment with systemic antibiotics for 2 weeks in uncomplicated cases to 4 to 6 weeks in deep-seated infections is optimal.

Infections caused by Gram-negative rods, such as Pseudomonas, E coli, and Acinetobacter, are associated with serious complications and a high rate of treatment failure when the catheter remains in place.[145] Removal of the catheter and administering parenteral antibiotics, such as a carbapenem, or third generation cephalosporin for 7 to 10 days is recommended, but if there are no access sites, systemic treatment with antibiotic lock therapy may be used. Catheter removal with generous debridement of infected tissue is also advisable for patients who have atypical mycobacterial infections.[146]

Irrespective of organism type catheter removal is indicated if the infection is recurrent or there is no response to antibiotics after 2 to 3 days of therapy. Evidence of a subcutaneous tunnel or periportal infection, septic emboli, hypotension with catheter use, septic shock, or deep seated infections are indications for removal along with prompt administration of antibiotics.[44]

In cases of catheter-related candidemia, guidelines recommend removal of the catheter and treatment with either amphotericin B or fluconazole for 14 days after the last blood culture. If C krusei is isolated then treatment with amphotericin B is required.[147] In a retrospective study of 416 subjects who had cancer, CVC retention was associated with poor outcome and higher rates of complications including endophthalmitis, hepatosplenic candidiasis, and peripheral abscess.[148]

Septic thrombosis is an intravascular infection commonly associated with high-grade and persistent bacteremia or fungemia. Persistently positive blood cultures after catheter removal suggests a diagnosis of septic thrombosis or endocarditis.[149] In general, S aureus is the most common infecting organism. Less common pathogens include Candida species and Gram-negative bacilli. In all cases, the involved catheter should be removed. Incision and drainage along with excision of the infected periph-eral vein and any involved tributaries should be done, especially when there is suppu-ration, persistent bacteremia or fungemia, or metastatic infection. Surgical excision and repair is needed in cases of peripheral arterial involvement with pseudoaneurysm formation.[150] Heparin should be used in the treatment of septic thrombosis of the great central veins and arteries and the duration of antimicrobial therapy is 4 to 6 weeks.

GENITOURINARY INFECTIONS

Genitourinary (GU) infections are an infrequent complication of cancer treatment. Nevertheless, patients who have cancer remain at risk because of the impairment of the immune defense mechanisms from the underlying disease, damaged urothelium, chemotherapy toxicity, impaired voiding caused by local or spinal disease, and mechanical obstruction, which promotes bacterial growth and resultant sepsis.[151] Bacteria are the most common pathogens causing GU infections, such as cystitis, pyelonephritis, prostatitis, and infection of urinary diversions, reconstructions, and stents. Patients who are neutropenic and have urinary tract infections are less likely to have dysuria and pyuria and are more likely to become bacteremic.[152]

Pyelonephritis

Pyelonephritis in patients who have cancer is most commonly caused by *E coli* fol-lowed by *Proteus, Klebsiella,* and *Staphylococcus saprophyticus*. It is usually an ascending infection from the urethra, rarely hematogenous, and causes significant ur-osepsis. Pyelonephritis in the setting of superimposed obstruction, such as hydro-nephrosis, may need urgent decompression with nephrostomies or stent placement in addition to IV antibiotics.[151]

Patients who have cancer and are immunocompromised are particularly suscep-tible to fungal pyelonephritis. *C albicans* is the most common pathogen followed by other *Candida* and *Aspergillus* species. The kidney is the most frequently involved organ in systemic candidiasis. Fungi are filtered by the glomerulus and become lodged in the distal tubules where they multiply and produce medullary and cortical abscesses. Systemic antifungal therapy is the mainstay of treatment. The mortality of renal fungal infection remains high.[153]

Infections of Urinary Diversions

Urinary diversions are indicated after radical cystectomy for the management of bladder carcinoma. Orthotopic bladder substitution uses a loop of small intestine, most frequently the ileum, to form a neobladder. Before surgery, antimicrobial treat-ment is used to minimize the bacterial population. However, these patients remain at increased risk for UTI because bacterial colonization remains. In addition, incom-plete emptying of the neobladder along with excessive mucus production promotes infection.[154] In patients who have orthotopic neobladder, the estimated 5-year prob-ability of urinary tract infection and urosepsis for patients who voided independently were 58% and 18%, respectively. Recurrent UTI was the only predictor for urosep-sis.[155] *E coli* is the most commonly implicated microorganism in patients who have neobladder-related UTI and was responsible for 59% of monobacterial infections. Other organisms cultured include *Klebsiella, Proteus mirabilis, Enterococcus, Pseudo-monas,* and *Citrobacter*.[156]

Ureteral Stents

Ureteral stents are placed to relieve obstruction caused by extrinsic compression that are caused by advanced cancer.[157] Many of these patients require chronic stent changes and are prone to developing infections. A retrospective review of 28 subjects who had a total of 201 stents placed, found that 18 developed UTI and 8 had urosepsis.[158]

SKIN AND SOFT TISSUE INFECTIONS
Necrotizing Fasciitis

Necrotizing fasciitis is a rare but potentially fatal, soft-tissue infection characterized by the necrosis of the subcutaneous fat and fascia. There are two clinical types of necrotizing fasciitis, the first type is a mixed infection caused by aerobic and anaerobic infection and occurs in patients who have diabetes and after surgical procedures. The second type is usually caused by Group A *Streptococcus* or methicillin-resistant Staphylococci. Prompt recognition is important, as delay in diagnosis is associated with high morbidity and mortality. Erythema, pain associated with skin discoloration and bullae might be some of the presenting signs. Diagnosis is clinical and high index of suspicion is needed in at-risk patients. Treatment consists of early and aggressive surgical debridement, intravenous antibiotics, and hemodynamic support. Treatment with intravenous immunoglobulin (IVIG) might be an effective adjunct for streptococcal toxic shock syndrome, possibly because of its ability to neutralize bacterial exotoxins.[159]

Gram-negative infections including *Pseudomonas, Aeromonas veronii,* and *E coli,* have been reported in patients, particularly young children who have acute leukemia during neutropenia.[160] Cytotoxic agents and steroids used in chemotherapeutic regimens further increase the risk for severe infections. Moreover, skin changes are not reliable in patients who are neutropenic because the inflammatory responses are blunted and clinical signs of systemic infection are absent early in the disease course. Therefore, severe local pain may be the only early sign of infection.[161]

Fournier's Gangrene

Fournier's gangrene is a fulminant, necrotizing fasciitis of the perineal, perirectal, or genital areas, which leads to gangrene caused by thrombosis of the small subcutaneous vessels. Surgical debridement is the mainstay of treatment along with intravenous antibiotics. Cases have been described where infections with Gram-negative bacilli including *Pseudomonas* are seen during the profound neutropenic stage after chemotherapy in leukemia patients.[162]

SPECIAL CONSIDERATIONS
Sepsis

Clinical trials for sepsis and septic shock frequently exclude patients who have active or metastatic cancer thereby making it difficult to determine the efficacy of new therapies in this population. Nonetheless, survival of patients who have cancer has improved during the same timeframe that treatment guidelines for severe sepsis have been implemented.[8] Current practice guidelines as outlined by the Surviving Sepsis campaign are generally applicable to patients who have cancer and provide a framework to manage patients who meet criteria for sepsis and septic shock.[163] Once sepsis has been recognized, appropriate antimicrobial therapy, fluid resuscitation, and source control should begin immediately. Special consideration should be made in oncologic patients when considering antibiotic selection, including suspicion for fungal pathogens in patients who have prolonged neutropenia or after HSCT.[42]

A targeted, structured approach to early goal directed therapy (EGDT) of patients who are septic in an emergency department has been shown to reduce ICU and 28-day mortality.[164] Because it is unclear which aspect of the EGDT protocol provided an improved outcome, all aspects of the algorithm should be employed. With that in mind, many patients who have cancer are anemic as result of underlying disease or chemotherapy. Thus, the use of packed red blood cells (PRBC) for the early part of resuscitation may improve oxygen delivery and provide volume support. However, it is not clear what the optimal hemoglobin target should be in patients who have cancer and PRBC transfusion should be guided by global indices of tissue perfusion and evidence of tissue hypoxia.

Drotrecogin alfa (activated) (Drot AA) (Xigris - Eli Lilly and Company, Indianapolis, IN) was approved in 2001 for patients who are at high risk of death from severe sepsis with an APACHE II score of 25 or more, or multiorgan failure.[165–167] In the PROWESS (Recombinant Human Activated Protein C Worldwide Evaluation in Severe Sepsis) trial, approximately 18% (303/1,690) of the study population had either prior or preexisting cancer; however, no specific survival benefit has been shown in this subgroup as a result of Drot AA administration.[165] Drot AA can be considered as adjunctive therapy; however, the bleeding risk needs to be balanced against the potential benefits in patients who have cancer who often have concomitant thrombocytopenia and coagulopathy. If Drot AA is to be administered in the setting of thrombocytopenia, the platelet count should be maintained above 50,000/mm^3 with transfusions throughout the duration of the 96-hour infusion.[168] Drot AA has been used in patients who develop severe sepsis soon after HSCT; however, efficacy is limited and bleeding risks are significant.[169,170] Additionally, subjects given Drot AA who underwent recent surgery (<30 days) with single-organ dysfunction had a higher mortality and more bleeding events.[167]

Patients who are septic and vasopressor-dependent may benefit from the administration of low-dose hydrocortisone for critical illness-related corticosteroid insufficiency (CIRCI).[171] However, large trials have generally excluded patients who have advanced cancer or underlying diseases with a poor prognosis. In the multicenter CORTICUS (Corticosteroid Therapy of Septic Shock) trial[172] and landmark trial by Annane and colleagues,[173] the study populations that had prior or preexisting cancer represented 16.8% and 13.7%, respectively. Again no specific benefit was determined as a result of steroid therapy for CIRCI in patients who had cancer with vasopressor-dependent septic shock. Patients who have cancer may have required corticosteroids as part of their cancer therapy and therefore replacement therapy may be warranted. However, the risk of further immunosuppression, especially in neutropenic or HSCT recipients, must be evaluated.

Targeting blood glucose values between 80 to 110 mg/dL in patients who are critically ill and have an insulin infusion has become common practice in many ICU's.[174,175] However, more recent data from the NICE-SUGAR (Normoglycemia in Intensive Care Evaluation-Survival Using Glucose Algorithm Regulation) trial suggests that maintaining a higher threshold of blood glucose values between 140 to180 mg/dL may have fewer episodes of hypoglycemia and lower mortality.[176] Though the effect of this practice in patients who have active cancer was not studied, it appears to be a reasonable target in these patients who are immunosuppressed.

Supportive Care

Colony-stimulating factors have been helpful in reducing the duration of neutropenia, the number of infectious episodes, and use of antibiotics after administration of myelosuppressive chemotherapy. Additionally, granulocyte-CSF(G-CSF) can enhance granulocyte function by increasing the production of superoxide radicals, phagocytosis, and antibody dependent cytotoxicity.[177] Although endogenous levels of G-CSF may be elevated in febrile neutropenic patients, exogenous administration is commonly used during these episodes.[178] The 2006 American Society of Clinical Oncology guidelines recommend use of colony-stimulating factor to reduce the risk of febrile neutropenia in high-risk patients, although there does not appear to be an influence on mortality.[116,179] The high mortality (54%) in patients who are neutropenic admitted to the ICU is caused by organ failure rather than the duration of neutropenia.[180] In critically ill patients who are neutropenic, data on the use of G-CSF or granulocyte-macrophage CSF is limited and did not shorten duration of neutropenia nor change survival as compared with historical controls.[180,181]

Granulocyte transfusions have been used since the 1960s for patients who have severe neutropenia and septicemia that was not responsive to antibiotics.[182] With the advent of colony-stimulating factors in the 1990s, granulocyte transfusions became less common. However, the use of G-CSF before donation allows for a greater yield by leukapheresis, thereby providing a larger dose of granulocytes for the recipient. This greater yield generated new enthusiasm for granulocyte transfusions in septic neutropenic patients.[177] A recent Cochrane review concluded that there was insufficient evidence to support or refute the use of granulocyte transfusions in patients who are neutropenic with severe infections. A possible survival benefit with using doses of granulocytes greater than 1×10^{10} was also suggested but further investigation is required.[183]

The administration of IVIG has shown benefit as prophylaxis in multiple myeloma and CLL and for treatment of severe VZV infections.[184,185] In critically ill patients who have severe sepsis or septic shock, meta-analyses show a survival benefit for patients given polyclonal IVIG when limited studies were evaluated. Because of the heterogeneity of the data analyzed a large, randomized placebo controlled trial is required to better understand the effect of this therapy in patients who have sepsis.[186–188]

Preventive Measures

Although a comprehensive approach to managing infections in this immunocompromised population is essential, prevention of nosocomial acquired infections is equally important and challenging. Simple measures including hand washing with alcohol based solutions, barrier precautions including donning of gown and gloves during patient interactions, and chlorhexidine baths can reduce the spread of resistant pathogens.[189,190] The implementation of bundles can similarly diminish the rates of nosocomial infections including CRBSI and VAP.[191] Novel interventions, such as the use of metal surfaces, invasive devices impregnated with antimicrobial agents, or subglottic aspiration of secretions, may help further reduce the spread and development of resistant infections in patients in the ICU.[192–197]

SUMMARY

Patients who have cancer are at a higher risk for infectious complications and frequently require ICU care. Although outcomes have improved, infection remains a significant cause for morbidity and mortality. Understanding the malignancy and concomitant immune dysfunction that occurs, either caused by the underlying disease or as a result of chemotherapy or radiotherapy, will help to guide the diagnostic workup. Although the infectious complications may be similar to the general population, the etiologies and clinical presentations are different. Patients who have cancer are also at risk for infection caused by otherwise nonpathogenic organisms. A high index of suspicion is required to properly diagnose and treat unique infections in this population. Management is based on recognizing distinct pathogens that occur with higher frequency in specific conditions seen in patients who have cancer. General supportive care to critically ill patients who have cancer is similar to other populations; however, specific therapies have not been well studied and may represent future areas of research. Preventative measures including bundling of proven interventions and novel techniques may help protect critically ill patients who have cancer.

REFERENCES

1. Martin GS, Mannino DM, Eaton S, et al. The epidemiology of sepsis in the United States from 1979 through 2000. N Engl J Med 2003;348:1546–54.
2. Danai PA, Moss M, Mannino DM, et al. The epidemiology of sepsis in patients with malignancy. Chest 2006;129:1432–40.
3. Safdar A, Armstrong D. Infectious morbidity in critically ill patients with cancer. Crit Care Clin 2001;17:531–70, vii–viii.
4. Angus DC, Linde-Zwirble WT, Lidicker J, et al. Epidemiology of severe sepsis in the United States: analysis of incidence, outcome, and associated costs of care. Crit Care Med 2001;29:1303–10.
5. Williams MD, Braun LA, Cooper LM, et al. Hospitalized cancer patients with severe sepsis: analysis of incidence, mortality, and associated costs of care. Crit Care 2004;8:R291–8.
6. American Cancer Society. Cancer facts & figures 2009. Atlanta (GA): American Cancer Society; 2009. Available at: http://www.cancer.org/downloads/STT/500809web.pdf. Accessed June 21, 2009.
7. Jemal A, Siegel R, Ward E, et al. Cancer statistics, 2009. CA Cancer J Clin 2009; 59:225–49.
8. Pene F, Percheron S, Lemiale V, et al. Temporal changes in management and outcome of septic shock in patients with malignancies in the intensive care unit. Crit Care Med 2008;36:690–6.
9. Taccone FS, Artigas AA, Sprung CL, et al. Characteristics and outcomes of cancer patients in European ICUs. Crit Care 2009;13:R15.
10. Hubel K, Hegener K, Schnell R, et al. Suppressed neutrophil function as a risk factor for severe infection after cytotoxic chemotherapy in patients with acute nonlymphocytic leukemia. Ann Hematol 1999;78:73–7.
11. Pickering LK, Ericsson CD, Kohl S. Effect of chemotherapeutic agents on metabolic and bactericidal activity of polymorphonuclear leukocytes. Cancer 1978; 42:1741–6.
12. Vaudaux P, Kiefer B, Forni M, et al. Adriamycin impairs phagocytic function and induces morphologic alterations in human neutrophils. Cancer 1984;54:400–10.
13. Bhatt V, Saleem A. Review: drug-induced neutropenia–pathophysiology, clinical features, and management. Ann Clin Lab Sci 2004;34:131–7.
14. Mac Manus M, Lamborn K, Khan W, et al. Radiotherapy-associated neutropenia and thrombocytopenia: analysis of risk factors and development of a predictive model. Blood 1997;89:2303–10.
15. Gallacher SJ, Thomson G, Fraser WD, et al. Neutrophil bactericidal function in diabetes mellitus: evidence for association with blood glucose control. Diabet Med 1995;12:916–20.

16. Turina M, Fry DE, Polk HC Jr. Acute hyperglycemia and the innate immune system: clinical, cellular, and molecular aspects. Crit Care Med 2005;33: 1624–33.
17. Chanock SJ, Pizzo PA. Infectious complications of patients undergoing therapy for acute leukemia: current status and future prospects. Semin Oncol 1997;24: 132–40.
18. Bodey GP, Buckley M, Sathe YS, et al. Quantitative relationships between circulating leukocytes and infection in patients with acute leukemia. Ann Intern Med 1966;64:328–40.
19. Deinard AS, Fortuny IE, Theologides A, et al. Studies on the neutropenia of cancer chemotherapy. Cancer 1974;33:1210–8.
20. Lalami Y, Paesmans M, Muanza F, et al. Can we predict the duration of chemotherapy-induced neutropenia in febrile neutropenic patients, focusing on regimen-specific risk factors? A retrospective analysis. Ann Oncol 2006;17: 507–14.
21. Marshall JC, Charbonney E, Gonzalez PD. The immune system in critical illness. Clin Chest Med 2008;29:605–16, vii.
22. Frank MM, Joiner K, Hammer C. The function of antibody and complement in the lysis of bacteria. Rev Infect Dis 1987;9(Suppl 5):S537–45.
23. Wadhwa PD, Morrison VA. Infectious complications of chronic lymphocytic leukemia. Semin Oncol 2006;33:240–9.
24. Paradisi F, Corti G, Cinelli R. Infections in multiple myeloma. Infect Dis Clin North Am 2001;15:373–84, vii–viii.
25. Fahey JL, Scoggins R, Utz JP, et al. Infection, antibody response and gamma globulin components in multiple myeloma and macroglobulinemia. Am J Med 1963;35:698–707.
26. Tabbara IA, Zimmerman K, Morgan C, et al. Allogeneic hematopoietic stem cell transplantation: complications and results. Arch Intern Med 2002;162:1558–66.
27. Notter DT, Grossman PL, Rosenberg SA, et al. Infections in patients with Hodgkin's disease: a clinical study of 300 consecutive adult patients. Rev Infect Dis 1980;2:761–800.
28. Plosker GL, Figgitt DP. Rituximab: a review of its use in non-Hodgkin's lymphoma and chronic lymphocytic leukaemia. Drugs 2003;63:803–43.
29. Martin SI, Marty FM, Fiumara K, et al. Infectious complications associated with alemtuzumab use for lymphoproliferative disorders. Clin Infect Dis 2006;43: 16–24.
30. Otahbachi M, Nugent K, Buscemi D. Granulomatous Pneumocystis jiroveci Pneumonia in a patient with chronic lymphocytic leukemia: a literature review and hypothesis on pathogenesis. Am J Med Sci 2007;333:131–5.
31. Wucherpfennig KW. T-cell immunity. In: Hoffman R, editor. Hematology: basic principles and practice. 5th edition. Philadelphia: Churchill Livingstone/Elsevier; 2009. p. 117–27.
32. Fisher RI, DeVita VT Jr, Bostick F, et al. Persistent immunologic abnormalities in long-term survivors of advanced Hodgkin's disease. Ann Intern Med 1980;92:595–9.
33. Mahieux R, Gessain A. HTLV-1 and associated adult T-cell leukemia/lymphoma. Rev Clin Exp Hematol 2003;7:336–61.
34. Bodey GP. Infection in cancer patients. A continuing association. Am J Med 1986;81:11–26.
35. Anaissie EJ, Kontoyiannis DP, O'Brien S, et al. Infections in patients with chronic lymphocytic leukemia treated with fludarabine. Ann Intern Med 1998;129: 559–66.

36. Mackall CL, Fleisher TA, Brown MR, et al. Lymphocyte depletion during treatment with intensive chemotherapy for cancer. Blood 1994;84:2221–8.
37. Schilling PJ, Vadhan-Raj S. Concurrent cytomegalovirus and pneumocystis pneumonia after fludarabine therapy for chronic lymphocytic leukemia. N Engl J Med 1990;323:833–4.
38. Su YB, Sohn S, Krown SE, et al. Selective CD4+ lymphopenia in melanoma patients treated with temozolomide: a toxicity with therapeutic implications. J Clin Oncol 2004;22:610–6.
39. Yu SK, Chalmers AJ. Patients receiving standard-dose temozolomide therapy are at risk of Pneumocystis carinii pneumonia. Clin Oncol (R Coll Radiol) 2007;19:631–2.
40. Sickles EA, Greene WH, Wiernik PH. Clinical presentation of infection in granulocytopenic patients. Arch Intern Med 1975;135:715–9.
41. Crawford J, Dale DC, Lyman GH. Chemotherapy-induced neutropenia: risks, consequences, and new directions for its management. Cancer 2004;100: 228–37.
42. Hughes WT, Armstrong D, Bodey GP, et al. 2002 guidelines for the use of antimicrobial agents in neutropenic patients with cancer. Clin Infect Dis 2002;34: 730–51.
43. Heussel CP, Kauczor HU, Heussel GE, et al. Pneumonia in febrile neutropenic patients and in bone marrow and blood stem-cell transplant recipients: use of high-resolution computed tomography. J Clin Oncol 1999;17: 796–805.
44. Mermel LA, Farr BM, Sherertz RJ, et al. Guidelines for the management of intravascular catheter-related infections. Clin Infect Dis 2001;32:1249–72.
45. Klastersky J. Antifungal therapy in patients with fever and neutropenia–more rational and less empirical? N Engl J Med 2004;351:1445–7.
46. Talcott JA, Siegel RD, Finberg R, et al. Risk assessment in cancer patients with fever and neutropenia: a prospective, two-center validation of a prediction rule. J Clin Oncol 1992;10:316–22.
47. Klastersky J, Paesmans M, Rubenstein EB, et al. The multinational association for supportive care in cancer risk index: a multinational scoring system for identifying low-risk febrile neutropenic cancer patients. J Clin Oncol 2000;18: 3038–51.
48. Wisplinghoff H, Seifert H, Wenzel RP, et al. Current trends in the epidemiology of nosocomial bloodstream infections in patients with hematological malignancies and solid neoplasms in hospitals in the United States. Clin Infect Dis 2003;36: 1103–10.
49. Rolston Kvi RI, Whimbey E, Bodey GP. The changing spectrum of bacterial infections in febrile neutropenic patients. In: Klastersky J, editor. Febrile neutropenia. New York: Springer-Verlag; 1997. p. 53–6, Berlin (Germany).
50. Elting LS, Bodey GP, Keefe BH. Septicemia and shock syndrome due to viridans streptococci: a case-control study of predisposing factors. Clin Infect Dis 1992; 14:1201–7.
51. Lecciones JA, Lee JW, Navarro EE, et al. Vascular catheter-associated fungemia in patients with cancer: analysis of 155 episodes. Clin Infect Dis 1992;14: 875–83.
52. Kontoyiannis DP, Bodey GP. Invasive aspergillosis in 2002: an update. Eur J Clin Microbiol Infect Dis 2002;21:161–72.
53. Morrison VA, Haake RJ, Weisdorf DJ. Non-Candida fungal infections after bone marrow transplantation: risk factors and outcome. Am J Med 1994;96:497–503.

54. Caillot D, Couaillier JF, Bernard A, et al. Increasing volume and changing characteristics of invasive pulmonary aspergillosis on sequential thoracic computed tomography scans in patients with neutropenia. J Clin Oncol 2001;19:253–9.

55. Cometta A, Calandra T, Gaya H, et al. Monotherapy with meropenem versus combination therapy with ceftazidime plus amikacin as empiric therapy for fever in granulocytopenic patients with cancer. The International Antimicrobial Therapy Cooperative Group of the European Organization for Research and Treatment of Cancer and the Gruppo Italiano Malattie Ematologiche Maligne dell'Adulto Infection Program. Antimicrob Agents Chemother 1996;40:1108–15.

56. Johnson MP, Ramphal R. Beta-lactam-resistant Enterobacter bacteremia in febrile neutropenic patients receiving monotherapy. J Infect Dis 1990;162:981–3.

57. Stroncek D, Shawker T, Follmann D, et al. G-CSF-induced spleen size changes in peripheral blood progenitor cell donors. Transfusion 2003;43:609–13.

58. Maschmeyer G, Link H, Hiddemann W, et al. Pulmonary infiltrations in febrile patients with neutropenia. Risk factors and outcome under empirical antimicrobial therapy in a randomized multicenter study. Cancer 1994;73:2296–304.

59. Crawford SW. Noninfectious lung disease in the immunocompromised host. Respiration 1999;66:385–95.

60. Jain P, Sandur S, Meli Y, et al. Role of flexible bronchoscopy in immunocompromised patients with lung infiltrates. Chest 2004;125:712–22.

61. Bodey GP, Rodriguez V, Chang HY, et al. Fever and infection in leukemic patients: a study of 494 consecutive patients. Cancer 1978;41:1610–22.

62. Bochud PY, Calandra T, Francioli P. Bacteremia due to viridans streptococci in neutropenic patients: a review. Am J Med 1994;97:256–64.

63. Jacobson KL, Miceli MH, Tarrand JJ, et al. Legionella pneumonia in cancer patients. Medicine (Baltimore) 2008;87:152–9.

64. Fujita J, Yamadori I, Xu G, et al. Clinical features of Stenotrophomonas maltophilia pneumonia in immunocompromised patients. Respir Med 1996;90:35–8.

65. Venditti M, Monaco M, Micozzi A, et al. In vitro activity of moxifloxacin against Stenotrophomonas maltophilia blood isolates from patients with hematologic malignancies. Clin Microbiol Infect 2001;7:37–9.

66. Safdar A, Rolston KV. Stenotrophomonas maltophilia: changing spectrum of a serious bacterial pathogen in patients with cancer. Clin Infect Dis 2007;45: 1602–9.

67. Traub WH, Leonhard B, Bauer D. Stenotrophomonas (Xanthomonas) maltophilia: in vitro susceptibility to selected antimicrobial drugs, single and combined, with and without defibrinated human blood. Chemotherapy 1998;44:293–304.

68. Martinez Tomas R, Menendez Villanueva R, Reyes Calzada S, et al. Pulmonary nocardiosis: risk factors and outcomes. Respirology 2007;12:394–400.

69. Shima T, Yoshimoto G, Miyamoto T, et al. Disseminated tuberculosis following second unrelated cord blood transplantation for acute myelogenous leukemia. Transpl Infect Dis 2009;11:75–7.

70. Blumberg HM, et al. Treatment of tuberculosis. MMWR Recomm Rep 2003;52: 1–77.

71. Reilly AF, McGowan KL. Atypical mycobacterial infections in children with cancer. Pediatr Blood Cancer 2004;43:698–702.

72. Meeuse JJ, Sprenger HG, van Assen S, et al. Rhodococcus equi infection after alemtuzumab therapy for T-cell prolymphocytic leukemia. Emerg Infect Dis 2007;13:1942–3.

73. Casetta M, Blot F, Antoun S, et al. Diagnosis of nosocomial pneumonia in cancer patients undergoing mechanical ventilation: a prospective comparison of the

plugged telescoping catheter with the protected specimen brush. Chest 1999; 115:1641–5.

74. Chemaly RF, Ghosh S, Bodey GP, et al. Respiratory viral infections in adults with hematologic malignancies and human stem cell transplantation recipients: a retrospective study at a major cancer center. Medicine (Baltimore) 2006;85: 278–87.

75. Whimbey E, Englund JA, Couch RB. Community respiratory virus infections in immunocompromised patients with cancer. Am J Med 1997;102:10–8 [discussion: 25–6].

76. Torres HA, Aguilera EA, Mattiuzzi GN, et al. Characteristics and outcome of respiratory syncytial virus infection in patients with leukemia. Haematologica 2007;92:1216–23.

77. Khanna N, Widmer AF, Decker M, et al. Respiratory syncytial virus infection in patients with hematological diseases: single-center study and review of the literature. Clin Infect Dis 2008;46:402–12.

78. Boeckh M, Berrey MM, Bowden RA, et al. Phase 1 evaluation of the respiratory syncytial virus-specific monoclonal antibody palivizumab in recipients of hematopoietic stem cell transplants. J Infect Dis 2001;184:350–4.

79. Nguyen Q, Estey E, Raad I, et al. Cytomegalovirus pneumonia in adults with leukemia: an emerging problem. Clin Infect Dis 2001;32:539–45.

80. Crawford SW, Bowden RA, Hackman RC, et al. Rapid detection of cytomegalovirus pulmonary infection by bronchoalveolar lavage and centrifugation culture. Ann Intern Med 1988;108:180–5.

81. de la Hoz RE, Stephens G, Sherlock C. Diagnosis and treatment approaches of CMV infections in adult patients. J Clin Virol 2002;25(Suppl 2):S1–12.

82. Schuller D, Spessert C, Fraser VJ, et al. Herpes simplex virus from respiratory tract secretions: epidemiology, clinical characteristics, and outcome in immunocompromised and nonimmunocompromised hosts. Am J Med 1993;94:29–33.

83. Connolly MG Jr, Baughman RP, Dohn MN, et al. Recovery of viruses other than cytomegalovirus from bronchoalveolar lavage fluid. Chest 1994;105:1775–81.

84. Pierangeli A, Gentile M, Di Marco P, et al. Detection and typing by molecular techniques of respiratory viruses in children hospitalized for acute respiratory infection in Rome, Italy. J Med Virol 2007;79:463–8.

85. Parody R, Rabella N, Martino R, et al. Upper and lower respiratory tract infections by human enterovirus and rhinovirus in adult patients with hematological malignancies. Am J Hematol 2007;82:807–11.

86. Kamboj M, Gerbin M, Huang CK, et al. Clinical characterization of human metapneumovirus infection among patients with cancer. J Infect 2008;57:464–71.

87. Kamble RT, Bollard C, Demmler G, et al. Human metapneumovirus infection in a hematopoietic transplant recipient. Bone Marrow Transplant 2007;40:699–700.

88. Lin SJ, Schranz J, Teutsch SM. Aspergillosis case-fatality rate: systematic review of the literature. Clin Infect Dis 2001;32:358–66.

89. Subira M, Martino R, Franquet T, et al. Invasive pulmonary aspergillosis in patients with hematologic malignancies: survival and prognostic factors. Haematologica 2002;87:528–34.

90. Reichenberger F, Habicht JM, Gratwohl A, et al. Diagnosis and treatment of invasive pulmonary aspergillosis in neutropenic patients. Eur Respir J 2002; 19:743–55.

91. Buchheidt D, Baust C, Skladny H, et al. Clinical evaluation of a polymerase chain reaction assay to detect Aspergillus species in bronchoalveolar lavage samples of neutropenic patients. Br J Haematol 2002;116:803–11.

92. Ascioglu S, Rex JH, de Pauw B, et al. Defining opportunistic invasive fungal infections in immunocompromised patients with cancer and hematopoietic stem cell transplants: an international consensus. Clin Infect Dis 2002;34: 7–14.
93. Zedek DC, Miller MB. Use of galactomannan enzyme immunoassay for diagnosis of invasive aspergillosis in a tertiary-care center over a 12-month period. J Clin Microbiol 2006;44:1601.
94. Walsh TJ, Pappas P, Winston DJ, et al. Voriconazole compared with liposomal amphotericin B for empirical antifungal therapy in patients with neutropenia and persistent fever. N Engl J Med 2002;346:225–34.
95. Prentice HG, Hann IM, Herbrecht R, et al. A randomized comparison of liposomal versus conventional amphotericin B for the treatment of pyrexia of unknown origin in neutropenic patients. Br J Haematol 1997;98:711–8.
96. Herbrecht R, Denning DW, Patterson TF, et al. Voriconazole versus amphotericin B for primary therapy of invasive aspergillosis. N Engl J Med 2002;347:408–15.
97. Walsh TJ, Raad I, Patterson TF, et al. Treatment of invasive aspergillosis with posaconazole in patients who are refractory to or intolerant of conventional therapy: an externally controlled trial. Clin Infect Dis 2007;44:2–12.
98. Maertens J, Raad I, Petrikkos G, et al. Efficacy and safety of caspofungin for treatment of invasive aspergillosis in patients refractory to or intolerant of conventional antifungal therapy. Clin Infect Dis 2004;39:1563–71.
99. Todeschini G, Murari C, Bonesi R, et al. Invasive aspergillosis in neutropenic patients: rapid neutrophil recovery is a risk factor for severe pulmonary complications. Eur J Clin Invest 1999;29:453–7.
100. Vento S, Cainelli F, Temesgen Z. Lung infections after cancer chemotherapy. Lancet Oncol 2008;9:982–92.
101. Morris A, Lundgren JD, Masur H, et al. Current epidemiology of Pneumocystis pneumonia. Emerg Infect Dis 2004;10:1713–20.
102. Torres HA, Chemaly RF, Storey R, et al. Influence of type of cancer and hematopoietic stem cell transplantation on clinical presentation of Pneumocystis jiroveci pneumonia in cancer patients. Eur J Clin Microbiol Infect Dis 2006;25: 382–8.
103. Limper AH, Offord KP, Smith TF, et al. Pneumocystis carinii pneumonia. Differences in lung parasite number and inflammation in patients with and without AIDS. Am Rev Respir Dis 1989;140:1204–9.
104. Morris A. Is there anything new in Pneumocystis jiroveci pneumonia? Changes in P. jirovecii pneumonia over the course of the AIDS epidemic. Clin Infect Dis 2008;46:634–6.
105. Pagano L, Fianchi L, Mele L, et al. Pneumocystis carinii pneumonia in patients with malignant haematological diseases: 10 years' experience of infection in GIMEMA centres. Br J Haematol 2002;117:379–86.
106. Green H, Paul M, Vidal L, et al. Prophylaxis for Pneumocystis pneumonia (PCP) in non-HIV immunocompromised patients. Cochrane Database Syst Rev 2007;(3):CD005590.
107. Keiser PB, Nutman TB. Strongyloides stercoralis in the Immunocompromised Population. Clin Microbiol Rev 2004;17:208–17.
108. Davila ML. Neutropenic enterocolitis: current issues in diagnosis and management. Curr Infect Dis Rep 2007;9:116–20.
109. Urbach DR, Rotstein OD. Typhlitis. Can J Surg 1999;42:415–9.
110. Gorschluter M, Mey U, Strehl J, et al. Neutropenic enterocolitis in adults: systematic analysis of evidence quality. Eur J Haematol 2005;75:1–13.

111. Baerg J, Murphy JJ, Anderson R, et al. Neutropenic enteropathy: a 10-year review. J Pediatr Surg 1999;34:1068–71.
112. Gorschluter M, Mey U, Strehl J, et al. Invasive fungal infections in neutropenic enterocolitis: a systematic analysis of pathogens, incidence, treatment and mortality in adult patients. BMC Infect Dis 2006;6:35.
113. Baden LR, Maguire JH. Gastrointestinal infections in the immunocompromised host. Infect Dis Clin North Am 2001;15:639–70, xi.
114. Kirkpatrick ID, Greenberg HM. Gastrointestinal complications in the neutropenic patient: characterization and differentiation with abdominal CT. Radiology 2003; 226:668–74.
115. Cartoni C, Dragoni F, Micozzi A, et al. Neutropenic enterocolitis in patients with acute leukemia: prognostic significance of bowel wall thickening detected by ultrasonography. J Clin Oncol 2001;19:756–61.
116. Smith TJ, Khatcheressian J, Lyman GH, et al. 2006 update of recommendations for the use of white blood cell growth factors: an evidence-based clinical practice guideline. J Clin Oncol 2006;24:3187–205.
117. Leffler DA, Lamont JT. Treatment of Clostridium difficile-associated disease. Gastroenterology 2009;136:1899–912.
118. Rupnik M, Wilcox MH, Gerding DN. Clostridium difficile infection: new developments in epidemiology and pathogenesis. Nat Rev Microbiol 2009;7: 526–36.
119. Gorschluter M, Glasmacher A, Hahn C, et al. Clostridium difficile Infection in patients with Neutropenia. Clin Infect Dis 2001;33:786–91.
120. Fenner L, Widmer AF, Goy G, et al. Rapid and reliable diagnostic algorithm for detection of Clostridium difficile. J Clin Microbiol 2008;46:328–30.
121. Johnson S, Gerding DN. Clostridium difficile–associated diarrhea. Clin Infect Dis 1998;26:1027–34, quiz 35–6.
122. Gerding DN, Muto CA, Owens RC Jr. Treatment of Clostridium difficile infection. Clin Infect Dis 2008;46(Suppl 1):S32–42.
123. Kontoyiannis DP, Luna MA, Samuels BI, et al. Hepatosplenic candidiasis. A manifestation of chronic disseminated candidiasis. Infect Dis Clin North Am 2000;14:721–39.
124. Pappas PG. Invasive candidiasis. Infect Dis Clin North Am 2006;20:485–506.
125. Pappas PG, Kauffman CA, Andes D, et al. Clinical practice guidelines for the management of candidiasis: 2009 update by the Infectious Diseases Society of America. Clin Infect Dis 2009;48:503–35.
126. DeAngelis LM, Posner JB. Central nervous system infections. In: DeAngelis LM, Posner JB, editors. Neurologic complications of cancer. 2nd edition. Oxford (UK)/New York: Oxford University Press; 2009. p. 369–416.
127. Pruitt AA. Central nervous system infections in cancer patients. Semin Neurol 2004;24:435–52.
128. Safdieh JE, Mead PA, Sepkowitz KA, et al. Bacterial and fungal meningitis in patients with cancer. Neurology 2008;70:943–7.
129. Pruitt AA. Nervous system infections in patients with cancer. Neurol Clin 2003; 21:193–219.
130. Huang SH, Jong AY. Cellular mechanisms of microbial proteins contributing to invasion of the blood-brain barrier. Cell Microbiol 2001;3:277–87.
131. Mylonakis E, Hohmann EL, Calderwood SB. Central nervous system infection with Listeria monocytogenes. 33 years' experience at a general hospital and review of 776 episodes from the literature. Medicine (Baltimore) 1998;77: 313–36.

132. Lukes SA, Posner JB, Nielsen S, et al. Bacterial infections of the CNS in neutropenic patients. Neurology 1984;34:269–75.
133. Schwartz S, Thiel E. Clinical presentation of invasive aspergillosis. Mycoses 1997;40(Suppl 2):21–4.
134. Quadri TL, Brown AE. Infectious complications in the critically ill patient with cancer. Semin Oncol 2000;27:335–46.
135. de Gans J, van de Beek D. Dexamethasone in adults with bacterial meningitis. N Engl J Med 2002;347:1549–56.
136. van de Beek D, de Gans J, McIntyre P, et al. Steroids in adults with acute bacterial meningitis: a systematic review. Lancet Infect Dis 2004;4:139–43.
137. Polsky B, Depman MR, Gold JW, et al. Intraventricular therapy of cryptococcal meningitis via a subcutaneous reservoir. Am J Med 1986;81:24–8.
138. Gottfredsson M, Perfect JR. Fungal meningitis. Semin Neurol 2000;20:307–22.
139. Raad I, Hanna HA. Long-term central venous catheters. In: Seifert H, Jansen B, Farr BM, editors. Catheter-related infections (infectious disease and therapy). 2nd edition. New York: Marcel Dekker; 2005. p. 425–44.
140. Sherertz RJ, Heard SO, Raad II. Diagnosis of triple-lumen catheter infection: comparison of roll plate, sonication, and flushing methodologies. J Clin Microbiol 1997;35:641–6.
141. Maki DG, Mermel LA. Infections due to infusion therapy. In: Bennett JV, Brachman PS, editors. Hospital infections. 4th edition. Philadelphia: Lippincott-Raven; 1998. p. 689–724.
142. Blot F, Nitenberg G, Chachaty E, et al. Diagnosis of catheter-related bacteraemia: a prospective comparison of the time to positivity of hub-blood versus peripheral-blood cultures. Lancet 1999;354:1071–7.
143. Capdevila JA, Planes AM, Palomar M, et al. Value of differential quantitative blood cultures in the diagnosis of catheter-related sepsis. Eur J Clin Microbiol Infect Dis 1992;11:403–7.
144. Raad I. Management of intravascular catheter-related infections. J Antimicrob Chemother 2000;45:267–70.
145. Elting LS, Bodey GP. Septicemia due to Xanthomonas species and non-aeruginosa Pseudomonas species: increasing incidence of catheter-related infections. Medicine (Baltimore) 1990;69:296–306.
146. Raad II, Vartivarian S, Khan A, et al. Catheter-related infections caused by the Mycobacterium fortuitum complex: 15 cases and review. Rev Infect Dis 1991;13:1120–5.
147. Rex JH, Walsh TJ, Sobel JD, et al. Practice guidelines for the treatment of candidiasis. Infectious Diseases Society of America. Clin Infect Dis 2000;30:662–78.
148. Anaissie EJ, Rex JH, Uzun O, et al. Predictors of adverse outcome in cancer patients with candidemia. Am J Med 1998;104:238–45.
149. Raad I, Narro J, Khan A, et al. Serious complications of vascular catheter-related Staphylococcus aureus bacteremia in cancer patients. Eur J Clin Microbiol Infect Dis 1992;11:675–82.
150. Verghese A, Widrich WC, Arbeit RD. Central venous septic thrombophlebitis–the role of medical therapy. Medicine (Baltimore) 1985;64:394–400.
151. Nambirajan T, O'Sullivan JM. Genitourinary tract infections in cancer patients. In: Spence RAJ, Hay RJ, Johnston PG, editors. Infection in the cancer patient: a practical guide. 1st edition. Oxford (UK)/New York: Oxford University Press; 2006. p. 101–12.
152. DeVita VT, Lawrence TS, Rosenberg SA. DeVita, Hellman, and Rosenberg's cancer: principles & practice of oncology. 8th edition. Philadelphia: Wolters Kluwer/Lippincott Williams & Wilkins; 2008.

153. Stunell H, Buckley O, Feeney J, et al. Imaging of acute pyelonephritis in the adult. Eur Radiol 2007;17:1820–8.
154. Falagas ME, Vergidis PI. Urinary tract infections in patients with urinary diversion. Am J Kidney Dis 2005;46:1030–7.
155. Wood DP Jr, Bianco FJ Jr, Pontes JE, et al. Incidence and significance of positive urine cultures in patients with an orthotopic neobladder. J Urol 2003;169:2196–9.
156. Keegan SJ, Graham C, Neal DE, et al. Characterization of Escherichia coli strains causing urinary tract infections in patients with transposed intestinal segments. J Urol 2003;169:2382–7.
157. Ganatra AM, Loughlin KR. The management of malignant ureteral obstruction treated with ureteral stents. J Urol 2005;174:2125–8.
158. Rosenberg BH, Bianco FJ Jr, Wood DP Jr, et al. Stent-change therapy in advanced malignancies with ureteral obstruction. J Endourol 2005;19:63–7.
159. Kaul R, McGeer A, Norrby-Teglund A, et al. Intravenous immunoglobulin therapy for streptococcal toxic shock syndrome–a comparative observational study. The Canadian Streptococcal Study Group. Clin Infect Dis 1999;28:800–7.
160. Lo WT, Cheng SN, Wang CC, et al. Extensive necrotising fasciitis caused by Pseudomonas aeruginosa in a child with acute myeloid leukemia: case report and literature review. Eur J Pediatr 2005;164:113–4.
161. Duncan BW, Adzick NS, deLorimier AA, et al. Necrotizing fasciitis in two children with acute lymphoblastic leukemia. J Pediatr Surg 1992;27:668–71.
162. Mantadakis E, Pontikoglou C, Papadaki HA, et al. Fatal Fournier's gangrene in a young adult with acute lymphoblastic leukemia. Pediatr Blood Cancer 2007;49:862–4.
163. Dellinger RP, Levy MM, Carlet JM, et al. Surviving Sepsis Campaign: international guidelines for management of severe sepsis and septic shock: 2008. Crit Care Med 2008;36:296–327.
164. Rivers E, Nguyen B, Havstad S, et al. Early goal-directed therapy in the treatment of severe sepsis and septic shock. N Engl J Med 2001;345:1368–77.
165. Bernard GR, Vincent JL, Laterre PF, et al. Efficacy and safety of recombinant human activated protein C for severe sepsis. N Engl J Med 2001;344:699–709.
166. Bernard GR, Margolis BD, Shanies HM, et al. Extended evaluation of recombinant human activated protein C United States Trial (ENHANCE US): a single-arm, phase 3B, multicenter study of drotrecogin alfa (activated) in severe sepsis. Chest 2004;125:2206–16.
167. Abraham E, Laterre PF, Garg R, et al. Drotrecogin alfa (activated) for adults with severe sepsis and a low risk of death. N Engl J Med 2005;353:1332–41.
168. Bernard GR, Macias WL, Joyce DE, et al. Safety assessment of drotrecogin alfa (activated) in the treatment of adult patients with severe sepsis. Crit Care 2003;7:155–63.
169. Pastores SM, Papadopoulos E, van den Brink M, et al. Septic shock and multiple organ failure after hematopoietic stem cell transplantation: treatment with recombinant human activated protein C. Bone Marrow Transplant 2002;30:131–4.
170. Pastores SM, Shaw A, Williams MD, et al. A safety evaluation of drotrecogin alfa (activated) in hematopoietic stem cell transplant patients with severe sepsis: lessons in clinical research. Bone Marrow Transplant 2005;36:721–4.
171. Marik PE, Pastores SM, Annane D, et al. Recommendations for the diagnosis and management of corticosteroid insufficiency in critically ill adult patients:

consensus statements from an international task force by the American College of Critical Care Medicine. Crit Care Med 2008;36:1937–49.

172. Sprung CL, Annane D, Keh D, et al. Hydrocortisone therapy for patients with septic shock. N Engl J Med 2008;358:111–24.

173. Annane D, Sebille V, Charpentier C, et al. Effect of treatment with low doses of hydrocortisone and fludrocortisone on mortality in patients with septic shock. JAMA 2002;288:862–71.

174. Van den Berghe G, Wilmer A, Hermans G, et al. Intensive insulin therapy in the medical ICU. N Engl J Med 2006;354:449–61.

175. van den Berghe G, Wouters P, Weekers F, et al. Intensive insulin therapy in the critically ill patients. N Engl J Med 2001;345:1359–67.

176. Finfer S, Chittock DR, Su SY, et al. Intensive versus conventional glucose control in critically ill patients. N Engl J Med 2009;360:1283–97.

177. Sulis ML, Lauren H, Cairo MS. Granulocyte transfusions in the neonate and child. In: Hillyer CD, Strauss RG, Luban NLC, editors. Handbook of pediatric transfusion medicine. Oxford (UK): Academic Press; 2004. p. 167–80.

178. Cebon J, Layton JE, Maher D, et al. Endogenous haemopoietic growth factors in neutropenia and infection. Br J Haematol 1994;86:265–74.

179. Heuser M, Ganser A, Bokemeyer C. Use of colony-stimulating factors for chemotherapy-associated neutropenia: review of current guidelines. Semin Hematol 2007;44:148–56.

180. Darmon M, Azoulay E, Alberti C, et al. Impact of neutropenia duration on short-term mortality in neutropenic critically ill cancer patients. Intensive Care Med 2002;28:1775–80.

181. Bouchama A, Khan B, Djazmati W, et al. Hematopoietic colony-stimulating factors for neutropenic patients in the ICU. Intensive Care Med 1999;25: 1003–5.

182. Freireich EJ, Levin RH, Whang J, et al. The function and fate of transfused leukocytes from donors with chronic myelocytic leukemia in leukopenic recipients. Ann N Y Acad Sci 1964;113:1081–9.

183. Stanworth SJ, Massey E, Hyde C, et al. Granulocyte transfusions for treating infections in patients with neutropenia or neutrophil dysfunction. Cochrane Database Syst Rev 2005;(3):CD005339.

184. Chapel HM, Lee M. The use of intravenous immune globulin in multiple myeloma. Clin Exp Immunol 1994;97(Suppl 1):21–4.

185. Morell A, Barandun S. Prophylactic and therapeutic use of immunoglobulin for intravenous administration in patients with secondary immunodeficiencies associated with malignancies. Pediatr Infect Dis J 1988;7:S87–91.

186. Turgeon AF, Hutton B, Fergusson DA, et al. Meta-analysis: intravenous immunoglobulin in critically ill adult patients with sepsis. Ann Intern Med 2007;146: 193–203.

187. Laupland KB, Kirkpatrick AW, Delaney A. Polyclonal intravenous immunoglobulin for the treatment of severe sepsis and septic shock in critically ill adults: a systematic review and meta-analysis. Crit Care Med 2007;35:2686–92.

188. Kreymann KG, de Heer G, Nierhaus A, et al. Use of polyclonal immunoglobulins as adjunctive therapy for sepsis or septic shock. Crit Care Med 2007;35: 2677–85.

189. Warren DK, Fraser VJ. Infection control measures to limit antimicrobial resistance. Crit Care Med 2001;29:N128–34.

190. Climo MW, Sepkowitz KA, Zuccotti G, et al. The effect of daily bathing with chlorhexidine on the acquisition of methicillin-resistant Staphylococcus aureus,

vancomycin-resistant Enterococcus, and healthcare-associated bloodstream infections: results of a quasi-experimental multicenter trial. Crit Care Med 2009;37:1858–65.

191. Kollef M. SMART approaches for reducing nosocomial infections in the ICU. Chest 2008;134:447–56.

192. Noyce JO, Michels H, Keevil CW. Potential use of copper surfaces to reduce survival of epidemic meticillin-resistant Staphylococcus aureus in the healthcare environment. J Hosp Infect 2006;63:289–97.

193. Weaver L, Michels HT, Keevil CW. Survival of Clostridium difficile on copper and steel: futuristic options for hospital hygiene. J Hosp Infect 2008;68:145–51.

194. Johnson JR, Kuskowski MA, Wilt TJ. Systematic review: antimicrobial urinary catheters to prevent catheter-associated urinary tract infection in hospitalized patients. Ann Intern Med 2006;144:116–26.

195. Kollef MH, Afessa B, Anzueto A, et al. Silver-coated endotracheal tubes and incidence of ventilator-associated pneumonia: the NASCENT randomized trial. JAMA 2008;300:805–13.

196. Ramritu P, Halton K, Collignon P, et al. A systematic review comparing the relative effectiveness of antimicrobial-coated catheters in intensive care units. Am J Infect Control 2008;36:104–17.

197. Bouza E, Perez MJ, Munoz P, et al. Continuous aspiration of subglottic secretions in the prevention of ventilator-associated pneumonia in the postoperative period of major heart surgery. Chest 2008;134:938–46.

Critical Care Issues in Oncological Surgery Patients

Sanam Ahmed, MD, John M. Oropello, MD*

KEYWORDS

• Cancer • Chemotherapy • Cytoreductive • ICU

Although progress has been made in reducing incidence and mortality rates and improving survival, cancer still accounts for more deaths than heart disease in persons younger than 85 years. A total of 1,479,350 new cancer cases and 562,340 deaths from cancer are projected to occur in the United States in 2009.[1] The intensive care unit (ICU) mortality rate for cancer patients may be decreasing due to advances in medicine and better selection of those most likely to benefit[2]; however, there are few published data on the specific characteristics of surgical oncologic patients in the ICU, with most of the data deriving from purely nonsurgical or mixed medical-surgical ICU settings. Surgery may be for primary or metastatic disease, or surgical complications of chemotherapy, radiotherapy, or previous surgery. In a mixed medical-surgical ICU setting, 15% of cancer patients had a prolonged length of stay (LOS) of 21 days or longer with a hospital mortality rate of about 50% regardless of the LOS.[3] The main outcome predictors included the number of organ failures, poor performance status, and older age. As in nononcological populations, the most frequent complications included infection, respiratory failure, and hemodynamic instability requiring vasopressors.

As life expectancy increases and advances in cancer treatment more often convert deadly conditions into more chronic diseases, the surgical intensivist can expect to be faced with greater numbers of oncology patients undergoing aggressive surgical treatments for curative intent, prolonging survival, or primarily palliation by alleviating obstruction, infection, bleeding, or pain. Many of these patients are immunocompromised and prone to infection, poor wound healing, and organ dysfunction due to preexisting diseases as well as perioperative adjuvant therapies, which may include combinations of systemic or regional

The authors state that they do not have any conflicts of interest.

Division of Critical Care Medicine, Department of Surgery, The Mount Sinai School of Medicine, 1 Gustave L. Levy Place, New York, NY 10029, USA

* Corresponding author.

E-mail address: john.oropello@mountsinai.org (J.M. Oropello).

Crit Care Clin 26 (2010) 93–106

doi:10.1016/j.ccc.2009.10.004

0749-0704/09/$ – see front matter © 2010 Elsevier Inc. All rights reserved.

criticalcare.theclinics.com

chemotherapy, radiotherapy, tumor ablation (radiofrequency, cryogenic, heat-focused lasers, microwaves), hormonal therapy, immunotherapy, or emerging gene therapy.

Just as critical illnesses take place in patients that differ in regards to the baseline function and susceptibility of their underlying organ systems, cancer is not a single disease entity but hundreds of different diseases that differ at the cellular level. Specific surgical oncology topics are wide-ranging and beyond the scope of this article, which focuses on major critical care issues concerning patients with advanced metastatic disease undergoing cytoreductive surgery (CRS) and heated intraperitoneal chemotherapy (HIPEC), which is a paradigm for the emerging field of multimodal aggressive oncological surgery. A discussion of the CRS/HIPEC technique is followed by a discussion of postoperative complications and critical care issues.

CYTOREDUCTIVE SURGERY AND HEATED INTRAPERITONEAL CHEMOTHERAPY

CRS with HIPEC is emerging as a therapeutic option for advanced, locally metastatic abdominal cavity cancer or peritoneal carcinomatosis. In peritoneal cancer, intravenous chemotherapy is ineffective. CRS encompasses extensive tumor debulking with visceral and parietal peritonectomy, resection of omentum, and resections of involved abdominal viscera such as stomach, small bowel, colon, spleen, liver, gall bladder, pancreas, bladder, diaphragm, and abdominal wall.[4–6] HIPEC is the intraoperative instillation of chemotherapeutic agents directly into the abdominal cavity along with a heating system. The goal of CRS is to completely eradicate macroscopic peritoneal disease; that of HIPEC is to eliminate microscopic tumor not visible to the naked eye, or to treat small residual deposits (eg, <0.5 cm) of tumor.

HIPEC is performed at the time of the CRS, before closure of the peritoneum and abdomen, thus avoiding entrapment of malignant cells in anastomoses and adhesions. However, gastrointestinal anastomoses must be performed before the chemotherapy is administered. The major advantage of intraperitoneal chemotherapy is the high local concentration of cytotoxic agents (20–1000 times higher than plasma levels) due to the peritoneal-plasma barrier, thereby maximizing the destruction of malignant cells and minimizing the systemic effects of chemotherapy. The added benefits of hyperthermia are the direct cytotoxic effects of heat on the cancer cells while sparing uninvolved cells, and the greater depth of drug penetration into the involved areas. HIPEC also destroys viable neutrophils, monocytes, and platelets from the peritoneal cavity. This process may diminish the promotion of tumor growth associated with the wound healing process.[7]

HIPEC is typically administered into a closed abdomen via sterile circuit. Cytotoxic solution flows through a pump and heat exchanger before entering the abdomen. Temperature probes are positioned in the circuit and peritoneum. Subdiaphragmatic and deep pelvic drains are connected to a heating unit that elevates the temperature of the solution to approximately 41° to 42°C. Although an open abdomen technique with skin traction allowing the surgeon to uniformly distribute the solution and cause less intra-abdominal hypertension and hemodynamic instability[8] may also be used, the advantages of a closed system include achievement of higher, more uniform temperatures within a shorter time period, and less theoretical exposure of the staff to aerosolization and direct contact with toxic chemotherapeutic agents.[9] Cytotoxic drugs (mitomycin C—the current standard for gastrointestinal malignancies, oxaliplatin, cisplatin, doxorubicin, 5-fluorouracil, or others depending on the tissue type) is infused for about 90 minutes (range, 60–120 minutes). After the procedure is complete, the abdomen is lavaged, drained, and closed.

The operation and procedure usually last about 10 hours (range, 6–14 hours), and the amount of blood loss ranges between 0.5 and 2 L or greater. Due to the aggressive surgical debulking and length of the procedure, large fluid shifts and sometimes massive blood loss can occur, and the majority requires blood transfusion.[10,11] Patients with peritoneal carcinomatosis frequently have discomfort and pain before and after CRS and HIPEC. In patients without contraindication, perioperative pain is managed by epidural anesthesia, which provides better pain control with less respiratory and hemodynamic complications.[12]

In patients with recurrent advanced ovarian cancer, CRS combined with HIPEC can lead to a substantial increase in subsequent rates of disease-free and overall survival.[13] This success coupled with the dismal prognosis of peritoneal cancer has led to investigations of CRS with HIPEC for other tumors such as appendiceal (pseudomyxoma peritonei),[14,15] colorectal, locally advanced gastric, small intestinal, and mesothelial peritoneum tumors,[16] as well as endometrial cancer.[17] Adding HIPEC to tumor debulking may lengthen survival and improve quality of life in these patients, who have a very limited life expectancy and high recurrence rate.[18]

Thus far, most of the reports are retrospective or nonrandomized prospective single-center phase 2 trials, with only one phase 3 randomized trial in peritoneal carcinomatosis of colorectal origin. The median survival of peritoneal carcinomatosis from colorectal cancer is 6 to 9 months,[19] whereas in this phase 3 trial comparing standard treatment consisting of systemic chemotherapy (fluorouracil-leucovorin) with or without palliative surgery versus aggressive CRS with HIPEC, the median survival was 12.6 months in the standard therapy group versus almost double (22.3 months) that in the HIPEC arm (log-rank test, $P = .032$).[20]

HIPEC therapy is not without limitations or issues. The specifics of the HIPEC administration lack uniformity, and the debate on the best method to deliver HIPEC is still open.[7] There are a wide range of inclusion and exclusion criteria, chemotherapeutic agents, temperatures, and methods of delivering the heated chemotherapy.[21] Furthermore, various classification systems have been used, which makes comparison of the different techniques, complications, and results almost impossible. Efforts at standardization of reporting are being made, but currently there are no clear data confirming benefit.[22]

Complications are more common in patients with negative outcome predictors, fairly consistent in all the reports,[11,23–27] and include diffuse abdominal region involvement, incomplete cytoreduction with limited or extensive residual disease, presence of malignant ascites, recurrent disease, or poorly differentiated chemotherapy resistant tumors. Morbidity is significantly associated with 3 clinical factors: male sex, high intra-abdominal temperature during HIPEC, and duration of the surgical procedure.[28] Irrespective of age, patients with good performance status, optimal cytoreduction, and well-differentiated tumor type are more likely to benefit from this treatment.[23] Extensive surgery (duration and number of peritonectomy procedures) and high intra-abdominal temperature represent the major risk factors for postoperative morbidity and mortality.[28]

In selected patients with primary gastric cancer and carcinomatosis, the 5-year survival of patients in whom a complete cytoreduction was possible was approximately 10%, with a median survival of 12 months.[29] Postoperative complications can be attributed to the effects of the surgical manipulation per se, the toxic effects of the heated intraoperative chemotherapy, and preexisting comorbidities. The treatment-related mortality rate for aggressive CRS and HIPEC ranges from 0 to 8%[20,28,29] and morbidity is frequent, in the range of at least 25% to 41%.[10,28,30,31]

CRITICAL ISSUES
Airway Management

In critically ill patients, tracheal intubation is considerably more difficult due to factors such as encephalopathy, respiratory dysfunction, oropharyngeal secretions, hemodynamic instability, bleeding, vomiting, and airway edema. As the number of laryngoscopic intubation attempts increase, complications such as hypoxemia, aspiration, bradycardia, and cardiac arrest increase significantly.[32]

Traditional endotracheal intubation performed via direct laryngoscopy using devices such as the Macintosh blade has been around for more than 65 years. Recent advances in indirect optical laryngoscopy are revolutionizing the technique of tracheal intubation, allowing less experienced personnel to rapidly achieve proficiency and assisting experienced operators to facilitate difficult airway management. The advantages of optical laryngoscopy include the need for less severe positioning of the head and neck, with better visualization of the vocal cords, facilitating a faster, less traumatic intubation that requires less sedation. Unlike direct laryngoscopy, whereby only the operator sees the airway, a visual display allows a supervisor to provide feedback, assistance, and assurance of proper endotracheal tube location.

It takes a first-year anesthesia resident performing direct laryngoscopy in the relatively controlled setting of the operating room about 47 tracheal intubations to achieve a 90% probability of a success.[33] This number would be expected to be higher in the ICU setting. Untrained operators, intubating noncritically ill patients with normal airways, had a success rate of 51% using direct laryngoscopy with the Macintosh blade, whereas these same operators using GlideScope optical laryngoscopy had a first-attempt success rate of more than 90%.[34]

Surgical oncology patients with head and neck masses or previous radiotherapy-induced fibrosis present particular challenges. In patients with upper airway tumors, optical laryngoscopes, when compared with direct laryngoscopy, were found to improve visualization of the vocal cords as assessed by Cormack and Lehane grades by approximately 80%.[35] Optical laryngoscopes are valuable tools for ICU airway management, and will become the new standard for tracheal intubation.

Respiratory Failure

The nature of extensive surgery involving tumor debulking, gastrointestinal anastomoses, and heated chemotherapy leads to extensive peritoneal inflammation and a systemic inflammatory response. Uncomplicated cases after CRS and HIPEC are usually extubated within 24 hours postoperatively, but complicated cases either fail extubation or remain mechanically ventilated.

The cause of respiratory failure in the postsurgical state is often noncardiogenic pulmonary edema, either subtle acute lung injury (ALI) or more severe acute respiratory distress syndrome (ARDS). The appearance of alveolar infiltrates may be subtle and overlooked on chest radiograph (CXR). Although respiratory failure is often attributed to pneumonia in postsurgical patients with fever and infiltrates on CXR, ALI is more commonly the cause of pulmonary infiltrates and is probably under-recognized, although the incidence, risk factors, and outcome have not been prospectively studied.[36] ALI is likely due to a systemic inflammatory response to tissue injury and trauma of the surgical procedure, and may also be caused by sepsis, hemorrhage, and blood transfusion, and be exacerbated by perioperative fluid resuscitation, especially in hemodynamically unstable patients.

Aspiration is another important cause of pneumonia and ALI that can occur intraoperatively, but is more common postoperatively in patients with encephalopathy and gastrointestinal dysfunction after abdominal surgery, who have had their nasogastric tube removed and have either frankly vomited or are discovered to have regurgitated when suctioned during tracheal intubation.

In patients who appear to be in the process of developing respiratory distress after CRS and HIPEC, concern for ruling out a pulmonary embolism (PE) is high because these patients are in a higher risk group for thromboembolic disease; however, the cause for respiratory failure is more often due to other causes such as aspiration or sepsis, often secondary to an intra-abdominal source. For this reason transport to radiology for a computed tomography (CT) angiogram to rule out PE should not take priority over pulmonary toilet, supplemental oxygen, endotracheal intubation if needed, and insertion of a nasogastric tube to decompress the stomach and prevent aspiration. If a patient is stabilized for transport to chest CT angiogram, it may be prudent to include an abdominal and pelvic CT so as to avoid multiple transports from the ICU that are unsafe for the critically ill patient.

Other causes of respiratory failure include encephalopathy (severe agitation unable to protect airway or breathe adequately without ventilator support), atelectasis, cardiogenic pulmonary edema, pneumothorax, empyema, and critical illness poly-myoneuropathy. Other preexisting lung diseases such as asthma, chronic obstructive lung disease, and the effects of previous radiotherapy and chemotherapy including pneumonitis, pleuritis, interstitial fibrosis, and pulmonary hemorrhage will increase respiratory complications and prolong time on the ventilator. With CRS, patients often undergo diaphragmatic stripping of tumor or diaphragm resection or reconstruction, and may develop pneumothorax, pleural effusions, or hemothorax. Chest tubes may be inserted intraoperatively, depending on the extent of surgery and entry into the pleural space or lung. These patients are more prone to extrapulmonary failure due to diaphragmatic dysfunction, depending on the extent of diaphragmatic injury and the degree of concurrent pulmonary dysfunction.

Failure to wean from the ventilator is sometimes attributed to pleural effusions, especially if they are moderate or large. The effects of thoracentesis on respiratory mechanics and gas exchange in patients receiving mechanical ventilation result in a significant decrease in work performed by the ventilator and in pleural liquid pressure, but indices of gas exchange are not significantly altered.[37] Ultrasound is useful for detecting effusions and guiding diagnostic and therapeutic thoracentesis.[38] Ultrasound may also allow rapid bedside detection of complex exudative effusions by identifying echogenic material and strands within the fluid; however, a completely anechoic effusion may be transudative or exudative, and laboratory analysis is needed to distinguish them. Unless there is an empyema that requires a standard larger bore chest tube drainage, smaller pigtail catheters placed under ultrasound guidance seem to be safe and as effective as the larger chest tubes in the drainage of postoperative pleural effusions in the ICU.[39] The smaller bore is an added benefit for oncology patients who frequently have coagulopathies.

In general, patients who are not weaned from the ventilator after 7 to 10 days of intensive care, with no impending extubation possibility, undergo tracheostomy.

Hemodynamic Instability

Many patients undergoing CRS and HIPEC have significant intravascular volume losses from the peritoneal surface as well as bleeding during the prolonged surgery, which can be massive. An inflammatory response caused by CRS and HIPEC can exacerbate the development of third-space distribution of fluids.[12] Significant losses of fluid from peritoneal inflammation continue postoperatively, and it is important to monitor the output of the intra-abdominal drains to detect bleeding as well as the quantity of ascites that should be replaced. Postoperative fluid loss of greater than 5 L per day is possible.

In addition to volume loss from the surgery, patients undergoing HIPEC also experience systemic vasodilation and a hyperdynamic state, leading to hypotension and tachycardia. If the intravascular volume is adequate after intraoperative resuscitation, the blood pressure may be normal and the stroke volume increased. Sinus tachycardia in the 100 to 140 beats per minute range is not uncommon in the immediate postoperative state, and is either related to intravascular volume depletion or is a consequence of the hyperdynamic state. If intravascular volume is adequate, the blood pressures may be relatively at baseline, and the bedside echocardiogram (ECHO) will demonstrate normal preload, and normal or hyperdynamic contractility, while dynamic indices of preload responsiveness such as the systolic blood pressure variability will be low. These patients do not usually respond nor require fluid challenges, and if there are no complications the tachycardia gradually resolves over a 24- to 72-hour period. It is still important, however, to continue adequate maintenance fluids to keep up with insensible and peritoneal fluid losses.

If preload is decreased, a trial of fluid challenges may be started and continued if there is hemodynamic improvement, for example, reduction in tachycardia, hypotension, or lactate. In patients with significant hypotension, elevated or rising postoperative lactate levels, or any respiratory or hemodynamic instability, a rapid physical examination looking for signs of pneumothorax, lung collapse, bleeding from wounds or drains, and elevated intra-abdominal pressure, concurrent with or followed by rapid bedside ultrasound, is recommended.

Ultrasound of the lung can rapidly rule out a pneumothorax (presence of lung sliding), detect atelectasis (shift of heart, echogenic lung appearance), and detect early interstitial disease such as pulmonary edema (vertical B-lines). Bedside ECHO can rapidly rule out significant pericardial effusion and assess both right and left ventricular preload and contractility.[38] If PE is suspected, a transesophageal ECHO should be performed to visualize the proximal pulmonary arteries; if a thrombus is detected, the diagnosis is immediately confirmed without the need to transport an unstable patient to CT scan. However, if negative it does not rule out a more distal embolus.

A bedside ECHO is also valuable for detection of a condition called dynamic left ventricular outflow tract obstruction (DLVOTO). DLVOTO is a reversible condition manifested by tachycardia, hypotension, and shock, which does not respond to increasing the dosage or number of inotropic agents that may be added because of worsening hypotension or, if a pulmonary artery catheter is in place, because of low cardiac output with a markedly elevated pulmonary artery occlusion pressure. In addition, pulmonary edema may develop as well as ST segment elevations on the electrocardiogram. In DLVOTO, instead of demonstrating the expected hypocontractile dilated heart, the ECHO shows severely reduced preload with end-systolic obliteration of the left ventricle, hyperdynamic contractility, and systolic anterior motion (SAM) of the anterior mitral valve leaflet. The SAM prevents the systemic ejection of blood via the aortic outflow tract. The treatment is rapid fluid challenge and withdrawal of the inotropes whereby the outflow tract obstruction disappears, hence the designation "dynamic." DLVOTO is under-recognized in the ICU,[40] and is one of the advantages of bedside ECHO over the pulmonary artery catheter for hemodynamic assessment.

It is important to ensure adequate intravascular volume resuscitation before resorting to vasopressors that may worsen organ perfusion and function, especially in the setting of nephrotoxic chemotherapeutic agents or intravenous contrast. On the other hand, in a patient with impending or developing renal failure with worsening hypoxemia due to ALI or ARDS, it may be prudent to prevent volume overload and limit volume resuscitation to what is necessary to ensure adequate perfusion. Bedside ECHO or noninvasive measures of dynamic indices of fluid responsiveness can be helpful to guide management.[41] Central venous pressure measurement is not reflective of intravascular volume, right ventricular preload, or fluid responsiveness, and it should not be used to guide fluid management.[42] Serial lactate measurements are an excellent measure of the response and adequacy of resuscitation, and decreasing lactate is associated with lower mortality.[43] If the lactate is not decreasing or increasing postoperatively, especially in the face of adequate resuscitation and cardiac function, an intra-abdominal source such as mesenteric ischemia must be entertained.

Although central or mixed venous oxygen is advocated to assess the adequacy of resuscitation, in the critically ill patient with sepsis, liver dysfunction, and arteriovenous shunting the venous oxygen level can be misleadingly normal or even elevated in the face of regional hypoperfusion, and does not correlate with cardiac output. The central or mixed venous carbon dioxide (CO_2) levels and the venous-arterial (V-A) CO_2 difference correlate with perfusion and cardiac output[44] and, if elevated (normal V-A CO_2 is <6), may indicate a low cardiac output, hypermetabolic state, or ongoing regional hypoperfusion.[45]

Bleeding and Coagulopathy

In one report of 356 CRS plus HIPEC procedures in patients with appendiceal mucinous neoplasms, the most common complications were hematological (28%).[46] Due to the extensive CRS, intra-abdominal bleeding is common and sometimes massive. HIPEC also induces fluid losses, as noted earlier. Volume resuscitation and blood transfusion can cause dilution of platelets and coagulation factors,[10] and worsen blood loss. Although the local peritoneal instillation of chemotherapy reduces systemic toxicity, mild to moderate thrombocytopenia and leukopenia secondary to mitomycin C–related myelosuppression may also occur.[26] Neutrophil counts may decrease about 5 to 10 days after HIPEC; however, granulocyte cell stimulating factor is not initiated unless the decrease is significant. Elevated International Normalized Ratio (INR) and thrombocytopenia are not treated with transfusion unless there is active bleeding or impending surgery. In such cases the target for platelet level is usually greater than 50,000 and the INR less than 2.0, depending on the procedure and preferences of the surgeon.

Close monitoring is needed for signs of ongoing or recurrent postoperative bleeding, which may manifest as respiratory distress, hemodynamic instability, brisk flow of hemorrhagic fluid or frank blood in the drains, increased abdominal distention and hypertension, bleeding from the wound, or combinations of these. Frank gastrointestinal bleeding may be detected from the nasogastric tube, ostomy, or rectum. Serial hemoglobin measurements are eventually decreased or fail to increase appropriately with transfusion but this may be delayed, especially if the bleeding is acute. Communication between the intensivist and surgeon is necessary to avoid delays in operative interventions that may be needed to identify and control the bleeding source.

The incidence of gastrointestinal bleeding due to stress-related mucosal ulceration in high-risk critically ill oncology patients in a mixed medical-surgical ICU receiving either histamine-2 receptor antagonists or proton pump inhibitor has been reported to be low.[47]

Percutaneous Venous Access

Percutaneous venous access is often more challenging in the surgical oncology patient for a variety of factors, including limited insertion site availability due to thrombosis, preexisting implanted catheters, tracheostomy site, surgical sites, open wounds, difficult anatomy due to tissue distortion from head, neck, and proximal extremity tumors, previous radiotherapy fibrosis, and increased bleeding risks due to coagulopathy.

Although the internal jugular and subclavian vein sites are preferred over the femoral vein because of probable lower thrombosis and infection risks, the final choice is dictated by the available sites that offer the safest and most rapid access. On rare occasions, usually due to extensive widespread thromboses and superior vena cava syndrome, central access may become impossible, requiring interventional radiologist insertion of percutaneous catheters into the vena cava or portal vein system.

Larger bore, limited length catheters that allow rapid infusion are preferred in critically ill patients and especially in the surgical oncology patient. Triple-lumen or quad-lumen catheters allow multiple medications to be simultaneously infused and also allow for blood sampling. With the increased incidence of venous thromboembolic disease, it is more common to encounter patients who have inferior vena cava filters, and care must be taken not to overinsert the guidewire beyond about 15 cm into the vessel to avoid entrapment of the wire in the filter.

There has been recent increased use of peripherally inserted central catheters (PICC), which can deliver medications centrally but whose peripheral insertion usually in the brachial, basilica, or cephalic upper extremity veins does not carry the risk of pneumothorax, hemithorax, or neck hematoma. The main limitation of PICCs in acutely ill patients is their small bore and long length that make the rapid infusion of fluids and blood products impossible.

Due to the aforementioned difficulties with central venous access, the incidence of mechanical complications such as pneumothorax, hemothorax, malposition, hematoma, and arterial puncture are higher in this patient population. The complication rate increases with the number of percutaneous punctures, with a rate of 54% when more than 2 punctures are required.[48] Ultrasound has been found to decrease the number of needle punctures and increase the rate of first-stick success, and decrease the time it takes to complete the procedure.[49] In addition, prescanning can help identify the most promising sites (largest veins with arteries away from the projected needle path) and eliminate those with absent or thrombosed vessels. The evidence that the subclavian site is less prone to infection is not conclusive,[50] and the advantages of vessel compressibility and easier real-time visualization under ultrasound make the internal jugular site or femoral site more attractive in the severely coagulopathic patient.

The main determinant of bleeding complications secondary to percutaneous central line insertion is not the INR, activated partial thromboplastin time, or platelet count, but the experience of the operator using proper insertion techniques.[51] One series of 76 patients with disorders of hemostasis undergoing central line insertion reported that only a single patient, with a platelet count of 6000/mL, required therapeutic blood product administration.[52] These findings indicate that the use of blood components for correction of coagulopathy before the procedure is not necessary, except in those patients who have the most severe hemostatic abnormalities.[53] The use of ultrasound can further reduce risks of bleeding complications. Therefore, the prophylactic correction of coagulation by transfusion of blood products or coagulation factors is not necessary before central venous catheter insertion.[54]

In the severely coagulopathic patient, oozing of blood at the insertion site is common. Continued bleeding requiring frequent dressing changes can occasionally be a significant problem. This problem can be alleviated or prevented by not using a scalpel before advancing the skin dilator. If this is not possible, then the smallest skin cut possible that allows dilator passage should be made. If significant oozing occurs, local hemostatic agents may be useful in reducing insertion site bleeding.

Meticulous care of the catheter sites, use of chlorhexidine, maximal sterile barrier precautions, insertion by an experienced team, avoiding routine replacement of central catheters, and using antibiotic or antiseptic impregnated short-term central venous catheters if the rate of central line associated bacteremia (CLAB) is high are all important in minimizing CLABs.[55] Use of a chlorhexidine gluconate-impregnated sponge in intravascular catheter dressings may further reduce catheter-related infections.[56]

Venous Thromboembolism

Perioperative venous thromboembolism (VTE) would be expected to be more common in patients with peritoneal carcinomatosis after CRS and HIPEC as they have significant surgical and oncologic risks of thrombus formation. PE after CRS and HIPEC has been reported in about 5% of patients.[28,57] One recent study of 60 patients after CRS and HIPEC reported that 10% had VTE as manifested by pulmonary embolism, superior mesenteric vein thrombosis, or deep vein thrombosis.[58] Only 33% of patients experienced clinical symptoms.

Surgical Complications, the Acute Abdomen, and Source Control

The most common surgical complications resulting from CRS and HIPEC are anastomotic leaks, intestinal perforation, abscesses, and intra-abdominal bleeding.[6,11,20,28] In one report of 356 CRS plus HIPEC procedures in patients with appendiceal mucinous neoplasms, gastrointestinal complications were reported in 26% and 11.1% of patients returned to the operating room.[46] Intestinal perforations may be due to inadvertent surgical injury, and patients with prior radiation exposure, chemotherapy, steroids, malnutrition, or inflammatory conditions are more prone. Intraperitoneal chemotherapy and hyperthermia leads to edema of the bowel, and perforations at the site of surgical anastomoses or distant intestinal sites may occur. Anastomotic leaks and intestinal fistulae occur in patients with a significantly higher number of peritonectomy procedures and longer operations.[28]

The increased risk of intra-abdominal contamination, even in the absence of an anastomotic leak or intestinal perforation, can manifest as peritonitis, wound infection, or the development of intra-abdominal abscesses. Residual blood or hematomas, and packing left in place to control massive intraoperative intra-abdominal bleeding are media for the growth of bacteria, which significantly increase the risk of intra-abdominal sepsis. Other important complications include prolonged ileus, bile leak, pancreatitis, abdominal wound dehiscence,[28] acalculous cholecystitis, mesenteric ischemia from low flow secondary to sepsis itself, mesenteric vein thrombosis or incarcerated bowel, and mechanical intestinal obstruction.

The most common cause of mortality in general surgical ICUs is sepsis leading to multiple organ failure, and these patients are at particularly higher risk due to the extensive CRS and HIPEC in the setting of recurrent, disseminated peritoneal cancer, previous chemotherapy, radiotherapy, surgery, long- or short-term central venous catheters, and parenteral nutrition, often coupled with preexisting medical conditions such as diabetes, chronic obstructive lung disease, coronary artery disease, peripheral vascular disease, renal insufficiency, and malnutrition.

The challenge in the critically ill surgical oncology patient is to ensure that source control is not overlooked and is rapidly identified and treated, because no matter how appropriate the antibiotics and hemodynamic support, if source control is lacking the patient will not recover. The intensivist must determine whether the source of sepsis is a medical complication, for example, a hospital acquired infection such as ventilator-associated pneumonia, aspiration, parapneumonic effusion, empyema, catheter infection, or *Clostridium difficile* colitis without toxic megacolon, or is caused by an intra-abdominal or surgical complication. This detection is often a very difficult process made even more challenging by the blunting of physiologic responses to injury and inflammation in critically ill patients who frequently have no nausea, vomiting, or abdominal pain, and only subtle nonspecific or no peritoneal signs of the classic acute abdomen. Encephalopathy, sedation, intubation, hemodynamic instability, immunosuppression from drugs or disease, advanced age, and diabetes have each been associated with "benign" abdominal examinations in the face of acute intra-abdominal crises.

The classic ICU presentation of intra-abdominal sepsis may be any one or a combination of unexplained encephalopathy, worsening gas exchange, ALI or ARDS, persistent respiratory failure/inability to tolerate a spontaneous breathing trial, labile blood pressure or the inability to tolerate diuresis, deteriorating renal function, or persistent positive fluid balance, with a soft and nontender abdomen. Leukocytosis and fever are not present in many cases and, unless decreases in white cell count and temperature are consistent with a truly improving clinical course, they should not be relied on to indicate resolving sepsis.

A careful search for sources of sepsis includes a thorough physical examination, including inspection of the oropharynx for ulcers or plaque-like lesions of herpes or thrush, of the skin and surgical wounds for signs of induration and erythema of bacterial cellulitis or necrotizing fasciitis, of catheter sites for erythema, tenderness, or discharge, and of the abdominal drains for increasing output (eg, leaks), quality (bile stained, pus, blood, foul smelling), appearance of ostomies, changes in the degree of distention, pliability to palpation, and tenderness. Standard laboratory testing includes complete blood cell count, liver and renal function tests, urine analysis, and blood cultures. In patients with ascites, if diagnostic paracentesis is performed it should be under ultrasound guidance to decrease the risk of complications in this postsurgical population.

Because the abdominal physical findings are often blunted or absent, and abdominal plain films nondiagnostic, the role of computerized axial tomography (CT scan) has assumed increasing importance in the identification of free fluid collections, peritoneal or visceral abscesses, hematomas, ileus, sites of gastrointestinal obstruction, free air, gas in the intestinal wall (pneumatosis intestinalis) or portal vein, and mesenteric vascular thrombus. Diagnostic bedside ultrasound, although not as sensitive as CT scan, is an option in a patient too unstable for transport to radiology. Often the source of sepsis is not clear, CT scans are negative or equivocal, and a decision must be made about surgical reexploration. If the patient is deteriorating or in a plateau state failing to improve with aggressive intensive care, the intensivist needs to maintain a high index of suspicion for intra-abdominal sepsis and an open channel of communication with the surgeon to determine whether reexploration is indicated.

Nutrition

Patients undergoing CRS and HIPEC are usually malnourished before surgery due to the catabolic effect of the tumor itself and complications of bowel obstruction. The enteral route is preferred to preserve gut integrity and to simplify glycemic management[59]; however, peritoneal carcinomatosis and gastrointestinal surgery often delay enteral feeding due to postoperative ileus, sepsis, waiting for gastrointestinal anastomoses to heal, and intra-abdominal complications such as anastomotic leaks, obstruction, and fistulas. If prolonged delays in oral intake are anticipated, an enteric feeding tube placed at the time of surgery is valuable. Most critically ill patients require between 20 and 30 kcal/kg ideal body weight to meet their daily energy expenditure. Under conditions of severe stress, requirements may approach 30 kcal/kg ideal body weight.[60] Because these patients are already malnourished, if delays in enteral feeding of greater than 2 to 3 days postoperatively are anticipated, early postoperative parenteral nutrition is initiated and can also be helpful in maintaining electrolyte and acid-base balance.

SUMMARY

As life expectancy increases and advances in cancer treatment more often convert deadly conditions into more chronic diseases, the surgical intensivist can expect to be faced with greater numbers of oncology patients undergoing aggressive surgical treatments for curative intent, prolonging survival, or primary palliation by alleviating obstruction, infection, bleeding, or pain. CRS and HIPEC are a paradigm for the emerging field of multimodal aggressive oncological surgery. A discussion of the CRS/HIPEC technique is followed by a discussion of postoperative complications and critical care issues. The most common surgical complications resulting from CRS and HIPEC are anastomotic leaks, intestinal perforation, abscesses, and intra-abdominal bleeding. The most common cause of mortality is sepsis leading to multiple organ failure, and these patients are at particularly higher risk due to the extensive CRS and HIPEC. The intensivist must be vigilant to ensure that source control is not overlooked. This process is a very difficult one, made even more challenging by the blunting of physiologic responses and the frequent absence of the classic acute abdomen.

REFERENCES

1. Jemal A, Siegel R, Ward E, et al. Cancer statistics, 2009. CA Cancer J Clin 2009; 59:225–49.
2. Darmon M, Azoulay E. Critical care management of cancer patients: cause for optimism and need for objectivity. Curr Opin Oncol 2009;21:318–26.
3. Soares M, Salluh JI, Torres VB, et al. Short- and long-term outcomes of critically ill patients with cancer and prolonged ICU length of stay. Chest 2008;134:520–6.
4. Sugarbaker PH. Peritonectomy procedures. Ann Surg 1995;221:29–42.
5. De Roover A, Detroz B, Detry O, et al. Adjuvant hyperthermic intraperitoneal peroperative chemotherapy (HIPEC) associated with curative surgery for locally advanced gastric carcinoma. An initial experience. Acta Chir Belg 2006;106: 297–301.
6. Jaehne J. Cytoreductive procedures-strategies to reduce postoperative morbidity and management of surgical complications with special emphasis on anastomotic leaks. J Surg Oncol 2009;100:302–5.
7. Esquivel J. Technology of hyperthermic intraperitoneal chemotherapy in the United States, Europe, China, Japan, and Korea. Cancer J 2009;15:249–54.
8. Esquivel J, Angulo F, Bland RK, et al. Hemodynamic and cardiac function parameters during heated intraoperative intraperitoneal chemotherapy using the open "coliseum technique". Ann Surg Oncol 2000;7:296–300.
9. Foltz P, Wavrin C, Sticca R. Heated intraoperative intraperitoneal chemotherapy—the challenges of bringing chemotherapy into surgery. AORN J 2004;80:1055–63 [quiz 65–8].
10. Schmidt C, Creutzenberg M, Piso P, et al. Peri-operative anaesthetic management of cytoreductive surgery with hyperthermic intraperitoneal chemotherapy. Anaesthesia 2008;63:389–95.

11. Fujimura T, Yonemura Y, Nakagawara H, et al. Subtotal peritonectomy with che-mohyperthermic peritoneal perfusion for peritonitis carcinomatosa in gastrointes-tinal cancer. Oncol Rep 2000;7:809–14.
12. Schmidt C, Moritz S, Rath S, et al. Perioperative management of patients with cy-toreductive surgery for peritoneal carcinomatosis. J Surg Oncol 2009;100: 297–301.
13. Pavlov MJ, Kovacevic PA, Ceranic MS, et al. Cytoreductive surgery and modified heated intraoperative intraperitoneal chemotherapy (HIPEC) for advanced and recurrent ovarian cancer—12-year single center experience. Eur J Surg Oncol 2009;35:1186–91.
14. Spratt JS, Adcock RA, Muskovin M, et al. Clinical delivery system for intraperito-neal hyperthermic chemotherapy. Cancer Res 1980;40:256–60.
15. Katayama K, Yamaguchi A, Murakami M, et al. Chemo-hyperthermic peritoneal perfusion (CHPP) for appendiceal pseudomyxoma peritonei. Int J Clin Oncol 2009;14:120–4.
16. Hesdorffer ME, Chabot JA, Keohan ML, et al. Combined resection, intraperitoneal chemotherapy, and whole abdominal radiation for the treatment of malignant peri-toneal mesothelioma. Am J Clin Oncol 2008;31:49–54.
17. Helm CW, Toler CR, Martin RS 3rd, et al. Cytoreduction and intraperitoneal heated chemotherapy for the treatment of endometrial carcinoma recurrent within the peritoneal cavity. Int J Gynecol Cancer 2007;17:204–9.
18. Piso P, Glockzin G, von Breitenbuch P, et al. Quality of life after cytoreductive surgery and hyperthermic intraperitoneal chemotherapy for peritoneal surface malignancies. J Surg Oncol 2009;100:317–20.
19. Chu DZ, Lang NP, Thompson C, et al. Peritoneal carcinomatosis in nongynecologic malignancy. A prospective study of prognostic factors. Cancer 1989;63:364–7.
20. Verwaal VJ, van Ruth S, de Bree E, et al. Randomized trial of cytoreduction and hyperthermic intraperitoneal chemotherapy versus systemic chemotherapy and palliative surgery in patients with peritoneal carcinomatosis of colorectal cancer. J Clin Oncol 2003;21:3737–43.
21. Esquivel J, Elias D, Baratti D, et al. Consensus statement on the loco regional treatment of colorectal cancer with peritoneal dissemination. J Surg Oncol 2008;98:263–7.
22. Younan R, Kusamura S, Baratti D, et al. Morbidity, toxicity, and mortality classifi-cation systems in the local regional treatment of peritoneal surface malignancy. J Surg Oncol 2008;98:253–7.
23. van Leeuwen BL, Graf W, Pahlman L, et al. Swedish experience with peritonec-tomy and HIPEC. HIPEC in peritoneal carcinomatosis. Ann Surg Oncol 2008; 15:745–53.
24. Bijelic L, Jonson A, Sugarbaker PH. Systematic review of cytoreductive surgery and heated intraoperative intraperitoneal chemotherapy for treatment of perito-neal carcinomatosis in primary and recurrent ovarian cancer. Ann Oncol 2007; 18:1943–50.
25. Shehata M, Chu F, Saunders V, et al. Peritoneal carcinomatosis from colorectal cancer and small bowel cancer treated with peritonectomy. ANZ J Surg 2006; 76:467–71.
26. Loggie BW, Fleming RA, McQuellon RP, et al. Cytoreductive surgery with intraper-itoneal hyperthermic chemotherapy for disseminated peritoneal cancer of gastro-intestinal origin. Am Surg 2000;66:561–8.
27. Sugarbaker PH, Chang D. Results of treatment of 385 patients with peritoneal surface spread of appendiceal malignancy. Ann Surg Oncol 1999;6:727–31.

28. Jacquet P, Stephens AD, Averbach AM, et al. Analysis of morbidity and mortality in 60 patients with peritoneal carcinomatosis treated by cytoreductive surgery and heated intraoperative intraperitoneal chemotherapy. Cancer 1996;77:2622–9.

29. Sugarbaker PH, Yonemura Y. Clinical pathway for the management of resectable gastric cancer with peritoneal seeding: best palliation with a ray of hope for cure. Oncology 2000;58:96–107.

30. Witkamp AJ, de Bree E, Van Goethem R, et al. Rationale and techniques of intra-operative hyperthermic intraperitoneal chemotherapy. Cancer Treat Rev 2001;27:365–74.

31. Glockzin G, Schlitt HJ, Piso P. Peritoneal carcinomatosis: patients selection, peri-operative complications and quality of life related to cytoreductive surgery and hyperthermic intraperitoneal chemotherapy. World J Surg Oncol 2009;7:5.

32. Mort TC. Emergency tracheal intubation: complications associated with repeated laryngoscopic attempts. Anesth Analg 2004;99:607–13.

33. Mulcaster JT, Mills J, Hung OR, et al. Laryngoscopic intubation: learning and performance. Anesthesiology 2003;98:23–7.

34. Nouruzi-Sedeh P, Schumann M, Groeben H. Laryngoscopy via Macintosh blade versus GlideScope: success rate and time for endotracheal intubation in untrained medical personnel. Anesthesiology 2009;110:32–7.

35. Lange M, Frommer M, Redel A, et al. Comparison of the Glidescope and Airtraq optical laryngoscopes in patients undergoing direct microlaryngoscopy. Anaes-thesia 2009;64:323–8.

36. Fernandez-Perez ER, Sprung J, Afessa B, et al. Intraoperative ventilator settings and acute lung injury after elective surgery: a nested case control study. Thorax 2009;64:121–7.

37. Doelken P, Abreu R, Sahn SA, et al. Effect of thoracentesis on respiratory mechanics and gas exchange in the patient receiving mechanical ventilation. Chest 2006;130:1354–61.

38. Mayo PH, Beaulieu Y, Doelken P, et al. American College of Chest Physicians/La Societe de Reanimation de Langue Francaise statement on competence in crit-ical care ultrasonography. Chest 2009;135:1050–60.

39. Liang SJ, Tu CY, Chen HJ, et al. Application of ultrasound-guided pigtail catheter for drainage of pleural effusions in the ICU. Intensive Care Med 2009;35:350–4.

40. Chockalingam A, Dorairajan S, Bhalla M, et al. Unexplained hypotension: the spectrum of dynamic left ventricular outflow tract obstruction in critical care settings. Crit Care Med 2009;37:729–34.

41. Marik PE. Techniques for assessment of intervascular volume in critically ill patients. J Intensive Care Med 2009;24:329–37.

42. Marik PE, Baram M, Vahid B. Does central venous pressure predict fluid respon-siveness? A systematic review of the literature and the tale of seven mares. Chest 2008;134:172–8.

43. Marecaux G, Pinsky MR, Dupont E, et al. Blood lactate levels are better prog-nostic indicators than TNF and IL-6 levels in patients with septic shock. Intensive Care Med 1996;22:404–8.

44. Cuschieri J, Rivers EP, Donnino MW, et al. Central venous-arterial carbon dioxide difference as an indicator of cardiac index. Intensive Care Med 2005;31:818–22.

45. van Beest PA, Hofstra JJ, Schultz MJ, et al. The incidence of low venous oxygen saturation on admission to the intensive care unit: a multi-center observational study in The Netherlands. Crit Care 2008;12:R33.

46. Sugarbaker PH, Alderman R, Edwards G, et al. Prospective morbidity and mortality assessment of cytoreductive surgery plus perioperative intraperitoneal

chemotherapy to treat peritoneal dissemination of appendiceal mucinous malignancy. Ann Surg Oncol 2006;13:635–44.

47. Bruno JJ, Canada TW, Wakefield CD, et al. Stress-related mucosal bleeding in critically ill oncology patients. J Oncol Pharm Pract 2009;15:9–16.

48. Eisen LA, Narasimhan M, Berger JS, et al. Mechanical complications of central venous catheters. J Intensive Care Med 2006;21:40–6.

49. Denys BG, Uretsky BF, Reddy PS. Ultrasound-assisted cannulation of the internal jugular vein. A prospective comparison to the external landmark-guided technique. Circulation 1993;87:1557–62.

50. Gowardman JR, Robertson IK, Parkes S, et al. Influence of insertion site on central venous catheter colonization and bloodstream infection rates. Intensive Care Med 2008;34:1038–45.

51. Foster PF, Moore LR, Sankary HN, et al. Central venous catheterization in patients with coagulopathy. Arch Surg 1992;127:273–5.

52. Doerfler ME, Kaufman B, Goldenberg AS. Central venous catheter placement in patients with disorders of hemostasis. Chest 1996;110:185–8.

53. DeLoughery TG, Liebler JM, Simonds V, et al. Invasive line placement in critically ill patients: do hemostatic defects matter? Transfusion 1996;36:827–31.

54. Weigand K, Encke J, Meyer FJ, et al. Low levels of prothrombin time (INR) and platelets do not increase the risk of significant bleeding when placing central venous catheters. Med Klin (Munich) 2009;104:331–5.

55. O'Grady NP, Alexander M, Dellinger EP, et al. Guidelines for the prevention of intravascular catheter-related infections. Centers for Disease Control and Prevention. MMWR Recomm Rep 2002;51:1–29.

56. Timsit JF, Schwebel C, Bouadma L, et al. Chlorhexidine-impregnated sponges and less frequent dressing changes for prevention of catheter-related infections in critically ill adults: a randomized controlled trial. JAMA 2009;301:1231–41.

57. Helm CW, Randall-Whitis L, Martin RS 3rd, et al. Hyperthermic intraperitoneal chemotherapy in conjunction with surgery for the treatment of recurrent ovarian carcinoma. Gynecol Oncol 2007;105:90–6.

58. Lanuke K, Mack LA, Temple WJ. A prospective evaluation of venous thromboembolism in patients undergoing cytoreductive surgery and hyperthermic intraperitoneal chemotherapy. Can J Surg 2009;52:18–22.

59. August DA, Huhmann MB. American Society for Parenteral and Enteral Nutrition A.S.P.E.N. clinical guidelines: nutrition support therapy during adult anticancer treatment and in hematopoietic cell transplantation. JPEN J Parenter Enteral Nutr 2009;33:472–500.

60. Braga M, Ljungqvist O, Soeters P, et al. ESPEN guidelines on parenteral nutrition: surgery. Clin Nutr 2009;28:378–86.

Hematological Issues in Critically Ill Patients with Cancer

Karen S. Carlson, MD, PhD[a], Maria T. DeSancho, MD, MSc[b],*

KEYWORDS

• Cancer • Thrombosis • Hemostasis • Critical illness

Patients with solid and hematologic malignancies including patients undergoing hematopoietic stem cell transplantation are at risk for bleeding and thrombotic complications. The diagnosis of cancer is often made in the context of a new bleeding diathesis or an unprovoked venous thromboembolism. Patients presenting with major bleeding or thrombotic complications usually require admission to an intensive care unit (ICU). These complications can also be the life-ending event in a cancer patient's clinical course, making their diagnosis and management even more important for the intensivist. Given the significant advances in the diagnosis and treatment of almost all types of cancers in recent years, the intensivist is likely to encounter an ever-increasing number of cancer patients in the ICU setting with these complications.

Abnormal hemostasis can occur as a consequence of both the pathology and treatment of cancer. Because cancer can have multiple effects on hemostatic equilibrium, treatment of these complications can be more complex than in the general population. This article reviews the physiology of coagulation and fibrinolysis, with special attention to those aspects that are most frequently altered in the setting of malignancy. The pathophysiology of bleeding and thrombotic complications specific to critically ill cancer patients are then detailed, and the diagnostic and therapeutic strategies are discussed. Special emphasis is placed on new cancer medications that have an effect on hemostasis, and on novel clotting and anticoagulant agents that are available to the intensivist for the management of these patients.

PHYSIOLOGY OF NORMAL HEMOSTASIS

Hemostasis is the process that maintains the integrity of a closed, high-pressure circulatory system after vascular damage.[1] Hemostasis is a balanced series of protease

[a] Department of Medicine, New York Presbyterian Hospital of Weill Cornell Medical College, 525 E 68th Street, Payson 3, New York, NY 10065, USA
[b] Department of Medicine, New York Presbyterian Hospital of Weill Cornell Medical College, 525 E 68th Street, Starr Building, 3rd Floor, Room 341, New York, NY 10065, USA
* Corresponding author.
E-mail address: mtd2002@med.cornell.edu (M.T. DeSancho).

Crit Care Clin 26 (2010) 107–132
doi:10.1016/j.ccc.2009.09.006
0749-0704/09/$ – see front matter © 2010 Elsevier Inc. All rights reserved.
criticalcare.theclinics.com

cascades and cellular interactions that ultimately control initiation of thrombin formation, propagation of thrombin activation, activation of endogenous anticoagulants, and fibrinolysis (**Fig. 1**).[1]

Platelet Thrombus Formation

Under physiologic circumstances, thrombus formation is initiated by injury to a vessel wall and the inner endothelial lining, exposing the subendothelial extracellular matrix. This process results in exposure of collagen, fibronectin, von Willebrand factor, and tissue factor (TF) to circulating platelets.[2–5] These proteins bind platelet receptors, localizing platelets to the site of injury, and initiating a cascade of events resulting in

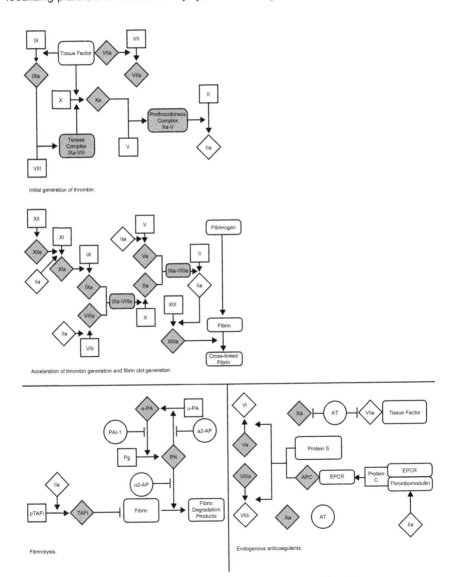

Fig. 1. Physiology of normal coagulation. Pg, plasminogen; PN, plasmin.

platelet activation. The end result is assembly and activation of the platelet receptor glycoprotein IIb-IIIa (GPIIb-IIIa) on the platelet cell membrane.[2,6] GP IIb-IIIa is able to bind both von Willebrand factor and fibrinogen, resulting in irreversible platelet adhesion and aggregation and ultimately in rapid formation of a platelet plug at the site of vessel wall injury.[2,5,6] Exposed TF initiates the generation of thrombin, which not only converts fibrinogen to fibrin but also activates platelets.

Fibrin Generation

Blood coagulation is initiated by TF, culminating in the generation of thrombin and fibrin. TF, a membrane protein expressed on fibroblasts and pericytes in the adventitia and medial smooth muscle cells of the vessel wall, binds activated factor VII (VIIa). TF-VIIa activates factors X and IX. Activated factor IX (factor IXa) then combines with factor VIIIa, which is activated from factor VIII by thrombin, to form a second pathway to activate factor X. Factor Xa complexes with factor Va and prothrombin to form the prothrombinase complex, which then cleaves prothrombin (factor II) to form thrombin (factor IIa), the key enzyme in hemostasis. Fibrin is ultimately generated by cleavage of fibrinogen by thrombin to form fibrin monomers, which then polymerize to form the fibrin clot. This polymer is covalently cross-linked by factor XIIIa (generated from factor XIII by thrombin) to form a chemically stable clot. Thrombin also feeds back to activate cofactors V, VIII, and XI, further amplifying the coagulation system (see **Fig. 1**).

Natural Anticoagulant Mechanisms

Fibrin deposition is limited by an endogenous anticoagulant system. Antithrombin (AT) is a plasma protein member of the serpins (serine protease inhibitors) family that inhibits the activities of all of the activated protease enzymes. Protein C is a vitamin K-dependent protein that proteolyses factor Va and factor VIIIa to inactive fragments. Protein C binds to an endothelial cell protein C receptor (EPCR)[7] and is activated by thrombin bound to thrombomodulin, another endothelial cell membrane-based protein, in a reaction that is modulated by a cofactor, protein S. TF pathway inhibitor is a plasma protein that forms a quaternary complex with tissue factor, factor VIIa, and factor Xa, thereby inhibiting the extrinsic coagulation pathway (see **Fig. 1**).[8]

Fibrinolysis

Fibrinolysis is the protease cascade that leads to breakdown of a fibrin clot (see **Fig. 1**). The 2 physiologic initiating enzymes are tissue-type and urokinase plasminogen activator (t-PA and u-PA, respectively). Both proteases are capable of activating plasminogen to the active protease, plasmin, which then degrades fibrin into fibrin degradation products (FDP).

t-PA and plasminogen bind to specific lysine residues within fibrin, and to annexin II on the surface of endothelial cells, monocytes, myeloid lineage cells, and smooth muscle cells. Fibrin binding not only localizes both proteases to the clot but also increases the catalytic efficiency of the single-chain active zymogen form of t-PA. There is convincing evidence that the initiating event for t-PA–mediated fibrinolysis is in fact generation of the fibrin clot itself (see **Fig. 1**).

In contrast, urokinase is not incorporated into a developing fibrin clot, but is instead localized to the surface of endothelial cells, monocytes, fibroblasts, and many tumor cells via binding to the urokinase-type plasminogen activator receptor (uPAR). As with t-PA, fibrin interactions, binding of single-chain u-PA to uPAR, results in a significant increase in urokinase catalytic efficiency and thus potential for cell surface plasmin generation.[9]

Fibrinolysis is negatively regulated by the serine protease inhibitors (serpins) plasminogen activator inhibitor-1 (PAI-1), PAI-2, and α2-antiplasmin, and by thrombin-activatable fibrinolysis inhibitor (TAFI).[10] When excess plasmin in the blood has saturated all the available α2-antiplasmin, a slower acting inhibitor, α2-macroglobulin, acts as a second-line defense.[11]

RELATIONSHIP OF THE COAGULATION SYSTEM AND CANCER

The relationship between the coagulation system and malignancy was first recognized by Bouillaud in 1823 when he described 3 patients with malignancy and fibrin clots,[12] and later by Trousseau in 1865 when he further described the link between cancer and thrombosis.[13,14] In 1878, Billroth demonstrated cancer cells within a thrombus and theorized that tumor cells spread by thromboembolism.[15] Cancer can affect all 3 aspects of Virchow's triad, namely changes in blood flow or stasis by physical occlusion of vessels by tumor mass or by increased intravascular cell mass, alteration of the normal hemostatic balance toward a hypercoagulable state, and direct injury to blood vessel endothelium.[16]

Several procoagulant molecules are specifically upregulated in cancer, including TF and cancer procoagulant (CP). TF expression is closely regulated, and present on the surface of endothelium and monocytes or macrophages only with vessel injury. However, cancer produces a proinflammatory state that triggers release of cytokines such as tumor necrosis factor-α (TNF-α) and interleukin-1β (IL-1β) that upregulate TF expression in these cell types.[16] CP is a procoagulant vitamin-K independent molecule thought to be specifically expressed by cancer cells, capable of direct factor X activation.[17,18] In addition to the upregulation of procoagulant molecules, TNF-α and IL-1β also downregulate thrombomodulin,[19] therefore decreasing activation of protein C, and thus the endogenous anticoagulant system, and they also upregulate PAI-1 expression,[20] which decreases effective fibrinolysis.

The propensity toward venous thromboembolism (VTE) in cancer patients is startling. Correcting for all other risk factors, cancer patients have an approximately six- to sevenfold higher risk of VTE than their cancer-free counterparts,[14,21,22] and 1 in 7 cancer patients who dies in the hospital will die from a pulmonary embolism.[14,23] Furthermore, an unprovoked VTE may be a herald sign of malignancy. Recent evidence suggests that patients with splanchnic venous thromboembolism should be tested for JAK2V617F mutation as an early screen for Ph-myeloproliferative disease.[24] A recent meta-analysis indicated that extensive workup for malignancy including abdominal and pelvic imaging may be warranted in cases of otherwise unprovoked VTE.[25] Finally, several reports suggest that prolonged treatment with warfarin may reduce the incidence of certain cancers.[26,27]

Pathophysiology and Management of Bleeding and Thrombosis in Cancer

Changes in hemostasis often occur with cancer patients, and can be catastrophic, which may result in their admission to the ICU. The mechanisms by which bleeding and thrombosis occur are related both to the effects of tumors on normal organ systems, as a direct effect of altered protein expression by malignant cells, and to the cancer treatment including surgery, chemotherapy, antiangiogenic agents, radiotherapy, and hormonal therapy (**Box 1**).[28]

Bleeding complications

Bleeding in the cancer patient may present as a localized bleeding, mainly as a direct result of tumor invasion to blood vessels, or as a generalized bleeding diathesis. The latter is usually due to severe thrombocytopenia, thrombocytopathies, coagulation

---

Box 1
Hemostatic abnormalities in patients with cancer

Platelet abnormalities

Quantitative—thrombocytopenia, thrombocytosis

Qualitative—thrombocytopathies, acquired von Willebrand syndrome, uremia

Increase in coagulation factors and coagulation activation markers

Factors V, VIII, IX, XI, fibrinogen

Fibrinogen/fibrin degradation products, D-dimer

Prothrombin fragment 1 + 2

Elevated thrombin-antithrombin complexes (TAT)

Altered fibrinolysis

Increased secretion of plasminogen activators

Decreased levels of plasminogen activator inhibitors

Overexpression of annexin II in APL

Decreased hepatic synthesis of anticoagulant proteins

Antithrombin

Protein C

Protein S

---

factor consumption or deficiencies, hyperfibrinolysis, or a combination of all the mentioned factors. Proper management of bleeding in the critically ill patient with cancer depends on the underlying disorder responsible for the bleeding. This article focuses on disorders that can lead to clinically significant or major bleeding in the cancer patient admitted to the ICU.

Thrombocytopenia Thrombocytopenia is the most frequently noted hemostatic disorder in patients with cancer, occurring in approximately 10% of cases before ever receiving chemotherapy.[29] In the critical care setting, thrombocytopenia can be the underlying cause for a life-threatening hemorrhage, and can be the reason for delay of administration of therapy. Thrombocytopenia is best understood and treated by consideration of the underlying mechanisms, including (1) decreased platelet production, (2) increased platelet destruction or consumption, and (3) splenic sequestration (**Box 2**).[28,30]

To differentiate between these 3 mechanisms of thrombocytopenia, it is important to obtain a detailed history of a patient's medical history including the time course of development of thrombocytopenia, current medications, presence and type of associated bleeding, and concurrent medical issues. The peripheral smear is of critical importance, as it will facilitate verification of the extent of thrombocytopenia and assist with differentiation between the multiple causes of a low platelet count (**Fig. 2**). For instance, a spurious low platelet count can be seen with automatic cytometers when there is platelet clumping, platelet satellitism, or platelets of unusual shape or size. Detection of schistocytes or microspherocytes will suggest a microangiopathic process. In cases where there is clinically significant bleeding, it is more likely that thrombocytopenia is a result of impaired platelet production rather than immune mediated peripheral destruction of platelets.[31]

Box 2
Differential diagnosis of thrombocytopenia in patients with cancer

Decreased platelet production

Metastasis to bone marrow

Acute and chronic leukemias

Lymphomas

Plasma cell dyscrasias

Cytotoxic chemotherapy

Radiation therapy

Platelet destruction

Medications

Immune mediated

Bacterial sepsis

Viral, fungal, and protozoal infections

Thrombotic thrombocytopenic purpura/hemolytic uremic syndrome

Splenic sequestration

Myeloproliferative disorders

Lymphomas

Chronic lymphocytic leukemias

Combination of these mechanisms

Decreased platelet production Impaired thrombopoiesis is reliant on hematopoietic stem cell (HSC) differentiation into megakaryocytes under the regulation of thrombopoietin (TPO) acting on the Mpl receptor in conjunction with interleukin (IL)-6, IL-2, and IL-11.[32,33] As HSCs differentiate into myeloid progenitor cells and eventually to megakaryocytes, they migrate from the bone marrow stem cell compartment to the marrow sinusoids where specific stromal cells produce stromal derived factor-1α (SDF-1α) and fibroblast growth factor-4 (FGF-4),[34] which are critical for platelet production. Any process such as marrow infiltration with malignant cells or chemotherapy that prevents normal maturation of HSCs to mature megakaryocytes, either by altering the bone marrow stroma or preventing precursor cell migration, can alter platelet production. Thrombocytopenia due to decreased platelet production is most

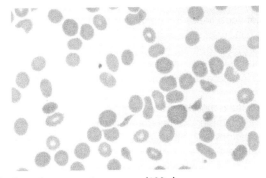

Fig. 2. Thrombotic thrombocytopenic purpura (100×).

commonly seen with hematological malignancies. However, bone marrow infiltration from solid tumors such as breast, prostate, and small cell lung cancers also occurs.

Platelet destruction and splenic sequestration Increased peripheral destruction of platelets may be drug-induced or sepsis-mediated, and also occurs within the context of disseminated intravascular coagulation (DIC) and thrombocytopenic purpura/ hemolytic uremic syndrome (TTP/HUS).[31] Thrombocytopenia secondary to splenic sequestration is usually observed with myeloproliferative disorders, and less commonly with lymphomas and chronic lymphocytic leukemia (CLL). Clinically evident bleeding episodes are more likely to occur when thrombocytopenia is caused by diminished production of megakaryocytes rather than by immune destruction.

The most common clinical manifestation of thrombocytopenia is mucocutaneous bleeding, which can occur in the form of petechiae, ecchymoses, epistaxis, oral, gastrointestinal, or genitourinary bleeding. Spontaneous bleeding usually does not occur unless the platelet count is less than $10,000/mm^3$. However, in the presence of sepsis, uremia, trauma, or surgery, bleeding complications with a higher platelet count may occur.

ACUTE MANAGEMENT OF THROMBOCYTOPENIA

The treatment of bleeding associated with thrombocytopenia in the cancer patient is often managed empirically, even when a specifically defined cause cannot be identified. Prophylactic transfusion of platelets is not indicated in patients who are asymptomatic for bleeding unless the platelet count is less than $5000/mm^3$. However, in cancer patients undergoing chemotherapy and those with leukemia, prophylactic platelet transfusions are generally beneficial in decreasing the risk of bleeding when the platelet count is less than $10,000/mm^3$. For cancer patients undergoing major surgery or invasive procedures such as central venous catheterization, bronchial or endoscopic biopsy, lumbar puncture, thoracentesis, thoracostomy tube placement, and abdominal paracentesis, it is generally recommended that platelet transfusions should be administered in thrombocytopenic patients to a target level of greater than $50,000/mm^3$ (see **Box 2**).[35] For minor invasive procedures such as arterial puncture or cannulation, prophylactic transfusion is not necessary if the platelet count is at least $20,000/mm^3$ and local pressure is applied at the puncture site until hemostasis is achieved. Platelet transfusions are usually indicated in thrombocytopenic patients to keep the platelet count greater than $50,000/mm^3$ when evidence of microscopic or gross bleeding is detected, as manifested by either occult blood on stool guaiac tests and mucocutaneous bleeding. The risk of central nervous system bleeding is generally low and bleeding depends on several factors such as underlying causes of thrombocytopenia, coagulation abnormalities, impaired renal or hepatic function, severe sepsis, trauma, and the use of mechanical ventilation. In the event of an intracerebral bleed, a platelet count greater than $100,000/\mu l$ is advised (**Table 1**).[36,37] Comparative studies have shown that platelets derived from single or random donors produce similar posttransfusion increments, hemostatic benefits, and side effects.[35] If a platelet transfusion fails to adequately control bleeding or increase the measured platelet count as anticipated, there are several factors to be considered, including (1) continued bleeding or platelet consumption, (2) alloimmunization, and (3) hypersplenism. In addition to consideration of the clinical scenario, it is helpful to measure platelet count 1 hour and 24 hours following transfusion. If the platelet count increases at 1 hour but is not maintained at 24 hours after transfusion, ongoing bleeding or a platelet consumptive process such as DIC or sepsis is most likely the cause. However, if the

Table 1 Critical platelet counts and recommendations for transfusion in cancer patients	
Platelet count threshold	
Mucocutaneous or gastrointestinal bleeding	>50,000
Leukemias	
Preinduction chemotherapy	>20,000
Acute promyelocytic leukemia	>5,000 to 10,000
Prophylaxis	
Asymptomatic	>5,000
Major surgery	>50,000
Invasive procedures	
Major	>50,000
Minor	>20,000

These recommendations are intended to serve as general guidelines. Actual treatment will vary depending on specific circumstances.

platelet count fails to increase at 1 hour, hypersplenism and alloimmunization are more likely contributing factors. If platelet refractoriness is on the working differential, platelet antibody testing should be performed to look for human leukocyte antigen (HLA) antibodies and appropriate cross-matched platelets obtained.[37]

THROMBOCYTOPATHIES

Changes in platelet function can also occur in the setting of malignancy, including development of an acquired von Willebrand syndrome, acquired factor VIII deficiency, uremic platelets, and other qualitative platelet defects seen in myeloproliferative disorders such as essential thrombocythemia and polycythemia vera where marked thrombocytosis can occur.

Acquired von Willebrand Syndrome

Several types of cancer have been reported in association with acquired von Willebrand syndrome (aVWS). Among the lymphoproliferative disorders, monoclonal gammopathy of undetermined significance (MGUS) is the condition most frequently associated with aVWS. MGUS can also be associated with multiple myeloma, Waldenstrom macroglobulinemia, CLL, hairy cell leukemia, and non-Hodgkin lymphoma. Among the myeloproliferative disorders, essential thrombocythemia is the most common, with polycythemia vera and chronic myeloid leukemia being less frequent. Solid tumors including Wilms tumors and carcinomas have also been associated with aVWS.[38–40]

The clinical manifestations of aVWS are similar to those seen in patients with the hereditary form of the disease, except for the notable absence of a family history or lifelong personal history for bleeding. Spontaneous mucocutaneous and gastrointestinal bleeding may be present; postsurgical bleeding may also occur. Laboratory screening tests generally reveal a prolonged activated partial thromboplastin time (aPTT) and a normal to borderline prolonged bleeding time. Plasma vWF antigen, vWF ristocetin cofactor activity, ristocetin-induced platelet aggregation, and vWF collagen binding activity are generally decreased. Laboratory tests usually fail to demonstrate inhibitory activity against vWF or factor VIII. Treatment is directed to the underlying malignancy and supportive measures including corticosteroids, deamino-8-D-arginine vasopressin (desmopressin acetate [DDAVP]), factor VIII/vWF concentrate, and intravenous immunoglobulin (IVIg).[38–40] Recombinant factor VII (rFVIIa, NovoSeven) has also been used.[41]

Acquired Factor VIII Inhibitors

Autoantibodies to factor VIII can develop in patients with lymphoproliferative and myeloproliferative[42] disorders, plasma cell dyscrasias, and solid tumors. The most common presentation is bleeding into the skin or muscles in patients with no previous history of bleeding diathesis. Most patients present with severe bleeding; life-threatening hemorrhage is more commonly seen in the first several weeks of presentation but can occur at any time if treatment is not initiated.[38–40] The hallmark laboratory finding is a prolongation of the aPTT in the presence of a normal prothrombin time (PT). Plasma mixing studies demonstrate an aPTT that remains prolonged after incubation at 37°C for 1 to 2 hours. Contamination of the blood sample with heparin, which frequently is the inadvertent result of instillation for maintaining vascular access line patency, may artifactually prolong the aPTT and affect the mixing tests. Heparin that has entered the sample may be removed with the enzyme reptilase or resin absorption, after which the plasma may be retested. A prolonged thrombin time in the presence of a normal reptilase time confirms the suspicion of heparin contamination. After a mixing study confirms the presence of an inhibitor and other nonspecific inhibitors have been ruled out, the factor VIII activity should be measured. If the factor VIII activity is low, the titer of the factor VIII antibody should be ascertained. The strength of an inhibitor can quantified by using the Bethesda assay, which measures residual factor VIII activity after incubation of normal plasma with serial dilutions of patient plasma for 2 hours at 37°C. The inhibitor titer in Bethesda units (BU) represents the reciprocal of the dilution of the patient's plasma that leads to 50% inhibition in the assay described. The goals in the treatment of acquired factor VIII inhibitors in patients with cancer are twofold: (1) management of the acute bleeding and (2) elimination of the autoantibody against factor VIII. The acute bleeding can be managed with desmopressin acetate if there is a low inhibitor titer (<5 BU) or with human or porcine factor VIII. Factor VIII bypassing agents such as recombinant human factor VIIa, or activated prothrombin complex concentrate are used in case of moderate- to high-titer inhibitor (>5 BU). Immunosuppressive therapy such as corticosteroids, cyclophosphamide, vincristine, cyclosporine, and intravenous immunoglobulin (IVIg) may be used in addition to the treatment of the underlying cancer. Rituximab should be considered in patients who are resistant to first-line therapy or cannot tolerate standard immunosuppressive therapy. It has been proposed that rituximab should be included as first-line therapy in combination with prednisone for patients with an inhibitor titer greater than 5 but less than 30, and in addition to prednisone and cyclophosphamide for those patients with a titer greater than 30.[40] Plasmapheresis may be helpful to transiently remove the autoantibody (typically IgG) from circulation.[31,43]

Uremia

Acute and chronic renal failure are frequent comorbidities in the critically ill cancer patient. Platelet dysfunction secondary to renal failure may cause significant bleeding. The pathophysiology of platelet dysfunction with uremia is multifactorial and includes dysfunctional vWF, increased levels of cyclic adenosine monophosphate and nitric oxide generated by platelets, uremic toxins, and anemia, which causes the platelets to be displaced from the vascular endothelium thereby decreasing their ability to adhere and aggregate in response to endothelial damage.[44] Treatment is recommended for patients with active bleeding or for those undergoing an invasive procedure, such as placement of a hemodialysis catheter. Patients usually respond to hemodialysis and administration of DDAVP at a dose of 0.3 μg/kg intravenous (IV); cryoprecipitate (10 units given IV over 30 minutes) and conjugated estrogens (0.6 mg/kg IV over 30–40 minutes once daily for 5 consecutive days) may occasionally be required. The time to onset of improvement with conjugated estrogens is as rapid as 6 hours, although peak effect occurs around 5 to 7 days after the start of treatment, and can be anticipated to last for up to 14 to 21 days. Erythropoietin-stimulating agents (ESA) such as recombinant human erythropoietin and darbepoetin have been shown to reduce and prevent bleeding in uremic patients, and have a more sustained effect than either DDAVP or conjugated estrogens.[45–47] The effect of ESA on uremic bleeding occurs around 7 days after start of treatment, and is maximally effective once the hematocrit reaches normal level. The potential mechanisms for erythropoietin-mediated improvement include increased red cell volume pushing platelets closer to the endothelium thus decreasing the effective time to platelet-response to vascular injury, increase in reticular (metabolically most active) platelets, improved platelet aggregation and adherence to exposed subendothelium, increased platelet signaling via tyrosine phosphorylation, and the effect of increased hemoglobin as a nitric oxide scavenger.[45,46,48–51]

THROMBOCYTOSIS

Cancer can cause both qualitative and quantitative changes in platelets. Significantly elevated platelet counts can occur with myeloproliferative disorders, mainly essential thrombocythemia (ET) and polycythemia vera (PV), and also in some solid tumors. The incidence of the recently described JAK2V617F7F mutation is found in virtually all patients with PV and approximately 50% of those with ET.[52] Risk factors for thrombosis in both of these disorders include advanced age (>60 years) and prior history of thrombosis.[52] Increased platelet turnover, TF, factor V and VIII activity, acquired activated protein C resistance, and decreased protein S have been shown to occur in patients with the JAK2 mutation and thrombosis.[53]

For patients with critically high platelet counts (>1,000,000/μl) who are at risk for thrombosis or bleeding, secondary to abnormal platelet function of the majority of platelets, plateletpheresis may be considered along with cytoreductive therapy to treat the underlying myeloproliferative disorder in the acute setting. More long-term management once a patient has stabilized include interferon therapy, hydroxyurea, anagrelide, and JAK2 inhibitors, with limited side effects.[54]

BLEEDING ASSOCIATED WITH COAGULATION FACTOR ABNORMALITIES

Critically ill cancer patients may develop various coagulation factor abnormalities as a result of vitamin K deficiency from malnutrition, diarrhea, liver disease, biliary obstruction, use of vitamin K antagonists, and antibiotic therapy. Patients with primary or metastatic hepatocellular carcinoma have deficiency of vitamin K-dependent factors (factors II, VII, IX, X, protein C, and protein S), similar to that seen with liver cirrhosis. These patients almost always have increased levels of fibrinogen, unlike patients with cirrhosis or acute liver failure who have decreased fibrinogen levels. Acquired inhibitors of coagulation factors are frequently seen in multiple myeloma and other plasma cell dyscrasias. Increased fibrinolysis is another cause of bleeding that may occur, especially in patients with acute promyelocytic leukemia where the leukemic cells overexpress annexin II, a t-PA cell surface receptor,[55] which results in increased t-PA dependent plasmin generation. In addition to annexin II overexpression, patients may also develop increased fibrinolysis as a result of impaired TAFI activation by thrombin or deficiency in α2-antiplasmin or PAI-1 as a result of impaired synthetic function.[56]

Acute Management of Coagulopathy

The treatment of cancer patients with coagulation factor deficiencies, aside from the treatment of the underlying malignancy and localized control of hemostasis with direct application of pressure, topical agents such as thrombin powder or fibrin glue, or surgical repair of injured vessels, is generally supportive and consists of vitamin K, fresh frozen plasma (FFP), and cryoprecipitate. Oral vitamin K is the treatment of choice; its administration is predictably effective and has the advantages of safety and convenience over parenteral routes. However, in the critically ill cancer patient a rapid response is necessary, and may be achieved by administering a slow IV infusion of 10 mg vitamin K over 15 to 30 minutes to minimize the risk of anaphylactic reactions and fat embolism resulting from the lipid emulsion. Intravenous vitamin K doses can be repeated up to every 12 hours until international normalized ratio (INR) or PT is normalized.[57]

FFP is plasma isolated from whole blood that is frozen within 6 hours of donation, containing 0.7 to 1 unit/mL of clotting factor activity for each clotting factor and 1 to 2 mg of fibrinogen per unit of 200 to 280 mL volume. The appropriate milliliter dose of FFP is calculated by multiplying the estimated patient plasma volume by the percentage increase in factor VII desired divided by 100. Factor VII has the shortest half-life, and so redosing of FFP is based on repletion of this factor. In clinical practice the usual dose of FFP used is 10 to 15 mL/kg by IV infusion. FFP should be transfused when immediate correction of coagulation factor deficiencies is required because of bleeding or in patients undergoing an invasive procedure; the dose may be higher in patients with massive bleeding. The complete dose should be given at least every 6 hours until hemostasis is achieved and clotting parameters are normalized. The drawback to factor repletion with FFP is the large fluid volume that must be administered. In patients in whom volume status is of concern, the amount of fluid needed to fully and continuously reverse a coagulopathy may not be feasible. Furthermore, because of the low concentration of clotting factors, the relative increase in factor activity once more than 1 liter of FFP is given with respect to a patient's total plasma volume will be minimal. In this circumstance, consideration of other blood products is necessary.[58]

Cryoprecipitate is the cryoglobulin fraction of plasma obtained by thawing a single donation of FFP. Cryoprecipitate is rich in factor VIII, von Willebrand factor, fibrinogen, fibronectin, and factor XIII; it is indicated for dysfibrinogenemia and hypofibrinogenemic states, and also for some patients with renal failure. Cryoprecipitate is generally administered at a dose of 1 unit of cryoprecipitate IV for every 5 kg of body weight.[37] Generally, 10 bags of cryoprecipitate are given if the fibrinogen level is between 50 and 100 mg/dL and 20 bags if it is less than 50 mg/dL. A fibrinogen level measured at 30 to 60 minutes after completion of the transfusion should be used to determine the need for additional doses. The therapeutic goal is to keep the plasma fibrinogen level above 100 mg/dL.

In recent years, new clotting factor concentrates have been approved for use in bleeding diathesis. These agents include purified or recombinant single factors such as recombinant factor VII (rFVIIa), and products that are physiologically relevant complexes of coagulation factors such as activated prothrombin complex concentrates (aPCCs), including factor VIII inhibitor bypassing activity (FEIBA). The hemostatic effect of rFVIIa depends on binding to TF and activated platelets.

rFVIIa (NovoSeven) is administered in hemophilia patients with inhibitors at a dose of 90 μg/kg IV every 2 to 3 hours until the bleeding has stopped. When using rFVIIa, the

PT, fibrinogen, and D-dimer should be carefully monitored to minimize the risk of thrombosis and DIC. The dose of rFVIIa may also need to be titrated downward based on a patient's underlying risk factors for thrombosis. rFVIIa has also been used to control bleeding in hematopoietic stem cell transplant patients with diffuse alveolar hemorrhage or hepatic veno-occlusive disease in whom acquired factor VII deficiency results from liver dysfunction,[59] and for hemorrhagic cystitis secondary to chemotherapy or radiation.[37] The main risk associated with rFVIIa use is thrombosis that has ranged from less than 1% to 7% depending on the underlying patient comorbidities.[37,60–62] DIC, myocardial infarction, stroke, and allergic reactions have also been described.

Activated PCCs are used in the treatment of patients with factor IX deficiency and in those with inhibitors to factor VIII. FEIBA is a plasma-derived isolate of prothrombin (factor II), factor VII, factor VIIa, factor IX, and factor X that is designed to bypass factor VIII to generate factor Xa when dosed at 50 to 100 U/kg IV every 6 to 12 hours. FEIBA depends on the presence of platelet-derived factor V to localize and initiate coagulation. The action of FEIBA largely depends on its thrombin content, probably accounting for its relatively long half-life of thrombin generation, several hours longer than that of rFVIIa.[63] In general, aPCCs must be used with caution as they can be associated with venous thromboembolism or DIC.

If a paraprotein is the suspected origin of a coagulopathy such as development of a factor VIII inhibitor or aVWD, additional treatment modalities such as IVIg at a dose of 1 g/kg daily for 2 doses and plasmapheresis should be considered. The main side effects of IVIg include allergic reaction, acute renal failure associated with the increased protein load and immune-complex formation, and hyperviscosity. IgA deficiency should be considered in patients with allergic reactions to IVIg.

If increased fibrinolysis is a contributing cause of bleeding, antifibrinolytic agents such as tranexamic acid or ϵ-aminocaproic acid (EACA) should be considered. Both are lysine analogues that effectively elute plasminogen from a fibrin clot by competing with the protease for binding to C-terminal lysine residues exposed during fibrin generation. EACA is dosed orally up to 50 mg/kg every 6 hours or IV starting with a slow 5 g IV bolus followed by a continuous infusion of 1 g/h. Tranexamic acid similarly is dosed orally at 25 mg/kg or 10 mg/kg IV every 8 hours.[37] These agents should not be administered to patients with DIC or in those receiving other clotting factor replacement or all-*trans* retinoic acid (used in the treatment of acute promyelocytic leukemia [APL]),[64] as this will increase the risk of thrombosis. In addition, the doses of these 2 antifibrinolytic agents should be continuously monitored and reduced with impaired renal function.

THROMBOTIC MANIFESTATIONS

Patients in the ICU are at high risk for venous thromboembolism (VTE), and the risk is higher if they have underlying cancer. VTE is a significant comorbidity for patients with cancer, identified in up to 15% of patients with cancer during their disease course,[65] and in up to 35% to 50% of cancer patients in postmortem studies.[66,67] Cancers with the highest incidence of VTE include pancreatic and gastrointestinal cancers, as well as lung, brain, prostate, breast, and ovary, and patients with acute promyelocytic leukemia and myeloproliferative disorders.[31] Patients with cancer have a higher risk of VTE recurrence and a higher risk of bleeding diathesis compared with those without cancer.[68] This finding highlights some of the difficulties that arise in treatment of cancer patients for VTE, including factors such as ongoing tumor activity, pharmacotherapy, end organ injury (especially hepatic and renal dysfunction), and malnutrition.

The pathogenesis of thrombotic complications in cancer patients is multifactorial. In addition to the common predisposing factors for thrombosis such as immobility, advanced age, history of previous thrombosis, venous stasis, sepsis, and the use of central venous catheters, tumor cells have unique prothrombotic characteristics. Transformed malignant cells can induce platelet abnormalities, abnormal activation of the coagulation cascade, decreased hepatic synthesis of anticoagulant and coagulant proteins, fibrinolytic abnormalities, acquired thrombophilias, and expression of inflammatory and angiogenic cytokines.[17]

Thrombotic manifestations in cancer patients may present as one of the following: migratory thrombophlebitis or Trousseau syndrome, VTE including catheter-related thrombosis, thrombotic microangiopathy (TTP/HUS), arterial thrombosis, and DIC.

Migratory Thrombophlebitis (Trousseau Syndrome)

Trousseau syndrome is a classically described variant form of venous thrombosis characterized by a recurrent and migratory pattern preferentially involving superficial veins of the arms, chest, and neck.[69] Trousseau syndrome is highly associated with mucin-producing adenocarcinomas.[25] The clinical manifestations of Trousseau syndrome also include chronic DIC associated with microangiopathy, verrucous endocarditis, and arterial emboli in patients with cancer.

Venous Thromboembolism

VTE, as manifested by deep vein thrombosis (DVT) and pulmonary embolism (PE), remains a leading cause of death in cancer patients.[69] VTE often complicates the care of cancer patients undergoing major surgery and of patients receiving chemotherapy or hormonal therapy. The risk of developing thrombosis in cancer patients is influenced by the age and hormonal status of the patient. Postmenopausal women with advanced breast cancer receiving tamoxifen in addition to adjuvant chemotherapy have a higher risk for thrombotic events than do premenopausal women with breast cancer.[70,71] Thromboembolic events have been also reported with angiogenesis inhibitors (thalidomide, lenalidomide, and bevacizumab).[72–74] The pathogenic mechanisms of thromboembolic events associated with thalidomide are thought to be related to the development of acquired activated protein C resistance and a reduction in thrombomodulin level.[72–74] Endothelial injury produced by the combination of thalidomide with chemotherapy and subsequent restoration of endothelial cell PAR-1 expression are probable factors that promote thrombosis.[72–74] Cancer patients receiving erythropoiesis-stimulating agents for anemia have also been reported to have increased thrombotic risk.[75]

Two major advances in the diagnosis of VTE include the development and validation of a standardized clinical model (Wells criteria) to determine the pretest probability of VTE, and the measurement of plasma D-dimer. The integration of these advances has resulted in the formulation of safe, diagnostic algorithms that decrease the need for serial or invasive testing.[76] In a clinical trial for which the Wells clinical model was combined with compression ultrasonography, the need for venography and serial compression ultrasonography testing was decreased.[77] D-dimer levels can be measured by enzyme-linked immunosorbent assay, latex agglutination assay, or by a rapid bedside whole blood assay. Of the 3 assays, the whole blood assay reportedly has the best predictive value, with sensitivity rates in symptomatic general medical patients ranging from 85% to 95% and specificity rates of 65% to 68%. The D-dimer test has a high negative predictive value (NPV) and sensitivity for PE in cancer patients and, if negative, can be used to exclude PE in this population.[78]

The majority of DVT in cancer patients originates in the ileofemoral venous system. Diagnostic imaging modalities for DVT include ascending contrast venography, compression ultrasonography, and magnetic resonance venography. Ascending contrast venography remains the gold standard for diagnosing DVT, but this procedure is invasive and requires contrast material, which is frequently irritating and may result in complications. The finding of an intraluminal filling defect caused by thrombus surrounded by contrast is diagnostic for DVT. Noncompressibility of a proximal lower limb vein on compression ultrasonography has a diagnostic sensitivity rate of 97% and a specificity rate of 94%.[79] Although compression ultrasonography is highly sensitive for detecting proximal DVT, it is not as accurate for diagnosing isolated calf DVT. Magnetic resonance venography, a relatively new imaging modality that does not use contrast, has sensitivity and specificity rates greater than 95% for proximal DVT. Magnetic resonance venography is potentially useful in diagnosing pelvic vein DVT, especially isolated iliac vein thrombosis, which is difficult to diagnose with compression ultrasonography.

Several studies conducted in cancer patients with suspected DVT have demonstrated that the combination of the following studies can reliably exclude DVT and decrease the need for invasive testing: a normal D-dimer level and a normal compression ultrasonogram, a low pretest probability and normal compression ultrasonogram,[77] and a low pretest probability and a normal D-dimer level.

The standard treatment of VTE is to initiate anticoagulation with either intravenous or subcutaneous unfractionated heparin (UFH), or subcutaneous low molecular weight heparin (LMWH) or fondaparinux (an indirect factor Xa inhibitor) at therapeutic doses followed by oral warfarin therapy for a minimum of 3 months, to achieve an INR between 2.0 and 3.0.[80] However, in patients with active cancer, continued anticoagulation is recommended following the first episode of VTE.[80] Intravenous UFH is usually started with an initial bolus of 80 U/kg followed by a continuous IV infusion of 18 U/kg/h, adjusted to maintain the aPTT at 1.5 to 2.5 times the control value.[80] Alternatively, low molecular weight heparins (LMWHs) can be administered in weight-adjusted, once- or twice-daily subcutaneous doses without the need for laboratory monitoring. LMWHs have several advantages over UFH, including improved bioavailability, more predictable dose response, and lesser incidence of heparin-induced thrombocytopenia (HIT). Currently approved LMWH agents in the United States are enoxaparin, dalteparin, and tinzaparin. However, in ICU patients who are morbidly obese or develop renal failure, dosing of LMWHs may be unpredictable and may lead to serious adverse consequences such as prolonged bleeding.[79] In addition, ICU patients often have significant edema that may impair the absorption of LMWHs administered subcutaneously. Thus, monitoring of anti–factor Xa levels 4 h after injection of the LMWH should be considered in these settings. Target therapeutic range for anti–factor Xa is 0.5 to 1.0 U/mL for patients on twice daily LMWH dosing and 1.0 to 2.0 U/mL for patients dosed once daily. Although LMWHs have been demonstrated to be as effective and safe as UFH in clinical trials of acute PE, these trials excluded patients with hemodynamically significant PE and patients who developed PE in the ICU. Protamine sulfate is less efficacious in reversing LMWH-related bleeding and because of the longer half-life of LMWH, a second dose of protamine may be required. The dose is 1 mg protamine per 1 mg of enoxaparin or 100 U of dalteparin or tinzaparin. Fondaparinux, a novel anti–factor Xa inhibitor, has also been recently shown to be as effective and safe as intravenous UFH in hemodynamically stable patients with PE, and may also be used in patients with HIT. This agent, however, is limited in its use for ICU patients due to its long half-life (approximately 17 hours), and renal elimination precludes its use in patients with severe renal failure (CrCl <30 mL/min).[79] Current guidelines recommend the use of LMWH for the first 3 to 6 months as long-term treatment of VTE in cancer patients.[80]

The use of thrombolytic agents such as streptokinase and t-PA should be restricted to patients with massive ileofemoral DVT or massive PE and hemodynamic instability, because of the significant risks of bleeding associated with thrombolysis.[80,81] Furthermore, despite the proven efficacy of thrombolytic agents in achieving more rapid resolution of radiologic and hemodynamic abnormalities, studies to date have not shown any survival benefit with thrombolysis. Catheter-directed thrombolysis for initial treatment of VTE should be confined to selected patients requiring limb salvage. In general, thrombolytic therapy is contraindicated in cancer patients with brain metastases who develop VTE because of their significant risk for intracranial bleeding.[82] However, risk stratification may help to identify subgroups of patients at high risk of death that might benefit from systemic thrombolysis.[82] Surgical thromboembolectomy is restricted to patients with massive PE who have contraindications to or who do not respond to thrombolysis, in centers that have the available resources.[80] For cancer patients with VTE who have contraindications to anticoagulant therapy or those with recurrent VTE despite anticoagulation, placement of a retrievable or permanent inferior vena cava (IVC) filter is generally recommended. However, IVC filters are associated with undesirable side effects, such as debilitating leg symptoms caused by filter-related thrombosis.[83] Wallace and colleagues[84] reported that IVC filters were safe and highly effective in preventing PE-related deaths in cancer patients with VTE. In addition, patients with a history of DVT and bleeding or metastatic/disseminated stage of disease had the lowest survival after IVC filter placement.

Perioperative cancer patients, particularly those with breast cancer undergoing chemotherapy or on selective estrogen receptor modulators, and patients with advanced cancers that are associated with high risk of VTE such as brain tumors, and colorectal, pancreatic, lung, renal cell, and ovarian adenocarcinomas, should receive antithrombotic prophylaxis with intermittent pneumatic compression devices or compression elastic stockings, and either subcutaneous UFH or LMWH. The recommended doses are low-dose UFH, 5000 U subcutaneous (SC) every 8 hours or LMWH, either dalteparin, 5000 U SC daily, or enoxaparin, 40 mg SC daily, or fondaparinux, 2.5 mg SC starting 8 to 12 hours postoperatively.[85] Two perioperative cancer trials reported that continuation of LMWH prophylaxis for 3 weeks after hospital discharge reduced the risk of late venographic DVT by 60%.[86-88]

Catheter-Related Thrombosis

Central venous catheters (CVCs) are frequently placed in ICU patients. The estimated thrombosis rate of CVCs ranges from 5% to 30%. Prophylaxis with low-dose warfarin (1 mg daily) or LMWH (dalteparin 2500 anti–factor Xa units daily) was previously shown to be efficacious in cancer patients with indwelling CVCs.[89,90] It seems, however, that the incidence of catheter-related thrombosis in cancer patients is much lower than previously reported.[91] Thus, routine prophylaxis with either warfarin, 1 mg daily or LMWH (dalteparin, 2500 IU SC once a day) is no longer recommended.[85] Alteplase, a recombinant t-PA, at a dose of 1 to 2 mg per catheter lumen is effective in restoring flow to indwelling catheters occluded by thrombus.[92]

Thrombotic Microangiopathies: Thrombotic Thrombocytopenic Purpura and Hemolytic Uremic Syndrome

TTP/HUS is a microangiopathic, hemolytic syndrome that is additionally characterized by thrombocytopenia, neurologic symptoms, renal dysfunction, and fever. Laboratory diagnosis of TTP is by examination of the peripheral smear for schistocytes and verification of thrombocytopenia, measurement of lactate dehydrogenase (LDH), and absence of other clinical presentation that could otherwise explain the pathology. Patients receiving mitomycin-C, bleomycin, cisplatin, and tamoxifen as well as the post–bone marrow transplant population are at increased risk for cancer treatment-related TTP/HUS as are patients with breast, gastric, lung, and prostate cancer,[93] and Hodgkin and non-Hodgkin lymphomas.[31] The pathophysiology of cancer-associated TTP/HUS is postulated to be similar to that of usual primary TTP/HUS. The pathophysiology involves injury to vascular endothelium with release of ultralarge von Willebrand factor (VFW) multimers, due to a deficiency of a vWF-cleaving protease (ADAMTS-13) causing platelet aggregation.[94,95] In cancer-related TTP, the activity of this enzyme seems to be decreased.[96] ADAMTS-13 activity has also been correlated with the extent of tumor dissemination and development of TTP with malignant processes.[97–99] The clinical manifestations of TTP/HUS in cancer patients are often not readily obvious because they tend to occur in complicated patients, often being treated with chemotherapy or radiation therapy with several comorbidities that may obscure the diagnosis. The microangiopathic hemolytic anemia and thrombocytopenia typically are severe, and reticulocytosis is usually present, with increased levels of LDH, reflecting intravascular hemolysis. The peripheral blood smear demonstrates numerous schistocytes. Renal failure and neurologic and pulmonary dysfunction are common. Neurologic signs and symptoms include headache, confusion, hemiplegia or hemiparesis, and coma. Severe acute respiratory distress syndrome rarely may occur late in the disease process and is usually fatal.

The cornerstone of TTP treatment is plasma exchange simultaneously to remove the ADAMTS-13 inhibitor and supply the patient with the active enzyme. If plasmapheresis is not immediately available, FFP at a dose of 30 mL/kg may be used as a temporizing measure. Other useful treatment modalities in refractory cases include vincristine, IVIg, rituximab, and splenectomy.[100,101] Platelet transfusions are usually contraindicated because infused platelets may amplify the extent and severity of the formation of microvascular thrombi. However, recent evidence suggests that the potential harmful effect of platelet transfusion in TTP is uncertain.[102] Regardless of treatment, the prognosis of cancer patients with TTP/HUS is generally poor.

Arterial Thrombosis

Unlike venous thrombosis, arterial thrombosis is much less common in cancer patients.[31] When it occurs, it is usually secondary to nonbacterial thrombotic endocarditis (NBTE) or associated with chemotherapeutic regimens containing cisplatin. NBTE represents a form of consumptive coagulopathy most commonly seen with lung and pancreatic adenocarcinomas. The diagnosis should be suspected in any cancer patient who presents with ischemic embolic events. Echocardiography is diagnostic with the finding of sterile thrombotic vegetations on cardiac valves. In addition to valvular vegetations, ventricular segmental wall motion abnormalities resulting from silent embolization to the coronary arteries has been reported in 18% of cancer patients with NBTE. Management is essentially supportive, and consists of treatment of the underlying cancer and anticoagulation therapy with unfractionated or LMWH.

Disseminated Intravascular Coagulation

DIC is a pathologic state in which nonspecific coagulation and secondary fibrinolysis are activated, resulting in consumption of clotting factors and natural anticoagulants. Although the initial phase of DIC is a thrombotic one, and all factors that predispose cancer patients to VTE are important in the initiation of DIC, eventually the systemic depletion in clotting factors, fibrinogen, and platelets, as well as increased fibrinolytic activity, result in hemorrhage.[16]

DIC is especially common in cancer patients with estimates of between 7% and 20% in those who develop overt DIC during their disease course.[16,103] Some investigators have suggested that almost all cancer patients have subclinical DIC.[16,104] Of note, cancer patients may experience both acute and chronic DIC. The thrombotic disorders associated with DIC include recurrent venous thrombosis, peripheral arterial thrombosis and cerebrovascular thrombosis, disseminated arterial disease with organ failure, peripheral limb ischemia, and gangrene. Chronic forms of DIC are characterized by less florid clinical findings and more subtle, but persistent, laboratory abnormalities. Metastatic cancer is a common cause of chronic DIC. Over time, approximately 25% of patients with metastatic cancer develop a thrombotic event. Acute DIC occurs when a large concentration of TF is released from the tumor over a short period of time, and although it may occur with solid tumors including prostate and mucin-secreting adenocarcinomas of the pancreas, gastrointestinal track, ovary, thyroid, and gallbladder, it is most frequently seen in the hematological malignancies including APL, acute and chronic myelocytic leukemias, acute lymphocytic leukemia, and lymphomas. Acute DIC may occur in the presence of excessive tumor burden, or when treatment is initiated in instances of tumor lysis syndrome. In both cases, procoagulant intracellular factors are rapidly released into circulation as the tumor cells die, and initiate systemic coagulation. In acute DIC, although thrombosis occurs initially, the more profound clinical manifestations are those of bleeding.

In cancer patients, the diagnosis of DIC is made clinically and is corroborated by a constellation of laboratory abnormalities.[105] There is no single laboratory test that can establish or exclude the diagnosis of DIC. In most cases, a combination of tests in a patient with a clinical condition that is associated with DIC can be used to diagnose the disorder with reasonable certainty. In the presence of an underlying disease associated with DIC, there is an initial platelet count of less than $100,000/mm^3$ or a rapid decline in the platelet count; prolongation of the PT and aPTT is seen in about 50% to 60% of cases of DIC; and fibrin(ogen) degradation products in plasma and D-dimers is present. Fibrinogen levels may remain in the normal range in the face of its consumption because of increased synthesis of this acute-phase reactant. A finding of hypofibrinogenemia is only useful diagnostically in very severe cases of DIC. The peripheral blood smear may also demonstrate the presence of red cell fragmentation or schistocytes, but rarely more than 10% of the red cells. There seems to be no added value in measuring the natural anticoagulants protein C or antithrombin.[106] The International Society of Thrombosis and Hemostasis (ISTH) scoring system for overt DIC[106] has a sensitivity and specificity of 91% and 97%, respectively.[107] It is important to repeat the tests to monitor the dynamically changing scenario based on the laboratory results and clinical manifestations.

In general, the treatment of DIC is directed against the underlying cancer, but supportive management for the bleeding or thrombotic manifestations is required. Cancer patients with DIC who are bleeding or at high risk for bleeding (patients undergoing surgery or invasive procedures) should receive platelet transfusions to maintain the platelet count above $50,000/\mu L$ and FFP (initial doses of 15 mL/kg, although a dose of 30 mL/kg produces a more complete correction of coagulation factor levels) if the PT or aPTT are prolonged. The administration of purified coagulation factor concentrates in DIC is not generally recommended unless patients are fluid overloaded and cannot receive FFP. Coagulation factor concentrates contain only specific factors, whereas in DIC there is a global deficiency in coagulation factors. Severe hypofibrinogenemia (<1 g/L) needs to be treated with cryoprecipitate or fibrinogen concentrates if available. A dose of 3 g would raise plasma fibrinogen by 1 g/L; this can be given as 2 cryoprecipitate pools (10 donor units) or as a 3 g of a fibrinogen concentrate. The response to transfusion therapy should be monitored clinically and with laboratory tests.[105] The bleeding associated with DIC in APL often responds dramatically to treatment with all-*trans* retinoic acid.[108]

Although there are no clinical, randomized controlled trials demonstrating that the use of heparin in patients with DIC results in improved clinical outcome, unfractionated heparin may be used in cancer patients with DIC-associated thrombosis for stabilization while the cancer is being treated unless moderate to severe thrombocytopenia or bleeding is present. Monitoring aPTT may be complicated but monitoring for signs of bleeding is important. In critically ill, nonbleeding patients with DIC, pharmacologic thromboprophylaxis with either UFH or LMWH is recommended.[105] In general, patients with DIC should not be treated with antifibrinolytic agents. However, in patients with DIC and bleeding secondary to primary fibrinolysis (eg, prostate cancer), the fibrinolytic inhibitor EACA can be administered with an initial loading dose of 4 to 6 g IV over 1 hour followed by an IV infusion of 1 g/h while monitoring the clinical response. The recommended oral dose of EACA is 50 to 60 mg/kg every 4 to 6 h.[109] However, in those patients with a primary thrombotic presentation and secondary fibrinolysis, fibrinolytic inhibitors should be avoided until the thrombotic process is controlled.[105]

The administration of purified coagulation factor concentrates in DIC is not generally recommended unless patients are fluid overloaded and cannot receive FFP. Coagulation factor concentrates contain only specific factors, whereas in DIC there is a global deficiency in coagulation factors. Severe hypofibrinogenemia (<1 g/L) needs to be treated with cryoprecipitate or fibrinogen concentrates if available. A dose of 3 g would raise plasma fibrinogen by 1 g/L. This dose can be given as 2 cryoprecipitate pools (10 donor units) or as 3 g of a fibrinogen concentrate.[105] The bleeding associated with DIC in APL often responds dramatically to treatment with all-*trans* retinoic acid.[108]

HEPARIN-INDUCED THROMBOCYTOPENIA

HIT is an immune-mediated thrombocytopenia that occurs in approximately 1% to 5% of patients receiving heparin.[110] HIT occurs when a patient develops IgG antibodies against the complex formed between heparin and platelet factor 4 (PF4). The resulting antibodies activate platelets via their FcγIIa receptors, ultimately resulting in increased thrombin generation and development of a hypercoagulable state. The platelet count typically drops to a nadir of around 60,000/μl or 50% of the initial platelet count within 5 to 10 days of starting heparin therapy.[111] This amount is in contrast to many drug- or malignancy-induced thrombocytopenias in which the platelet count decreases to an average of 10,000/μl.[112] HIT may develop within 24 hours if there has been exposure to heparin during the preceding 3 months. On occasion the platelet count starts to decrease only after heparin has been stopped (delayed-onset HIT). The thrombocytopenia of HIT is in part related to platelet consumption, and most patients with HIT develop concurrent thrombosis.[113] Major risk factors that predispose to the development of HIT include gender[114] (women have an increased incidence), type of heparin preparation (bovine UFH>porcine UFH>LMWH), the exposed patient population (postoperative>medical>pregnancy),[110] and duration of heparin use.[113] Venous or arterial thromboses including DVT, PE, limb artery thrombosis, thrombotic stroke, and myocardial infarction can occur. A clinical pretest probability score known as the 4 Ts (degree of thrombocytopenia, timing of thrombocytopenia, other etiologies of thrombocytopenia and thrombosis) is useful in clinical practice. HIT should be suspected and treatment rapidly instituted in a patient with an intermediate or high test probability.[115]

The "gold standard" test for laboratory diagnosis is the platelet serotonin release assay; however, this test is cumbersome and is performed only in a few specialized coagulation laboratories. In clinical practice, the laboratory diagnosis of HIT is made with a positive platelet factor 4-dependent immunoassay. Management consists of discontinuing all forms of heparin and using direct thrombin inhibitors (DTIs) such as lepirudin or argatroban, which do not have any cross-reactivity to HIT antibodies. Lepirudin is excreted by the kidney and should not be used in patients with severe renal failure (creatinine clearance <20 mL/min). The recommended doses are 0.4 mg/kg bolus followed by 0.15 mg/kg/h in HIT with thrombosis and 0.10 mg/kg/h without a bolus in HIT without thrombosis. Argatroban is metabolized by the liver, and the dose should be reduced in patients with hepatic impairment. The usual dose is 2 µg/kg/min to maintain the aPTT at 1.5 to 3 times baseline. The starting dose should be reduced by 75% in a patient with significant liver dysfunction. In countries where danaparoid (a heparanoid) is available, this agent may also be used for the prevention and treatment of HIT complicated by thrombosis.[110] Warfarin should be avoided during the acute HIT episode because it decreases the level of protein C and predisposes to microvascular thrombosis, including warfarin-induced venous limb gangrene and skin necrosis syndromes. For patients receiving warfarin at the time of diagnosis of HIT, reversal of warfarin anticoagulation with vitamin K is recommended.

NOVEL DRUGS FOR TREATMENT OF BLEEDING AND THROMBOTIC DISORDERS
Recombinant Factor VIIa

The expanding use of rFVIIa in the acute care setting in recent years merits brief further discussion. rFVIIa has been used in the acute management of life-threatening intracerebral bleeding, uncontrolled surgical bleeding (cardiac and hepatic surgery), trauma-related bleeding, and for reversal of anticoagulation-related bleeding due to LMWH and DTIs. The use of rFVIIa in nonapproved settings should be critically evaluated, given the high costs and significant risk of thrombosis associated with its use. It is likely that recommendations about the use of rFVIIa will change rapidly in the coming years as the results of clinical trials become available.

Novel Thrombopoietic Agents

IL-11 (oprelvekin) is a Food and Drug Administration approved cytokine molecule that promotes megakaryocyte differentiation, and may be used in solid tumor and lymphoma treatment associated thrombocytopenia, but not for thrombocytopenia associated with myeloid lineage malignancies.[116]

Cloning of Mpl (TPO-receptor) ligands have offered novel agents directed toward stimulating thrombocytopoiesis. The first generation of Mpl agonists showed initial promise, with dose-dependent improvement in chemotherapy-associated thrombocytopenia as well with poor platelet production associated with MDS. However, reports of autoantibody development against TPO with these agents resulting in severe thrombocytopenia have curtailed their further use.[117] Two second-generation TPO mimetics, romiplostim and eltrombopag, have been recently approved for the treatment of refractory chronic immune thrombocytopenia, and are also being evaluated for the treatment of chemotherapy-induced thrombocytopenia.

Of importance is that these novel thrombopoietic agents are not recommended for use in the acute management of critically low platelet counts with associated bleeding events, as they increase megakaryocyte differentiation over the course of weeks to months. Although some patients may have a durable improvement in platelet counts with these agents,[117] in many patients the platelet counts rapidly decrease with attendant bleeding risks when these agents are withdrawn, especially if the underlying cause for thrombocytopenia is unresolved.

Novel Anticoagulants

Oral direct factor Xa inhibitors such as rivaroxaban and apixaban, and oral DTIs such as dabigatran, are completing clinical trials for the prevention and treatment of VTE. These oral agents can be given in fixed doses without routine monitoring.[118] Rivaroxaban has a half-life of 9 hours and is eliminated by the renal and intestinal routes. Apixaban has a half-life of 12 hours and is cleared by the fecal and renal routes. Phase 2 trials of apixaban in cancer patients are currently ongoing. Dabigatran etexilate is a prodrug that, once absorbed, is converted to its active metabolite dabigatran. Peak plasma level occurs at 2 hours, and its half-life is 8 hours after a single dose administration and 17 hours after multiple doses. As 80% of dabigatran is excreted by the kidney, this agent is contraindicated in patients with renal failure.[119] Idraparinux is an indirect factor Xa inhibitor that binds with high affinity to antithrombin and has a plasma half-life of 80 hours, allowing for subcutaneous administration once a week. Idraparinux can cause excessive bleeding; therefore a biotinylated form of idraparinux has been developed that has the same pharmacokinetics and pharmacodynamic properties as idraparinux, but can be neutralized by avidin. Avidin binds biotin with high affinity, and the complex is cleared renally.[120] To the authors' knowledge, there are no clinical trials using these novel antithrombotic agents in critically ill patients.

SUMMARY

Cancer affects multiple organ systems, nearly all of which can severely impact the delicate balance of thrombosis and hemostasis. Although much progress has been made in the diagnosis and management of many types of cancers, a significant number of cancer patients still develop life-threatening bleeding and thrombotic complications requiring ICU admission. Cancer- and chemotherapy-related malnutrition, renal failure, and hepatic dysfunction all directly increase a patient's risk of developing thrombosis, significant bleeding, or both as occurs with DIC. Furthermore, the malignancy and its treatment may make diagnosis of these processes more complicated, for example, differentiating TTP-associated thrombocytopenia from a complication of chemotherapy. Fortunately, there is an ever-increasing assortment of diagnostic and therapeutic tools available for management of hemostatic complications in cancer patients that one hopes will allow for improved survival of these patients.

REFERENCES

1. Furie B, Furie BC. Mechanisms of thrombus formation. N Engl J Med 2008; 359(9):938–49.
2. Andrews RK, Shen Y, Gardiner EE, et al. Platelet adhesion receptors and (patho)physiological thrombus formation. Histol Histopathol 2001;16(3):969–80.
3. Reininger AJ. Function of von Willebrand factor in haemostasis and thrombosis. Haemophilia 2008;14(Suppl 5):11–26.
4. Varga-Szabo D, Pleines I, Nieswandt B. Cell adhesion mechanisms in platelets. Arterioscler Thromb Vasc Biol 2008;28(3):403–12.
5. Ruggeri ZM. Mechanisms initiating platelet thrombus formation. Thromb Haemost 1997;78(1):611–6.

6. Fullard JF. The role of the platelet glycoprotein IIb/IIIa in thrombosis and haemostasis. Curr Pharm Des 2004;10(14):1567–76.
7. Esmon CT. Inflammation and the activated protein C anticoagulant pathway. Semin Thromb Hemost 2006;32(Suppl 1):49–60.
8. Rosenberg RD, Aird WC. Vascular-bed-specific hemostasis and hypercoagulable states. N Engl J Med 1999;340(20):1555–64.
9. Manchanda N, Schwartz BS. Single chain urokinase. Augmentation of enzymatic activity upon binding to monocytes. J Biol Chem 1991;266(22):14580–4.
10. Wiman B. The fibrinolytic enzyme system. Basic principles and links to venous and arterial thrombosis. Hematol Oncol Clin North Am 2000;14(2): 325–38, vii.
11. McMahon B, Kwaan HC. The plasminogen activator system and cancer. Pathophysiol Haemost Thromb 2008;36(3–4):184–94.
12. Bouillaud S. De l-Obliteration des veines et de son influence sur la formation des hydropisies partielles: consideration sur la hydropisies passive et general. Arch Gen Med 1823;1:188–204 [in French].
13. Trousseau A. Phlegmasia alba dolens. In: Trousseau A, editor. Clinique medicinale de l'Hotel-Dieu de Paris. 2nd edition. Paris (France): Bailliere J.-B. et fils; 1865. p. 645–712.
14. Buller HR, van Doormaal FF, van Sluis GL, et al. Cancer and thrombosis: from molecular mechanisms to clinical presentations. J Thromb Haemost 2007; 5(Suppl 1):246–54.
15. Billroth T. Lectures on surgical pathology and therapeutics: a handbook for students and practitioners. In: Hackley CE, editor. New York (NY): D. Appelton and Company; 1877.
16. Saba HI, Morelli GA, Saba RI. Disseminated intravascular coagulation (DIC) in cancer. Cancer Treat Res 2009;148:137–56.
17. Kaplinska K, Mielicki WP. Direct analysis reveals an absence of gamma-carboxyglutamic acid in cancer procoagulant from human tissues. Blood Coagul Fibrinolysis 2009;20(5):315–20.
18. Kaplinska K, Rozalski M, Krajewska U, et al. Cancer procoagulant (CP) analysis in human WM 115 malignant melanoma cells in vitro. Thromb Res 2009;124(3): 364–7.
19. Moore KL, Esmon CT, Esmon NL. Tumor necrosis factor leads to the internalization and degradation of thrombomodulin from the surface of bovine aortic endothelial cells in culture. Blood 1989;73(1):159–65.
20. Nachman RL, Hajjar KA, Silverstein RL, et al. Interleukin 1 induces endothelial cell synthesis of plasminogen activator inhibitor. J Exp Med 1986;163(6):1595–600.
21. Heit JA, Mohr DN, Silverstein MD, et al. Predictors of recurrence after deep vein thrombosis and pulmonary embolism: a population-based cohort study. Arch Intern Med 2000;160(6):761–8.
22. Blom JW, Doggen CJ, Osanto S, et al. Malignancies, prothrombotic mutations, and the risk of venous thrombosis. JAMA 2005;293(6):715–22.
23. Shen VS, Pollak EW. Fatal pulmonary embolism in cancer patients: is heparin prophylaxis justified? South Med J 1980;73(7):841–3.
24. Dentali F, Squizzato A, Brivio L, et al. JAK2V617F mutation for the early diagnosis of Ph-myeloproliferative neoplasms in patients with venous thromboembolism: a meta-analysis. Blood 2009;113(22):5617–23.
25. Carrier M, Le Gal G, Wells PS, et al. Systematic review: the Trousseau syndrome revisited: should we screen extensively for cancer in patients with venous thromboembolism? Ann Intern Med 2008;149(5):323–33.

26. Tagalakis V, Tamim H, Blostein M, et al. Use of warfarin and risk of urogenital cancer: a population-based, nested case-control study. Lancet Oncol 2007; 8(5):395–402.
27. Tagalakis V, Blostein M, Robinson-Cohen C, et al. The effect of anticoagulants on cancer risk and survival: systematic review. Cancer Treat Rev 2007;33(4): 358–68.
28. Maria T, DeSancho JHR. Coagulopathic complications of cancer patients. In: Kufe DW, editor. Cancer medicine. 7th edition. Hamilton (ON) Canada: BC Decker; 2006.
29. Johnson MJ. Bleeding, clotting and cancer. Clin Oncol (R Coll Radiol) 1997;9(5): 294–301.
30. Marks PW. Coagulation disorders in the ICU. Clin Chest Med 2009;30(1): 123–9, ix.
31. DeSancho MT, Rand JH. Bleeding and thrombotic complications in critically ill patients with cancer. Crit Care Clin 2001;17(3):599–622.
32. Kaplan RN, Psaila B, Lyden D. Niche-to-niche migration of bone-marrow-derived cells. Trends Mol Med 2007;13(2):72–81.
33. Kaushansky K, Drachman JG. The molecular and cellular biology of thrombo-poietin: the primary regulator of platelet production. Oncogene 2002;21(21): 3359–67.
34. Avecilla ST, Hattori K, Heissig B, et al. Chemokine-mediated interaction of hema-topoietic progenitors with the bone marrow vascular niche is required for throm-bopoiesis. Nat Med 2004;10(1):64–71.
35. Slichter SJ. Evidence-based platelet transfusion guidelines. Hematology Am Soc Hematol Educ Program 2007;172–8.
36. Schiffer CA, Anderson KC, Bennett CL, et al. Platelet transfusion for patients with cancer: clinical practice guidelines of the American Society of Clinical Oncology. J Clin Oncol 2001;19(5):1519–38.
37. Green D. Management of bleeding complications of hematologic malignancies. Semin Thromb Hemost 2007;33(4):427–34.
38. Federici AB. Acquired von Willebrand syndrome: is it an extremely rare disorder or do we see only the tip of the iceberg? J Thromb Haemost 2008; 6(4):565–8.
39. Federici AB. Acquired von Willebrand syndrome: an underdiagnosed and mis-diagnosed bleeding complication in patients with lymphoproliferative and myeloproliferative disorders. Semin Hematol 2006;43(1 Suppl 1):S48–58.
40. Federici AB. Therapeutic approaches to acquired von Willebrand syndrome. Expert Opin Investig Drugs 2000;9(2):347–54.
41. Sucker C, Scharf RE, Zotz RB. Use of recombinant factor VIIa in inherited and acquired von Willebrand disease. Clin Appl Thromb Hemost 2009;15(1):27–31.
42. Fozza C, Bellizzi S, Piseddu G, et al. Acquired hemophilia in a patient affected by acute myeloid leukemia. Am J Hematol 2005;79(1):81–2.
43. Tiede A, Huth-Kuhne A, Oldenburg J, et al. Immunosuppressive treatment for acquired haemophilia: current practice and future directions in Germany, Austria and Switzerland. Ann Hematol 2009;88(4):365–70.
44. Brophy DF, Martin EJ, Carr SL, et al. The effect of uremia on platelet contractile force, clot elastic modulus and bleeding time in hemodialysis patients. Thromb Res 2007;119(6):723–9.
45. Cases A, Escolar G, Reverter JC, et al. Recombinant human erythropoietin treat-ment improves platelet function in uremic patients. Kidney Int 1992;42(3): 668–72.

46. Diaz-Ricart M, Etebanell E, Cases A, et al. Erythropoietin improves signaling through tyrosine phosphorylation in platelets from uremic patients. Thromb Haemost 1999;82(4):1312–7.
47. Hedges SJ, Dehoney SB, Hooper JS, et al. Evidence-based treatment recommendations for uremic bleeding. Nat Clin Pract Nephrol 2007;3(3):138–53.
48. Vigano G, Benigni A, Mendogni D, et al. Recombinant human erythropoietin to correct uremic bleeding. Am J Kidney Dis 1991;18(1):44–9.
49. Zwaginga JJ, IJsseldijk MJ, de Groot PG, et al. Treatment of uremic anemia with recombinant erythropoietin also reduces the defects in platelet adhesion and aggregation caused by uremic plasma. Thromb Haemost 1991;66(6):638–47.
50. Peng J, Friese P, Heilmann E, et al. Aged platelets have an impaired response to thrombin as quantitated by P-selectin expression. Blood 1994;83(1):161–6.
51. Tassies D, Reverter JC, Cases A, et al. Effect of recombinant human erythropoietin treatment on circulating reticulated platelets in uremic patients: association with early improvement in platelet function. Am J Hematol 1998;59(2):105–9.
52. Tefferi A, Elliott M. Thrombosis in myeloproliferative disorders: prevalence, prognostic factors, and the role of leukocytes and JAK2V617F. Semin Thromb Hemost 2007;33(4):313–20.
53. Arellano-Rodrigo E, Alvarez-Larran A, Reverter JC, et al. Platelet turnover, coagulation factors, and soluble markers of platelet and endothelial activation in essential thrombocythemia: relationship with thrombosis occurrence and JAK2 V617F allele burden. Am J Hematol 2009;84(2):102–8.
54. Finazzi G, Barbui T. Evidence and expertise in the management of polycythemia vera and essential thrombocythemia. Leukemia 2008;22(8):1494–502.
55. Menell JS, Cesarman GM, Jacovina AT, et al. Annexin II and bleeding in acute promyelocytic leukemia. N Engl J Med 1999;340(13):994–1004.
56. Tallman MS, Brenner B, Serna J de L, et al. Meeting report. Acute promyelocytic leukemia-associated coagulopathy, 21 January 2004, London, United Kingdom. Leuk Res 2005;29(3):347–51.
57. Ansell J, Hirsh J, Hylek E, et al. Pharmacology and management of the vitamin K antagonists: American College of Chest Physicians Evidence-Based Clinical Practice Guidelines (8th Edition). Chest 2008;133(Suppl 6):160S–98S.
58. DeLoughery TG. Critical care clotting catastrophies. Crit Care Clin 2005;21(3):531–62.
59. Richardson P. Hemostatic complications of hematopoietic stem cell transplantation: from hemorrhage to microangiopathies and VOD. Pathophysiol Haemost Thromb 2003;33(Suppl 1):50–3.
60. O'Connell KA, Wood JJ, Wise RP, et al. Thromboembolic adverse events after use of recombinant human coagulation factor VIIa. JAMA 2006;295(3):293–8.
61. Mayer SA, Brun NC, Begtrup K, et al. Recombinant activated factor VII for acute intracerebral hemorrhage. N Engl J Med 2005;352(8):777–85.
62. Aledort LM. Comparative thrombotic event incidence after infusion of recombinant factor VIIa versus factor VIII inhibitor bypass activity. J Thromb Haemost 2004;2(10):1700–8.
63. Hay CR. Thrombosis and recombinant factor VIIa. J Thromb Haemost 2004;2(10):1698–9.
64. Abraham S, Zhang W, Greenberg N, et al. Maspin functions as tumor suppressor by increasing cell adhesion to extracellular matrix in prostate tumor cells. J Urol 2003;169(3):1157–61.

65. Sun NC, McAfee WM, Hum GJ, et al. Hemostatic abnormalities in malignancy, a prospective study of one hundred eight patients. Part I. Coagulation studies. Am J Clin Pathol 1979;71(1):10–6.
66. Francis JL, Biggerstaff J, Amirkhosravi A. Hemostasis and malignancy. Semin Thromb Hemost 1998;24(2):93–109.
67. Rahr HB, Sorensen JV. Venous thromboembolism and cancer. Blood Coagul Fibrinolysis 1992;3(4):451–60.
68. Prandoni P, Lensing AW, Piccioli A, et al. Recurrent venous thromboembolism and bleeding complications during anticoagulant treatment in patients with cancer and venous thrombosis. Blood 2002;100(10):3484–8.
69. Babu B, Carman TL. Cancer and clots: all cases of venous thromboembolism are not treated the same. Cleve Clin J Med 2009;76(2):129–35.
70. Lee AY, Levine MN, Baker RI, et al. Low-molecular-weight heparin versus a coumarin for the prevention of recurrent venous thromboembolism in patients with cancer. N Engl J Med 2003;349(2):146–53.
71. Lee AY, Rickles FR, Julian JA, et al. Randomized comparison of low molecular weight heparin and coumarin derivatives on the survival of patients with cancer and venous thromboembolism. J Clin Oncol 2005;23(10):2123–9.
72. Cortes J, Saura C, Atzori F. Risk of venous thromboembolism with bevacizumab in cancer patients. JAMA 2009;301(14):1434–5 [author reply: 1435–6].
73. El Accaoui RN, Shamseddeen WA, Taher AT. Thalidomide and thrombosis. A meta-analysis. Thromb Haemost 2007;97(6):1031–6.
74. Zangari M, Elice F, Fink L, et al. Thrombosis in multiple myeloma. Expert Rev Anticancer Ther 2007;7(3):307–15.
75. Bokemeyer C, Aapro MS, Courdi A, et al. EORTC guidelines for the use of erythropoietic proteins in anaemic patients with cancer: 2006 update. Eur J Cancer 2007;43(2):258–70.
76. Wells PS, Hirsh J, Anderson DR, et al. Accuracy of clinical assessment of deep-vein thrombosis. Lancet 1995;345(8961):1326–30.
77. Wells PS, Anderson DR, Bormanis J, et al. Value of assessment of pretest probability of deep-vein thrombosis in clinical management. Lancet 1997;350(9094):1795–8.
78. King V, Vaze AA, Moskowitz CS, et al. D-dimer assay to exclude pulmonary embolism in high-risk oncologic population: correlation with CT pulmonary angiography in an urgent care setting. Radiology 2008;247(3):854–61.
79. Kearon C, Ginsberg JS, Hirsh J. The role of venous ultrasonography in the diagnosis of suspected deep venous thrombosis and pulmonary embolism. Ann Intern Med 1998;129(12):1044–9.
80. Kearon C, Kahn SR, Agnelli G, et al. Antithrombotic therapy for venous thromboembolic disease: American College of Chest Physicians Evidence-Based Clinical Practice Guidelines, 8th edition. Chest 2008;133(Suppl 6):454S–545S.
81. Pastores SM. Management of venous thromboembolism in the intensive care unit. J Crit Care 2009;24(2):185–91.
82. Han S, Chaya C, Hoo GW. Thrombolytic therapy for massive pulmonary embolism in a patient with a known intracranial tumor. J Intensive Care Med 2006;21(4):240–5.
83. Fox MA, Kahn SR. Postthrombotic syndrome in relation to vena cava filter placement: a systematic review. J Vasc Interv Radiol 2008;19(7):981–5.
84. Wallace MJ, Jean JL, Gupta S, et al. Use of inferior vena caval filters and survival in patients with malignancy. Cancer 2004;101(8):1902–7.

85. Geerts WH, Bergqvist D, Pineo GF, et al. Prevention of venous thromboembolism: American College of Chest Physicians Evidence-Based Clinical Practice Guidelines (8th Edition). Chest 2008;133(Suppl 6):381S–453S.

86. Agnelli G, Bergqvist D, Cohen AT, et al. Randomized clinical trial of postoperative fondaparinux versus perioperative dalteparin for prevention of venous thromboembolism in high-risk abdominal surgery. Br J Surg 2005;92(10): 1212–20.

87. Bergqvist D, Agnelli G, Cohen AT, et al. Duration of prophylaxis against venous thromboembolism with enoxaparin after surgery for cancer. N Engl J Med 2002; 346(13):975–80.

88. Rasmussen MS. Preventing thromboembolic complications in cancer patients after surgery: a role for prolonged thromboprophylaxis. Cancer Treat Rev 2002;28(3):141–4.

89. Bern MM, Lokich JJ, Wallach SR, et al. Very low doses of warfarin can prevent thrombosis in central venous catheters. A randomized prospective trial. Ann Intern Med 1990;112(6):423–8.

90. Monreal M, Alastrue A, Rull M, et al. Upper extremity deep venous thrombosis in cancer patients with venous access devices—prophylaxis with a low molecular weight heparin (Fragmin). Thromb Haemost 1996;75(2):251–3.

91. Walshe LJ, Malak SF, Eagan J, et al. Complication rates among cancer patients with peripherally inserted central catheters. J Clin Oncol 2002;20(15):3276–81.

92. Ponec D, Irwin D, Haire WD, et al. Recombinant tissue plasminogen activator (alteplase) for restoration of flow in occluded central venous access devices: a double-blind placebo-controlled trial—the Cardiovascular Thrombolytic to Open Occluded Lines (COOL) efficacy trial. J Vasc Interv Radiol 2001;12(8):951–5.

93. Chang JC, Naqvi T. Thrombotic thrombocytopenic purpura associated with bone marrow metastasis and secondary myelofibrosis in cancer. Oncologist 2003;8(4):375–80.

94. Tsai HM, Lian EC. Antibodies to von Willebrand factor-cleaving protease in acute thrombotic thrombocytopenic purpura. N Engl J Med 1998;339(22):1585–94.

95. Tripodi A, Chantarangkul V, Bohm M, et al. Measurement of von Willebrand factor cleaving protease (ADAMTS-13): results of an international collaborative study involving 11 methods testing the same set of coded plasmas. J Thromb Haemost 2004;2(9):1601–9.

96. Peyvandi F, Siboni SM, Lambertenghi Deliliers D, et al. Prospective study on the behaviour of the metalloprotease ADAMTS13 and of von Willebrand factor after bone marrow transplantation. Br J Haematol 2006;134(2):187–95.

97. Oleksowicz L, Bhagwati N, DeLeon-Fernandez M. Deficient activity of von Willebrand's factor-cleaving protease in patients with disseminated malignancies. Cancer Res 1999;59(9):2244–50.

98. Mannucci PM, Karimi M, Mosalaei A, et al. Patients with localized and disseminated tumors have reduced but measurable levels of ADAMTS-13 (von Willebrand factor cleaving protease). Haematologica 2003;88(4):454–8.

99. Blot E, Decaudin D, Veyradier A, et al. Cancer-related thrombotic microangiopathy secondary to Von Willebrand factor-cleaving protease deficiency. Thromb Res 2002;106(2):127–30.

100. Reddy PS, Deauna-Limayo D, Cook JD, et al. Rituximab in the treatment of relapsed thrombotic thrombocytopenic purpura. Ann Hematol 2005;84(4): 232–5.

101. Crowther MA, George JN. Thrombotic thrombocytopenic purpura: 2008 update. Cleve Clin J Med 2008;75(5):369–75.

102. Swisher KK, Terrell DR, Vesely SK, et al. Clinical outcomes after platelet transfusions in patients with thrombotic thrombocytopenic purpura. Transfusion 2009; 49(5):873–87.
103. Levi M. Cancer and DIC. Haemostasis 2001;31(Suppl 1):47–8.
104. Rickles FR, Falanga A. Molecular basis for the relationship between thrombosis and cancer. Thromb Res 2001;102(6):V215–24.
105. Levi M, Toh CH, Thachil J, et al. Guidelines for the diagnosis and management of disseminated intravascular coagulation. Br J Haematol 2009;145(1):24–33.
106. Toh CH, Hoots WK. The scoring system of the Scientific and Standardisation Committee on Disseminated Intravascular Coagulation of the International Society on Thrombosis and Haemostasis: a 5-year overview. J Thromb Haemost 2007;5(3):604–6.
107. Bakhtiari K, Meijers JC, de Jonge E, et al. Prospective validation of the International Society of Thrombosis and Haemostasis scoring system for disseminated intravascular coagulation. Crit Care Med 2004;32(12):2416–21.
108. Falanga A, Rickles FR. Pathogenesis and management of the bleeding diathesis in acute promyelocytic leukaemia. Best Pract Res Clin Haematol 2003; 16(3):463–82.
109. Mannucci PM, Levi M. Prevention and treatment of major blood loss. N Engl J Med 2007;356(22):2301–11.
110. Warkentin TE, Greinacher A, Koster A, et al. Treatment and prevention of heparin-induced thrombocytopenia: American College of Chest Physicians Evidence-Based Clinical Practice Guidelines, 8th edition. Chest 2008; 133(Suppl 6):340S–80S.
111. Warkentin TE, Roberts RS, Hirsh J, et al. An improved definition of immune heparin-induced thrombocytopenia in postoperative orthopedic patients. Arch Intern Med 2003;163(20):2518–24.
112. Warkentin TE. Drug-induced immune-mediated thrombocytopenia—from purpura to thrombosis. N Engl J Med 2007;356(9):891–3.
113. Warkentin TE. Heparin-induced thrombocytopenia. Hematol Oncol Clin North Am 2007;21(4):589–607, v.
114. Warkentin TE, Sheppard JA, Sigouin CS, et al. Gender imbalance and risk factor interactions in heparin-induced thrombocytopenia. Blood 2006;108(9):2937–41.
115. Lo GK, Juhl D, Warkentin TE, et al. Evaluation of pretest clinical score (4 T's) for the diagnosis of heparin-induced thrombocytopenia in two clinical settings. J Thromb Haemost 2006;4(4):759–65.
116. Cantor SB, Elting LS, Hudson DV Jr, et al. Pharmacoeconomic analysis of oprelvekin (recombinant human interleukin-11) for secondary prophylaxis of thrombocytopenia in solid tumor patients receiving chemotherapy. Cancer 2003; 97(12):3099–106.
117. Levy B, Arnason JE, Bussel JB. The use of second-generation thrombopoietic agents for chemotherapy-induced thrombocytopenia. Curr Opin Oncol 2008; 20(6):690–6.
118. Eriksson BI, Quinlan DJ, Weitz JI. Comparative pharmacodynamics and pharmacokinetics of oral direct thrombin and factor Xa inhibitors in development. Clin Pharmacokinet 2009;48(1):1–22.
119. Sanford M, Plosker GL. Dabigatran etexilate. Drugs 2008;68(12):1699–709.
120. Prandoni P, Tormene D, Perlati M, et al. Idraparinux: review of its clinical efficacy and safety for prevention and treatment of thromboembolic disorders. Expert Opin Investig Drugs 2008;17(5):773–7.

Critical Care of the Hematopoietic Stem Cell Transplant Recipient

Bekele Afessa, MD[a],*, Elie Azoulay, MD, PhD[b]

KEYWORDS

- Bone marrow transplantation • Intensive care units
- Mechanical ventilation • Mortality • Multiple organ failure
- Prognosis

An estimated 50,000 to 60,000 patients undergo hematopoietic stem cell transplantation (HSCT) worldwide annually.[1] Peripheral blood is the source of more than 95% of autologous transplantation in adults. The most common indications for HSCT are multiple myeloma and lymphoma, accounting for 56%. Multiple myeloma and acute leukemia are the most common indications for autologous and allogeneic transplantation, respectively. Among adults, 44% of allogeneic transplants are from unrelated donors, and bone marrow accounted for 28% of unrelated donor transplants between 2003 and 2006 compared with 66% between 1999 and 2000.[1] Very few adults receive umbilical-cord–blood transplants.

Because their innate and acquired immune systems are impaired, HSCT recipients frequently have infectious and noninfectious complications. The post-transplant recovery of the immune system depends on the underlying disorder, conditioning regimen, stem cell source, and on complications, such as graft-versus-host disease (GVHD). The post-transplant complications follow characteristic time patterns. The pretransplant conditioning regimen virtually eliminates all preexisting innate and acquired immunity.[2] After HSCT, the immune system recovers along predictable patterns depending on the underlying disorder, stem cell source, and complications such as GVHD. Recovery occurs faster in autologous recipients, in those who receive peripheral blood stem cell grafts, and after nonmyeloablative conditioning regimen.

The post-transplant period is divided into 3 phases: pre-engraftment, early post-transplant, and late post-transplant. The pre-engraftment phase (0 to 30 days) is

Grant support: None.

[a] Division of Pulmonary and Critical Care Medicine, Mayo Clinic College of Medicine, 200 First Street SW, Rochester, MN 55905, USA

[b] Service de Réanimation Médicale, Hôpital Saint-Louis, 1 Avenue Claude Vellefaux, Paris 75010, France

* Corresponding author.

E-mail address: afessa.bekele@mayo.edu (B. Afessa).

characterized by neutropenia and breaks in the mucocutaneous barriers. During this phase, the most prevalent pathogens are bacteria and *Candida* species and, if neutropenia persists, *Aspergillus* species. During the period of neutropenia, there is no significant difference in the type of infection between allogeneic and autologous HSCT recipients.[3] The early post-engraftment phase (30 to 100 days) is dominated by impaired cell-mediated immunity. The effect of this cell-mediated defect is determined by the development of GVHD and the immunosuppressant medications used to treat it. *Cytomegalovirus* (CMV), *Pneumocystis jiroveci* and *Aspergillus* species are the predominant pathogens during this phase. The late post-transplant phase (>100 days) is characterized by defects in cell-mediated and humoral immunity and in function of the reticuloendothelial system in allogeneic transplant recipients. During this phase, allogeneic HSCT recipients are at risk of viral infection and infection by encapsulated bacteria such as *Haemophilus influenzae* and *Streptococcus pneumoniae*. In endemic areas of the world, pulmonary tuberculosis occurs during the late post-transplant phase. After neutrophil engraftment, infections occur more frequently in allogeneic HSCT recipients.[3]

Some of the post-transplant complications may be life-threatening and require treatment in the intensive care unit (ICU). A recent publication has provided an excellent review of the critical care outcome of adult and pediatric HSCT recipients.[4] This article reviews the critical care support of adult HSCT recipients.

RATE AND REASONS OF ICU ADMISSION

The reported numbers of HSCT recipients admitted to the ICU range from less than 5% to more than 55%, with an overall rate of 15.7%.[5–15] In the studies of patients treated before 1995,[5–7,12,14,16] 272 of 1412 HSCT recipients (19.3%) were admitted to the ICU compared with 371 of 3037 patients (12.2%) after 1995[9,11,15,17,18] (P<.001). In one study that included only autologous HSCT recipients, less than 6% of them were admitted to the ICU.[15] In the only study of adult umbilical-cord–blood recipients, 57% of them were admitted to the ICU.[11]

The most common reason for ICU admission is respiratory (**Box 1**).[5–8,10,11,18,19] Among 844 HSCT recipients admitted to the ICU, the primary reason for admission was respiratory in 492 (58.3%).[6–8,12,14,15,17–21] Pneumonia and sepsis-induced acute lung injury (ALI)/ARDS are common causes of hypoxemic respiratory failure in HSCT recipients.[22] Airway compromise due to mucositis may also lead to ICU admission during the pre-engraftment period.[7,8,21] Several noninfectious pulmonary complications can lead to respiratory failure in HSCT patients leading to ICU admission. Among these complications, pulmonary edema, DAH, and PERDS usually occur during the first 30 days following transplant and IPS can occur at any time following transplant.[23–25]

Hemodynamic instability in HSCT recipients can be precipitated by hypovolemia and sepsis. Poor oral intake associated with mucositis and gastrointestinal bleeding associated with mucositis and thrombocytopenia can lead to hypovolemic shock with multiple organ dysfunction requiring ICU admission. Autologous and allogeneic HSCT recipients are at increased risk of sepsis during the neutropenic, pre-engraftment period. In allogeneic HSCT recipients, GVHD and its treatment lead to prolonged immunodeficiency with additional risk of sepsis. Hemodynamic compromise secondary to sepsis was the primary reason for ICU admission in 101 of 548 HSCT recipients (18.4%) described in the literature.[7,12,14,15,18–21] Some studies have described cardiac dysrhythmias to be the primary reason for admission to the ICU in 8% to 17% of HSCT recipients.[18,19,21] Thrombocytopenia and GVHD predispose HSCT recipients to hemorrhagic complications.[26] Intracranial bleeding is reported in

---

Box 1
Main reasons for intensive care unit (ICU) admissions of HSCT recipients

Respiratory system

  Airway

  Pneumonia

  Pulmonary edema

  Acute respiratory distress syndrome (ARDS)

  Idiopathic pneumonia syndrome (IPS)

  Diffuse alveolar hemorrhage (DAH)

  Per-engraftment respiratory distress syndrome (PERDS)

Cardiovascular system

  Septic shock

  Hypovolemic shock (dehydration and bleeding)

  Cardiogenic shock

  Obstructive shock

Central nervous system

  Seizure

  Intracranial bleeding

Gastrointestinal system

  Gastrointestinal bleeding

  Hepatic failure

  Neutropenic colitis

Renal failure

2% to 5% of HSCT recipients.[26,27] In one autopsy study of 180 HSCT recipients, intracranial hemorrhage was found in 32%.[28] Seizure and other central nervous manifestations are reported to be the primary reason for ICU admission in approximately 11% of HSCT recipients.[11,12,15,17–19,21] Although hemostatic complications leading to bleeding and thromboembolic events are common in HSCT recipients,[26] gastrointestinal bleeding has been reported to be the reason for ICU admission in only 15 of 326 (4.6%) patients.[7,11,12,15,21] Neutropenic colitis and acute intestinal GVHD can lead to ICU admission for perforation and bleeding.[7,11,12,15,21,29] Although acute renal failure is common in critically ill HSCT recipients,[10] it is reported to be the primary reason for ICU admission in less than 5%.[11,19,21]

ICU COURSE AND COMPLICATIONS

The ICU course of HSCT recipients is complicated with multiorgan dysfunction. Some of the organ dysfunctions occur at ICU admission whereas others develop during the ICU course. Single or multiorgan failure has been reported in 64% to 94% and multiorgan failure in 22% to 81% of HSCT recipients admitted to the ICU.[15,18,19,30] However, because of variations in organ failure definitions and incomplete reports, it is difficult to determine specific organ failure rates. Respiratory failure is the most common organ failure and develops in most patients. Afessa and colleagues[19] reported ARDS in 62% of their patients. ARDS and interstitial pneumonia were the most common cause of death in the study by Jackson and colleagues.[7] Naeem and colleagues[11] reported acute renal failure in 20 (80%) and hepatic failure in 13 (52%) of their 25 umbilical blood transplant recipients admitted to the ICU. A similarly high rate of acute renal failure, in 43 of 57 HSCT recipients (73.7%), was reported by Letourneau and colleagues.[10] However, other studies have reported these rates to be less than 20%.[13,21]

DIAGNOSTIC INTERVENTIONS

Various diagnostic and therapeutic procedures are performed in HSCT recipients admitted to the ICU. An earlier study had reported pulmonary artery catheterization to be performed in most HSCT recipients admitted to the ICU.[5] There are limited randomized clinical trials aimed at defining the role of pulmonary artery catheterization in the critically ill. A review by the Cochrane Collaboration group showed pulmonary artery catheterization to have no effect on patient outcome, including mortality and length of stay.[31] Most of the recent studies of critically ill HSCT recipients do not mention pulmonary artery catheterization or report a lower use rate.[13] The authors believe that the pulmonary artery catheter use rate in the critically ill HSCT recipient may have declined since the 1996 publication of a retrospective study showing potential harm associated with it.[32]

The patient's immune system dysfunction, post-transplant timing, epidemiologic history, noninvasively obtained microbiological and other laboratory values, and the pattern and rapidity of development of chest radiographic findings often help to narrow the differential diagnosis and initiate empiric therapy in the critically ill HSCT recipient presenting with pulmonary infiltrates. However, the atypical presentations of some common diagnoses, the occurrence of unusual diagnoses, the coexistence of multiple conditions responsible for the infiltrates, and the detrimental effect of missed diagnosis often lead to invasive diagnostic interventions, such as bronchoscopy, and rarely, surgical lung biopsy.[33–38] Unfortunately, such invasive procedures are not without complications in the critically ill HSCT recipient. In a study by Jackson and colleagues,[7] 11 patients had invasive mechanical ventilation (MV) initiated following bronchoscopy or open lung biopsy and 9 of them died.

Recently, Azoulay and colleagues[39] have described the role of diagnostic bronchoscopy in hematology and oncology patients, including HSCT recipients with acute respiratory failure. In this observational, prospective, multicenter study, bronchoscopy provided the only conclusive result in 33.7% of the patients who underwent the procedure.[39] However, the bronchoscopy was associated with respiratory deterioration in 22 of 45 (49%) patients who were not intubated during the procedure, leading to endotracheal intubation for MV support in 16 of them (36%). The noninvasive diagnostic strategies for evaluation of pulmonary conditions include blood cultures; serology for Aspergillus antigen; examination of spontaneously expectorated sputum for bacteria, Aspergillus, and other fungi; induced sputum for *P jiroveci*; urine antigen for *Legionella pneumophila*, and *S pneumoniae*; CMV circulating antigen; nasopharyngeal aspirations; and echocardiography.[39] Azoulay and colleagues[39] included 148 patients from 14 medical centers in their prospective, observational study; 141 (95.3%) had at least 1 noninvasive evaluation and 101 (68.2%) underwent bronchoscopy. The noninvasive diagnostic strategy led to 105 diagnoses in 94 (66.7%) patients and the bronchoscopy led to 58 diagnoses in 51 (50.5%) patients. Among the 148 diagnoses established in the study, 88 (60.3%) were made only by noninvasive tests, 41 (28.1%) only by bronchoscopy, and 17 (11.6%) by both types. There were no statistically significant difference in mortality between the bronchoscopy and noninvasive groups. This study highlights that the diagnosis of pulmonary infiltrates in hematology and oncology patients, including HSCT recipients with acute respiratory failure, can be established by following a noninvasive strategy. However, bronchoscopy plays a complementary role in selected patients.

ORGAN SUPPORT

Almost all critically ill HSCT recipients develop single or multiorgan failure. Pancytopenia is an expected consequence of the conditioning regimen in HSCT recipients. Neutropenia is a major risk factor for bacterial and fungal infections. Despite prophylaxis, preemptive and therapeutic use of antibiotics, and administration of colony-stimulating factors, infections are common in neutropenic HSCT recipients. The rate of infection depends on the degree and duration of neutropenia. Some recommend that certain minimal criteria be met before the initiation of granulocyte transfusion: an absolute neutrophil count lower than 500/μL and infection unresponsiveness to antibiotic therapy for at least 48 hours.[40] However, a retrospective, case-control feasibility study of candidates and recipients of HSCT showed no benefit associated with granulocyte transfusion.[41] Similarly, a Cochrane meta-analysis of 8 randomized clinical trials concluded that the available evidence was insufficient to either support or refute the generalized use of granulocyte transfusion therapy in most neutropenic patients, including HSCT recipients.[42]

Moreover, granulocyte transfusion is associated with multiple complications including fever and chills, respiratory failure due to sequestration of cells in the pulmonary vasculature, transfusion-associated GVHD, human leukocyte antigen (HLA) alloimmunization, and infection. There are limited data to guide clinicians on when to transfuse platelets to HSCT recipients. In a retrospective study of HSCT recipients that excluded patients at high risk of bleeding, an increased risk of bleeding could be established only if the platelet count dropped to less than 13,000/μL.[43] The American Society of Clinical Oncology clinical practice guidelines recommend a platelet threshold of 10,000/μL for transfusion.[44] However, platelet transfusion at higher levels may be necessary if there is active bleeding, rapid fall in platelet count, or coagulation abnormalities. In the absence of hemodynamic instability, active bleeding, or comorbidities, red blood cell transfusion is rarely needed if the hemoglobin is greater than 7 g/dL.[45] To minimize the complications that may arise from leukocyte contamination, leukoreduced red blood cells are used for transfusion. To avoid the occurrence of GVHD, red blood cells must be subjected to irradiation before transfusion. CMV-negative blood components should be administered to CMV seronegative HSCT recipients.

Vasopressor-requiring shock is a common occurrence in critically ill HSCT recipients. Of 499 HSCT recipients included in 6 studies, 236 (47.3%) required vasopressor support.[7,8,11,17,19,21] The most common reason for vasopressor administration is septic shock.[19] Shock and other factors predispose the critically ill HSCT recipient to acute renal failure.[10] Renal replacement therapy was instituted in 118 of 829 HSCT recipients (14.2%) included in 3 studies.[7,13,17]

MECHANICAL VENTILATION

Most HSCT recipients are admitted to the ICU for respiratory failure and some more develop respiratory failure after ICU admission. Older age, active malignancy at time of transplantation, and donor-recipient marrow HLA mismatch are independent risks for assisted MV after marrow transplantation.[46] Among HSCT recipients

Table 1
Rate of invasive MV and associated mortality in HSCT recipients admitted to the ICU

Study	Years	Total	Invasive MV	Mortality of Invasive MV
Torrecilla[14]	1981–1987	25	16 (64%)	15 (94%)
Denardo[6]	1979–1984	50	44 (88%)	40 (91%)
Faber-Langendoen[48]	1978–1990		191	173 (91%)
Afessa[5]	1982–1990	35	27 (77%)	25 (93%)
Crawford[46]	1986–1990		348	333 (96%)
Paz[12]	1984–1991	36	28 (78%)	27 (96%)
Epler[47]	1985–1991		71	64 (90%)
Paz[16]	1984–1993		25	24 (96%)
Jackson[7]	1988–1993	116	92 (79%)	76 (83%)
Huaringa[49]	1992–1993		60	55 (92%)
Kress[51]	1993–1996		20	11 (55%)
Price[21]	1994–1996	115	48 (42%)	39 (81%)
Khassawneh[30]	1991–1999		78	58 (74%)
Afessa[19]	1996–2000	112	62 (55%)	32 (52%)
Kew[8]	1992–2001	37	25 (68%)	20 (80%)
Soubani[18]	1998–2001	85	51 (60%)	41 (80%)
Scales[13]	1992–2002	504	258 (51%)	224 (87%)
Naeem[11]	1998–2003	25	12 (48%)	10 (83%)
Pene[17]	1997–2003	209	122 (58%)	103 (84%)
Trinkaus[15]	2001–2006	34	20 (59%)	11 (55%)
Total			805/1383 (58.2%)	1381/1598 (86.4%)

Abbreviation: MV, mechanical ventilation.

admitted to ICU, 42% to 88% receive invasive MV (**Table 1**).[5–8,11–15,17–19,21] The mortality rate associated with invasive MV exceeded 80% in most of the reported studies, with an overall survival rate of only 13.6% (see **Table 1**).[5–8,11–19,21,30,46–51]

There are conflicting data regarding the factors that influence the outcome of HSCT recipients receiving MV. Price and colleagues[21] reported peripheral blood stem cell source to be associated with lower mortality. However, this was not confirmed in the study by Afessa and colleagues.[19] The cause of the respiratory failure is likely to influence the prognosis of MV in HSCT recipients. Survival is better for patients intubated for DAH or pulmonary edema.[7,49] In the study by Huaringa and colleagues,[49] 5 of 26 patients with DAH, 4 of 33 patients with pneumonia, and all 4 patients who experienced congestive heart failure/pulmonary edema survived. However, of the 7 patients with idiopathic pneumonia syndrome, bronchiolitis obliterans organizing pneumonia, multisystem organ failure, or recurrent malignancy, none survived. The mortality rate was 100% in the patients who had CMV pneumonitis (n = 9), aspergillosis (n = 5), and respiratory syncytial virus (n = 4).[49]

Two studies had shown MV duration of more than 4 and 7 days to be associated with 100% mortality.[6,14] However, this was not confirmed by later findings.[7,18] In the study by Scales and colleagues,[13] 7% of the patients intubated for 10 days or more survived. In the study by Faber-Langendoen and colleagues,[48] 7 of the 16 30-day survivors received MV for 30 days or more and 2 for 3 months or more. Despite the high short-term mortality rate associated with invasive MV, some patients survive long-term. Two large transplant centers with 539 patients in total, each reported a 6-month survival rate of 3%.[46,48] In the study by Jackson and colleagues,[7] 9 of 92 patients (10%) were alive at a median of 55 months postextubation. In the study by Huaringa and colleagues,[49] 5% were alive at 6 months. In the study by Khassawneh and colleagues,[30] 13 of 78 (17%) were alive at 6 months. In the study by Scales and colleagues,[13] the 1-year mortality of MV recipients was 87%. In the study by Pene and colleagues,[17] 6-month and 1-year survival was 14% and 10.6%, respectively.

NONINVASIVE POSITIVE PRESSURE VENTILATION

Despite some improvement, the prognosis of HSCT recipients requiring endotracheal intubation and MV has remained dismal. The use of noninvasive positive pressure ventilation (NPPV) in patients with hematologic malignancy and acute respiratory failure improves gas exchange and reduces tachypnea.[52] A randomized clinical trial of 52 immunocompromised patients, including 17 HSCT recipients with pulmonary infiltrates had shown that NPPV reduces endotracheal intubation and serious complication rates, and it reduces mortality.[53] The success of NPPV requires its early application and experienced staff with dedicated time. In a study of 237 mechanically ventilated patients with cancer, including 42 HSCT recipients admitted to the ICU, Azoulay and colleagues[54] have documented improvement in mortality in recent years. Using multiple logistic regression analysis, they showed that NPPV was partly responsible for the improved survival. Selected HSCT recipients with quickly reversible acute respiratory failure are likely to benefit from NPPV. However, the available data are scarce. Afessa and colleagues[19] reported on 71 patients treated with positive-pressure MV: NPPV only in 9 (13%), invasive only in 47 (66%), and combined invasive and NPPV in 15 (21%). In the study by Pene and colleagues,[17] 66 patients (32%) were initially treated with NPPV for a median of 2 days, of whom 44 (66%) subsequently received invasive MV. The hospital mortality of the 22 patients treated only with NPPV was 55% compared with 82% receiving invasive MV.[17]

THE IMPORTANCE OF RECENT CLINICAL TRIALS IN CRITICAL CARE

After decades of failure and negative results, recent clinical trials in critical care have revealed that some interventions improve the outcome of the critically ill. In a randomized clinical trial, Van de Berghe and colleagues[55] showed intensive insulin therapy aimed at achieving blood glucose levels between 80 and 110 mg/dL reduces the mortality rate of critically ill surgical patients, a significant number of them receiving parenteral nutrition. However, the result could not be confirmed in other groups of patients.[56,57] Moreover, intensive insulin therapy may predispose critically ill septic patients to hypoglycemia-related adverse effects.[58]

The ARDS Network group has shown that tidal volume of 6 (vs 12) mL/kg of predicted weight is associated with reduced mortality and duration of MV in patients with ALI and ARDS.[59]

In a randomized clinical trial of patients with septic shock refractory to vasopressors, Annane and colleagues[60] showed that a 7-day treatment with low-dose hydrocortisone and fludrocortisone reduces mortality in a subgroup of patients with relative adrenal insufficiency. However, the finding was not confirmed by a later trial that used different inclusion criteria and treatment.[61] In a randomized clinical trial of 1690 patients with severe sepsis and septic shock, treatment with recombinant human activated protein C reduced mortality.[62] However, the potentially life-threatening complication of recombinant human activated protein C and the premature termination of subsequent studies have led to controversies and its limited use in clinical practice.[63] In the randomized clinical trial by Rivers and colleagues,[64] early goal-directed therapy reduced the mortality rate of patients with severe sepsis and septic shock from 46.5% to 30.5%. Although there may not be clarity about which component of the therapy is responsible for the mortality reduction, its application in clinical practice has led to significant reduction of sepsis-associated mortality worldwide.[65]

The International Surviving Sepsis Campaign Guidelines make several recommendations for the management of the critically ill, based on the Grades of Recommendation, Assessment, Development and Evaluation (GRADE) system to rate the available evidence and the strength of recommendation.[66] We have listed some of these recommendations in **Table 2**. However, we advise caution when applying these recommendations to the critically ill HSCT recipient. Although the Surviving Sepsis Campaign recommendations were based on the available clinical trials, HSCT recipients were inadequately represented or actively excluded from most of these trials. The authors believe that early goal-directed therapy for severe sepsis and septic shock and a lung protective strategy with low tidal volume for ALI/ARDS are likely to benefit critically ill HSCT recipients. It is advisable to avoid hypoglycemia and hyperglycemia. However, the available conflicting data do not provide strong support to make specific recommendations about the target glucose level for critically ill HSCT recipients. Although the role of short-term, low-dose corticosteroid for septic shock has not been specifically studied in HSCT recipients, the authors believe it is unlikely to have significant adverse effect. HSCT recipients were actively excluded from the original clinical trial evaluating the role of recombinant human activated protein C.[62] An open-label, multicenter, single-arm clinical trial to investigate the safety and efficacy of recombinant human activated protein C in HSCT recipients with severe sepsis was prematurely terminated due to low enrollment: 7 patients at 3 of the 15 sites.[67] Among 6 of the 7 patients who completed the

Table 2
Recommendations for the management of severe sepsis based on the 2008 International Surviving Sepsis Campaign Guidelines[66]

Recommendation	Level of Evidence
Fluid resuscitation targeting central venous pressure of 8 (12 if positive-pressure ventilation) mm Hg	1C
Vasopressors to maintain mean arterial pressure of 65 mm Hg	1C
If central venous oxygen saturation <70% or mixed venous oxygen saturation <65% despite fluid, and hematocrit <30%, consider red blood cell transfusion	2C
If central venous oxygen saturation <70% or mixed venous oxygen saturation <65% despite fluid and hematocrit $\geq$30%, consider dobutamine	2C
Consider low dose intravenous hydrocortisone for septic shock poorly responsive to fluid and vasopressors	2C
Consider recombinant human activated protein C for sepsis induced organ dysfunction with APACHE II score $\geq$25	2B
Target a tidal volume of 6 mL/kilogram of predicted weight when ventilating patients with ALI/ARDS	1B
Use intravenous insulin to control hyperglycemia in patients with severe sepsis	1B

Abbreviation: APACHE, Acute Physiology And Chronic Health Evaluation.

drug infusion, 2 experienced serious bleeding, a nonfatal DAH, and a fatal intracranial hemorrhage. The available evidence does not justify the use of recombinant human activated protein C in HSCT recipients.

MORTALITY

Several studies have reported the short-term mortality rate of HSCT recipients admitted to the ICU (**Table 3**).[5–8,12,14–21,68–70] Overall, 772 of 1193 (65%) patients died in the hospital or within 30 days of ICU discharge (see **Table 3**). Limited data are available with regard to long-term mortality rate. The 6- to 12-month mortality rates range between 67% and 96%, with overall rate 74% (see **Table 3**). The outcome of HSCT recipients admitted to the ICU has improved over the years. Of 267 patients treated in the ICU before 1995,[5–7,12,14,16] 212 (79.4%) died compared with 327 of 502 patients (62.9%) treated after 1995[8,11,15,17–19,69] ($P<.001$). This improvement of survival over time may be due to selection bias. The earlier literature reported a very high mortality rate. This may have led health care providers to refuse admission of selected critically ill HSCT recipients to the ICU and also caused reluctance among HSCT recipients to be admitted there.[48,71] Other possible explanations for the improved outcome include wider use of colony-stimulating factors for neutropenia, more frequent use of autologous transplant, use of peripheral blood stem cell transplantation, use of corticosteroids for respiratory failure due to DAH and PERDS, earlier application of noninvasive ventilation, lung protective strategies for acute lung injury, and early goal-directed therapy for severe sepsis.

Table 3
The mortality of HSCT recipients admitted to the ICU

Study	Year	Total	Hospital and 30-Day Death (%)	6-Month to 1-Year Death (%)
Denardo[6]	1979–1984	52	43 (83)	50 (96)
Torrecilla[14]	1981–1987	23	22 (96)	
Afessa[5]	1982–1990	35	27 (77)	
Paz 1[12]	1984–1991	36	24 (67)	
Paz 2[16]	1991–1993	10	7 (70)	
Jackson[7]	1988–1993	111	89 (80)	
Price[21]	1994–1996	115	62 (54)	
Groeger[68]	1994	253	141 (56)	
Staudinger[70]		38	30 (79)	36 (95)
Afessa 2[19]	1996–2000	112	58 (52)	
Kim[69]	1999–2001	18	17 (94)	
Kew[8]	1992–2001	37	23 (62)	29 (84)
Soubani[18]	1998–2001	85	50 (59)	55/76 (72)
Scales[13]	1992–2002	504		340 (67)
Naeem[11]	1998–2003	25	18 (72)	
Pene[17]	1997–2003	209	141 (67)	165 (79)
Trinkaus[15]	2001–2006	34	20 (59)	
Overall mortality			772/1193 (65)	675/916 (74)

PROGNOSTIC FACTORS

There are several prognostic factors that may influence the outcome of HSCT recipients admitted to the ICU (**Box 2**). Advanced age, coexisting comorbidities, and lower functional status have an adverse effect on survival. Allogeneic HSCT has higher 100-day mortality than autologous HSCT.[1] The 100-day post-transplant mortality of autologous HSCT recipients with multiple myeloma is less than 5%, whereas it exceeds 10% in acute leukemia not in remission.[1] In allogeneic transplant recipients with leukemia not in remission, the 100-day mortality exceeds 20%.[1] In autologous HSCT recipients, the most common cause of death is underlying disease relapse (70%), followed by infection (8%) and organ toxicity (6%).[1] In allogeneic HSCT recipients from HLA-identical sibling donors, the most common cause of death is underlying disease relapse (41%), followed by infection (17%), GVHD (13%), and organ toxicity (10%). In allogeneic HSCT recipients from unrelated donors, the most common cause of death is underlying disease relapse (34%), followed by infection (20%), GVHD (14%), and organ toxicity (10%). Except in patients with active disease, patients receiving allogeneic transplants after reduced-intensity conditioning have lower early mortality.[1]

In the studies that reported the type of transplant, the mortality rate of allogeneic HSCT recipients admitted to ICU was 70.0% (604 of 867) compared with 58.3% (319 of 588) of autologous HSCT recipients (P<.001).[5–8,11–13,15,18,19,68–70,72,73] GVHD is also a poor prognostic factor in the critically ill HSCT recipient.[17,49] The available data do not show clear association between ICU mortality and source of stem cell. In the study by Price and colleagues,[21] there was no significant difference in overall mortality between peripheral blood stem cell and bone marrow transplant recipients. However, in patients receiving MV, the mortality rate was lower in peripheral blood stem cell recipients. Subsequent studies have not found an association between stem cell source and ICU mortality.[17,19] There are limited data with regard to umbilical

---

Box 2
Prognostic factors influencing the outcome of the critically ill HSCT recipient

Pretransplant

    Age

    Functional status

    Underlying diagnosis

Transplant-related

    Disease status at transplant

    Conditioning regimen

    Transplant type

    Source of stem cell

ICU-related

    Reason for ICU

    Admission

    Organ failure

    Severity of critical illness

cord blood transplantation and ICU outcome. In one study that included only umbilical cord blood stem cell recipients, the short-term mortality rate was 72%, which is comparable to other sources.[11] Among the 209 allogeneic HSCT recipients reported by Pene and colleagues,[17] the stem cell source was bone marrow in 67%, peripheral blood in 28%, and umbilical cord blood in 5%. The stem cell source had no effect on mortality.

The reason for ICU admission and the timing of the admission may influence outcome. Some studies have shown the presence of pneumonia,[11] gram-negative infection,[15] and infection or gastrointestinal bleeding[21] at ICU admission to be associated with increased mortality. There are conflicting data addressing the effect of the timing of ICU admission after transplant on mortality. Some studies have shown that ICU admission during an earlier period following HSCT is associated with higher mortality rate,[21,48,74] whereas others have found to the contrary.[17,21] Several other studies have not found statistically significant association between timing of ICU admission and mortality.[7,19,49,71]

The authors have described earlier the dismal prognosis of respiratory failure requiring invasive MV. The development of nonrespiratory organ failure also correlates with increased mortality.[7,8,11,13–15,17,19,21] Jackson and colleagues[7] reported 100% mortality for patients admitted to ICU with multiorgan failure. In the study by Scales and colleagues,[13] the 1-year mortality rate of HSCT recipients who received hemodialysis in the ICU was 94%. In a study by Soubani and colleagues,[18] no patient with serum lactate of more than 6 survived.

ARDS and severe sepsis are frequent complications of critically ill HSCT recipients. In a study by Afessa and colleagues,[19] the 30-day mortality rate of patients with ARDS was 74% compared with 35% of those without ARDS, and the mortality rate of patients with sepsis was 70% compared with 23% of those without sepsis.

MORTALITY PREDICTION

The clinical decision-making process regarding the critically ill often requires the active participation of health care providers and patients and surrogates. This process is facilitated by knowledge of the patient's prognosis. Although they have no role in individual patient decision-making, there are several adult ICU prognostic models developed and validated to predict the probability of hospital death.[75] The adult ICU prognostic models are derived from age, comorbidities, lead time bias, ICU admission diagnosis and admission source, and physiologic variables. The latest versions of the adult ICU prognostic models are Simplified Acute Physiology Score (SAPS) 3,[76,77] Acute Physiology and Chronic Health Evaluation (APACHE) IV[78] and Mortality Prediction Model (MPM) III.[79] The pertinent comorbidities included in these models are immunosuppression/hematologic malignancy in APACHE IV,[78] hematological malignancies in SAPS 3,[76,77] and metastatic neoplasm in MPM III.[79] There are no data evaluating the performance of these new models in predicting the prognosis of the critically ill HSCT recipient. Although these models were based on data from tens and hundreds of thousands of patients, critically ill HSCT patients were not adequately represented. Among the older generation adult ICU prognostic models, APACHE II[80] and III,[81] SAPS II,[82] and MPM II[83] have been studied in the critically ill HSCT recipient. Several studies have shown nonsurvivors to have higher APACHE II[7,12,15,18,21] and APACHE III[19] scores, and MPM II predicted probability of death[18,21] compared with survivors. APACHE II, SAPS II, and MPM II models underestimate the mortality rate of the HSCT patient admitted to the ICU.[5,7,21] In the study by Jackson and colleagues,[7] mortality was 100% when APACHE II score exceeded 45. In a study of

414 patients with cancer, including 38 HSCT recipients admitted to the ICU, all patients with APACHE III score exceeding 80 died in the ICU.[70] Most of the studies addressing the role of the adult ICU prognostic models in HSCT recipients did not describe the discrimination and calibration of the models. In the study by Afessa and colleagues,[19] the observed and APACHE III-predicted hospital mortality rates were 46% and 42%, respectively, and the area under the receiver operating characteristic curve was 0.704 with good calibration (Hosmer-Lemeshow statistic 6.563, $P = .564$).

Accurate estimation of the risk of death is important in clinical trials, epidemiologic studies, and most importantly, in clinical practice. Because of the high human and financial costs, the accurate estimation of risk is most important in ICU patients. Because prediction models, including the adult ICU ones based on data from the general population, are unlikely to give us accurate estimation for the risk of HSCT recipient death, some have tried to develop disease-specific models. Parimon and colleagues[84] had reported a model for predicting the 2-year risk of death following allogeneic HSCT. However, this model is not specific for HSCT patients admitted to the ICU. Groeger and colleagues[68] developed and validated a model for predicting mortality of patients with cancer, including 253 HSCT recipients admitted to the ICU. The study included 1713 patients from 4 large cancer centers. The model included 16 predictor variables: PaO_2/FIO_2 ratio, platelet count, respiratory rate, systolic blood pressure, pre-ICU hospital days, intracranial mass effect, allogeneic bone marrow transplantation, recurrent or progressive cancer, albumin less than 2.5 g/dL, bilirubin 2 mg/dL or more, Glasgow Coma Scale score less than 6, prothrombin time more than 15 seconds, blood urea nitrogen more than 50 mg/dL, endotracheal intubation, performance status before hospitalization, and cardiopulmonary resuscitation.[68] The calibration was good for the development and validation models. The areas under the receiver operating characteristic curves were 0.812 and 0.802 for the development and validation models, respectively. Although other studies have also reported multiple logistic regression models based on variables obtained in HSCT recipients admitted to the ICU,[7,19,21] they are not as well described and validated as the model by Groeger and colleagues.[68]

TRIAGE FOR ICU ADMISSION

Intensivists and hematologists/oncologists often face the question of whether or not to transfer a clinically deteriorating HSCT recipient to the ICU. Because most of the intensivists do not participate in the pre- and post- ICU care of HSCT recipients, they are familiar only with the tip of the iceberg. Thiery and colleagues[85] reported that intensivists and hematologists/oncologists disagree 15% of the time on ICU admission triage decisions for patients with cancer. Appropriate triage for ICU admission is extremely important, especially in institutions with limited critical care resources, and it requires the active participation of intensivists, hematologists/oncologists, and patients and their surrogates for health care. There is a consensus in principle that patients too well or too sick to benefit from ICU support should be denied ICU admission. However, the intensivists' judgement in determining who is sick enough to benefit from ICU admission is far from perfect. In a prospective study of 206 patients with cancer considered for ICU admission, the intensivists considered 47 patients (22.8%) too well and 54 patients (26.2%) too sick to benefit from ICU admission.[85] Of the 47 patients considered too well, 13 (28%) were subsequently admitted to ICU. The 30-day mortality rate of the 54 patients considered too sick was 74%. One of the authors' institutions has implemented a triage policy for ICU admission of patients with cancer.[86] According

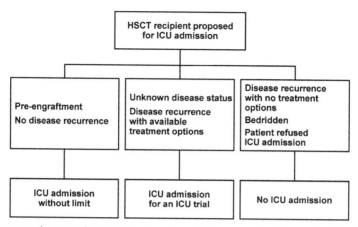

Fig. 1. Suggested approach in triaging hematopoietic stem cell recipients for ICU admission.

to the policy, patients with cancer who have previously untreated malignancy, acute tumor lysis syndrome, or a bulky or infiltrating tumor at the earliest phase of treatment, and patients in complete remission are admitted to the ICU for full, unlimited support. Bedridden patients and patients with palliative care as the only treatment option and those who refuse ICU admission are not admitted. All other groups of patients are admitted to ICU on a trial basis, with full ICU support for 4 days and reevaluation on day 5 for the appropriate level of care. In a prospective study, called the ICU Trial, Lecuyer and colleagues[86] reported their experience with such a policy. Among 188 patients (including 24 autologous HSCT recipients) admitted for ICU Trial, 85 (45.2%) died within the first 4 ICU days. Among the 103 5-day survivors, 14 had received and 31 were scheduled to receive autologous HSCT; all those who received MV, vasopressors, or dialysis beyond the third ICU day died.[86] With improving critical care support, there are several reports of HSCT recipients who survive 3 days of MV and other ICU organ support. Based on the available data, the authors recommend saying "yes" more often than "no" in considering HSCT recipients for ICU admission (**Fig. 1**).[87] Lowering the level of care after ICU trial is not an uncommon practice. In the study by DeNardo and colleagues,[6] do-not-resuscitate (DNR) orders were written in 26 of 50 HSCT recipients (52%) at a mean of 10 days after ICU admission. Similarly, in 2 studies from Mayo Clinic, DNR orders were written in 24 of 35 (68%) and 40 of 112 (36%) HSCT recipients.[5,19] In the study by Soubani and colleagues,[18] 22 of 33 ICU deaths followed life support withdrawal.

SUMMARY

HSCT recipients often develop life-threatening complications following transplant for lethal conditions. Although the mortality rate of HSCT recipients admitted to the ICU has declined over the last 2 decades, it still exceeds 80% in those receiving MV. With improvement in transplantation and critical care, we expect the prognosis of the critically ill to get better. Researchers need to continue their efforts to find better treatment modalities and describe the effect of the modalities on patient outcome. For appropriate use of limited ICU resources, reliable prognostication models need to be developed. When triaging HSCT recipients for ICU admission, the status of the patients' underlying disease, short- and long-term prognostic factors, and the patients' wishes should be incorporated into the decision-making process.

REFERENCES

1. Pasquini MC, Wang Z, Schneider L. Current use and outcome of hematopoietic stem cell transplantation: part I - CIBMTR Summary Slides. Available at: http://www.cibmtr.org/PUBLICATIONS/Newsletter/DOCS/2007Dec.pdf.   Accessed June 11, 2009.
2. Matulis M, High KP. Immune reconstitution after hematopoietic stem-cell transplantation and its influence on respiratory infections. Semin Respir Infect 2002; 17(2):130–9.
3. Ninin E, Milpied N, Moreau P, et al. Longitudinal study of bacterial, viral, and fungal infections in adult recipients of bone marrow transplants. Clin Infect Dis 2001;33(1):41–7.
4. McArdle JR. Critical care outcomes in the hematologic transplant recipient. Clin Chest Med 2009;30(1):155–67.
5. Afessa B, Tefferi A, Hoagland HC, et al. Outcome of recipients of bone marrow transplants who require intensive- care unit support. Mayo Clin Proc 1992; 67(2):117–22.
6. DeNardo SJ, Oye RK, Bellamy PE. Efficacy of intensive care for bone marrow transplant patients with respiratory failure. Crit Care Med 1989;17(1):4–6.
7. Jackson SR, Tweeddale MG, Barnett MJ, et al. Admission of bone marrow transplant recipients to the intensive care unit: outcome, survival and prognostic factors. Bone Marrow Transplant 1998;21(7):697–704.
8. Kew AK, Couban S, Patrick W, et al. Outcome of hematopoietic stem cell transplant recipients admitted to the intensive care unit. Biol Blood Marrow Transplant 2006;12(3):301–5.
9. Kim DH, Kim JG, Lee NY, et al. Risk factors for late cytomegalovirus infection after allogeneic stem cell transplantation using HLA-matched sibling donor: donor lymphocyte infusion and previous history of early CMV infection. Bone Marrow Transplant 2004;34(1):21–7.
10. Letourneau I, Dorval M, Belanger R, et al. Acute renal failure in bone marrow transplant patients admitted to the intensive care unit. Nephron 2002;90(4):408–12.
11. Naeem N, Eyzaguirre A, Kern JA, et al. Outcome of adult umbilical cord blood transplant patients admitted to a medical intensive care unit. Bone Marrow Transplant 2006;38(11):733–8.
12. Paz HL, Crilley P, Weinar M, et al. Outcome of patients requiring medical ICU admission following bone marrow transplantation. Chest 1993;104(2):527–31.
13. Scales DC, Thiruchelvam D, Kiss A, et al. Intensive care outcomes in bone marrow transplant recipients: a population-based cohort analysis. Crit Care 2008;12(3):R77.
14. Torrecilla C, Cortes JL, Chamorro C, et al. Prognostic assessment of the acute complications of bone marrow transplantation requiring intensive therapy. Intensive Care Med 1988;14(4):393–8.
15. Trinkaus MA, Lapinsky SE, Crump M, et al. Predictors of mortality in patients undergoing autologous hematopoietic cell transplantation admitted to the intensive care unit. Bone Marrow Transplant 2009;43(5):411–5.
16. Paz HL, Garland A, Weinar M, et al. Effect of clinical outcomes data on intensive care unit utilization by bone marrow transplant patients. Crit Care Med 1998; 26(1):66–70.
17. Pene F, Aubron C, Azoulay E, et al. Outcome of critically ill allogeneic hematopoietic stem-cell transplantation recipients: a reappraisal of indications for organ failure supports. J Clin Oncol 2006;24(4):643–9.

18. Soubani AO, Kseibi E, Bander JJ, et al. Outcome and prognostic factors of hematopoietic stem cell transplantation recipients admitted to a medical ICU. Chest 2004;126(5):1604–11.
19. Afessa B, Tefferi A, Dunn WF, et al. Intensive care unit support and Acute Physiology and Chronic Health Evaluation III performance in hematopoietic stem cell transplant recipients. Crit Care Med 2003;31(6):1715–21.
20. Naeem N, Reed MD, Creger RJ, et al. Transfer of the hematopoietic stem cell transplant patient to the intensive care unit: does it really matter? Bone Marrow Transplant 2006;37(2):119–33.
21. Price KJ, Thall PF, Kish SK, et al. Prognostic indicators for blood and marrow transplant patients admitted to an intensive care unit. Am J Respir Crit Care Med 1998;158(3):876–84.
22. Peters SG, Afessa B. Acute lung injury after hematopoietic stem cell transplantation. Clin Chest Med 2005;26(4):561–9.
23. Afessa B, Tefferi A, Litzow MR, et al. Outcome of diffuse alveolar hemorrhage in hematopoietic stem cell transplant recipients. Am J Respir Crit Care Med 2002;166(10):1364–8.
24. Afessa B, Tefferi A, Litzow MR, et al. Diffuse alveolar hemorrhage in hematopoietic stem cell transplant recipients. Am J Respir Crit Care Med 2002;166(5):641–5.
25. Afessa B, Peters SG. Major Complications following Hematopoietic Stem Cell Transplantation. Semin Respir Crit Care Med 2006;27(3):297–309.
26. Pihusch R, Salat C, Schmidt E, et al. Hemostatic complications in bone marrow transplantation: a retrospective analysis of 447 patients. Transplantation 2002;74(9):1303–9.
27. Nevo S, Swan V, Enger C, et al. Acute bleeding after bone marrow transplantation (BMT)- incidence and effect on survival. A quantitative analysis in 1,402 patients. Blood 1998;9(14):1469–77.
28. Bleggi-Torres LF, Werner B, Gasparetto EL, et al. Intracranial hemorrhage following bone marrow transplantation: an autopsy study of 58 patients. Bone Marrow Transplant 2002;29(1):29–32.
29. Chirletti P, Caronna R, Arcese W, et al. Gastrointestinal emergencies in patients with acute intestinal graft-versus-host disease. Leuk Lymphoma 1998;29(1–2):129–37.
30. Khassawneh BY, White P Jr, Anaissie EJ, et al. Outcome from mechanical ventilation after autologous peripheral blood stem cell transplantation. Chest 2002;121(1):185–8.
31. Harvey S, Young D, Brampton W, et al. Pulmonary artery catheters for adult patients in intensive care. Cochrane Database Syst Rev 2006;(3):CD003408.
32. Connors AF Jr, Speroff T, Dawson NV, et al. The effectiveness of right heart catheterization in the initial care of critically ill patients. SUPPORT Investigators. JAMA 1996;276(11):889–97.
33. Feinstein MB, Mokhtari M, Ferreiro R, et al. Fiberoptic bronchoscopy in allogeneic bone marrow transplantation: findings in the era of serum cytomegalovirus antigen surveillance. Chest 2001;120(4):1094–100.
34. Hofmeister CC, Czerlanis C, Forsythe S, et al. Retrospective utility of bronchoscopy after hematopoietic stem cell transplant. Bone Marrow Transplant 2006;38(10):693–8.
35. Kasow KA, King E, Rochester R, et al. Diagnostic yield of bronchoalveolar lavage is low in allogeneic hematopoietic stem cell recipients receiving immunosuppressive therapy or with acute graft-versus-host disease: the St. Jude experience, 1990–2002. Biol Blood Marrow Transplant 2007;13(7):831–7.

36. Patel NR, Lee PS, Kim JH, et al. The influence of diagnostic bronchoscopy on clinical outcomes comparing adult autologous and allogeneic bone marrow transplant patients. Chest 2005;127(4):1388–96.
37. Soubani AO, Qureshi MA, Baynes RD. Flexible bronchoscopy in the diagnosis of pulmonary infiltrates following autologous peripheral stem cell transplantation for advanced breast cancer. Bone Marrow Transplant 2001;28(10):981–5.
38. Springmeyer SC, Silvestri RC, Sale GE, et al. The role of transbronchial biopsy for the diagnosis of diffuse pneumonias in immunocompromised marrow transplant recipients. Am Rev Respir Dis 1982;126(5):763–5.
39. Azoulay E, Mokart D, Rabbat A, et al. Diagnostic bronchoscopy in hematology and oncology patients with acute respiratory failure: prospective multicenter data. Crit Care Med 2008;36(1):100–7.
40. Bishton M, Chopra R. The role of granulocyte transfusions in neutropenic patients. Br J Haematol 2004;127(5):501–8.
41. Hubel K, Carter RA, Liles WC, et al. Granulocyte transfusion therapy for infections in candidates and recipients of HPC transplantation: a comparative analysis of feasibility and outcome for community donors versus related donors. Transfusion 2002;42(11):1414–21.
42. Stanworth SJ, Massey E, Hyde C, et al. Granulocyte transfusions for treating infections in patients with neutropenia or neutrophil dysfunction. Cochrane Database Syst Rev 2005;(3):CD005339.
43. Holler E, Kolb HJ, Greinix H, et al. Bleeding events and mortality in SCT patients: a retrospective study of hematopoietic SCT patients with organ dysfunctions due to severe sepsis or GVHD. Bone Marrow Transplant 2009;43(6):491–7.
44. Schiffer CA, Anderson KC, Bennett CL, et al. Platelet transfusion for patients with cancer: clinical practice guidelines of the American Society of Clinical Oncology. J Clin Oncol 2001;19(5):1519–38.
45. Murphy MF, Wallington TB, Kelsey P, et al. Guidelines for the clinical use of red cell transfusions. Br J Haematol 2001;113(1):24–31.
46. Crawford SW, Petersen FB. Long-term survival from respiratory failure after marrow transplantation for malignancy. Am Rev Respir Dis 1992;145(3):510–4.
47. Epner DE, White P, Krasnoff M, et al. Outcome of mechanical ventilation for adults with hematologic malignancy. J Investig Med 1996;44(5):254–60.
48. Faber-Langendoen K, Caplan AL, McGlave PB. Survival of adult bone marrow transplant patients receiving mechanical ventilation: a case for restricted use. Bone Marrow Transplant 1993;12(5):501–7.
49. Huaringa AJ, Leyva FJ, Giralt SA, et al. Outcome of bone marrow transplantation patients requiring mechanical ventilation [see comments]. Crit Care Med 2000; 28(4):1014–7.
50. Ishida T, Arita M, Fujimori N. [Diffuse alveolar hemorrhage after allogeneic bone marrow transplantation]. Nihon Kyobu Shikkan Gakkai Zasshi 1996; 34(3):369–73 [in Japanese].
51. Kress JP, Christenson J, Pohlman AS, et al. Outcomes of critically ill cancer patients in a university hospital setting. Am J Respir Crit Care Med 1999; 160(6):1957–61.
52. Conti G, Marino P, Cogliati A, et al. Noninvasive ventilation for the treatment of acute respiratory failure in patients with hematologic malignancies: a pilot study. Intensive Care Med 1998;24(12):1283–8.
53. Hilbert G, Gruson D, Vargas F, et al. Noninvasive ventilation in immunosuppressed patients with pulmonary infiltrates, fever, and acute respiratory failure. N Engl J Med 2001;344(7):481–7.

54. Azoulay E, Alberti C, Bornstain C, et al. Improved survival in cancer patients requiring mechanical ventilatory support: impact of noninvasive mechanical ventilatory support. Crit Care Med 2001;29(3):519–25.
55. Van den Berghe G, Wouters P, Weekers F, et al. Intensive insulin therapy in the critically ill patients. N Engl J Med 2001;345(19):1359–67.
56. Van den Berghe G, Wilmer A, Hermans G, et al. Intensive insulin therapy in the medical ICU. N Engl J Med 2006;354(5):449–61.
57. Finfer S, Chittock DR, Su SY, et al. Intensive versus conventional glucose control in critically ill patients. N Engl J Med 2009;360(13):1283–97.
58. Brunkhorst FM, Engel C, Bloos F, et al. Intensive insulin therapy and pentastarch resuscitation in severe sepsis. N Engl J Med 2008;358(2):125–39.
59. Ventilation with lower tidal volumes as compared with traditional tidal volumes for acute lung injury and the acute respiratory distress syndrome. The Acute Respiratory Distress Syndrome Network. N Engl J Med 2000;342(18):1301–8.
60. Annane D, Sebille V, Charpentier C, et al. Effect of treatment with low doses of hydrocortisone and fludrocortisone on mortality in patients with septic shock. JAMA 2002;288(7):862–71.
61. Sprung CL, Annane D, Keh D, et al. Hydrocortisone therapy for patients with septic shock. N Engl J Med 2008;358(2):111–24.
62. Bernard GR, Vincent JL, Laterre PF, et al. Efficacy and safety of recombinant human activated protein C for severe sepsis. N Engl J Med 2001;344(10):699–709.
63. Eichacker PQ, Natanson C, Danner RL. Surviving sepsis–practice guidelines, marketing campaigns, and Eli Lilly. N Engl J Med 2006;355(16):1640–2.
64. Rivers E, Nguyen B, Havstad S, et al. Early goal-directed therapy in the treatment of severe sepsis and septic shock. N Engl J Med 2001;345(19):1368–77.
65. Ferrer R, Artigas A, Levy MM, et al. Improvement in process of care and outcome after a multicenter severe sepsis educational program in Spain. JAMA 2008;299(19):2294–303.
66. Dellinger RP, Levy MM, Carlet JM, et al. Surviving sepsis campaign: international guidelines for management of severe sepsis and septic shock: 2008. Crit Care Med 2008;36(1):296–327.
67. Pastores SM, Shaw A, Williams MD, et al. A safety evaluation of drotrecogin alfa (activated) in hematopoietic stem cell transplant patients with severe sepsis: lessons in clinical research. Bone Marrow Transplant 2005;36(8):721–4.
68. Groeger JS, Lemeshow S, Price K, et al. Multicenter outcome study of cancer patients admitted to the intensive care unit: a probability of mortality model. J Clin Oncol 1998;16(2):761–70.
69. Kim SW, Kami M, Urahama N, et al. Feasibility of acute physiology and chronic health evaluation (APACHE) II and III score-based screening in patients receiving allogeneic hematopoietic stem-cell transplantation. Transplantation 2003;75(4):566–70.
70. Staudinger T, Stoiser B, Mullner M, et al. Outcome and prognostic factors in critically ill cancer patients admitted to the intensive care unit. Crit Care Med 2000;28(5):1322–8.
71. Rubenfeld GD, Crawford SW. Withdrawing life support from mechanically ventilated recipients of bone marrow transplants: a case for evidence-based guidelines. Ann Intern Med 1996;125(8):625–33.
72. Alasaly K, Muller N, Ostrow DN, et al. Cryptogenic organizing pneumonia. A report of 25 cases and a review of the literature. Medicine (Baltimore) 1995;74(4):201–11.

73. Prince DS, Wingard JR, Saral R, et al. Longitudinal changes in pulmonary function following bone marrow transplantation. Chest 1989;96(2):301–6.

74. Ewig S, Torres A, Riquelme R, et al. Pulmonary complications in patients with haematological malignancies treated at a respiratory ICU. Eur Respir J 1998;12(1):116–22.

75. Afessa B, Gajic O, Keegan MT. Severity of illness and organ failure assessment in adult intensive care units. Crit Care Clin 2007;23(3):639–58.

76. Metnitz PG, Moreno RP, Almeida E, et al. SAPS 3–From evaluation of the patient to evaluation of the intensive care unit. Part 1: objectives, methods and cohort description. Intensive Care Med 2005;31(10):1336–44.

77. Moreno RP, Metnitz PG, Almeida E, et al. SAPS 3–From evaluation of the patient to evaluation of the intensive care unit. Part 2: development of a prognostic model for hospital mortality at ICU admission. Intensive Care Med 2005;31(10):1345–55.

78. Zimmerman JE, Kramer AA, McNair DS, et al. Acute Physiology and Chronic Health Evaluation (APACHE) IV: hospital mortality assessment for today's critically ill patients. Crit Care Med 2006;34(5):1297–310.

79. Higgins TL, Teres D, Copes WS, et al. Assessing contemporary intensive care unit outcome: an updated Mortality Probability Admission Model (MPM0-III). Crit Care Med 2007;35(3):827–35.

80. Knaus WA, Draper EA, Wagner DP, et al. APACHE II: a severity of disease classification system. Crit Care Med 1985;13(10):818–29.

81. Knaus WA, Wagner DP, Draper EA, et al. The APACHE III prognostic system. Risk prediction of hospital mortality for critically ill hospitalized adults. Chest 1991;100(6):1619–36.

82. Le Gall JR, Lemeshow S, Saulnier F. A new Simplified Acute Physiology Score (SAPS II) based on a European/North American multicenter study. JAMA 1993;270(24):2957–63.

83. Lemeshow S, Teres D, Klar J, et al. Mortality Probability Models (MPM II) based on an international cohort of intensive care unit patients. JAMA 1993;270(20):2478–86.

84. Parimon T, Au DH, Martin PJ, et al. A risk score for mortality after allogeneic hematopoietic cell transplantation. Ann Intern Med 2006;144(6):407–14.

85. Thiery G, Azoulay E, Darmon M, et al. Outcome of cancer patients considered for intensive care unit admission: a hospital-wide prospective study. J Clin Oncol 2005;23(19):4406–13.

86. Lecuyer L, Chevret S, Thiery G, et al. The ICU trial: a new admission policy for cancer patients requiring mechanical ventilation. Crit Care Med 2007;35(3):808–14.

87. Azoulay E, Afessa B. The intensive care support of patients with malignancy: do everything that can be done. Intensive Care Med 2006;32(1):3–5.

Acute Kidney Injury in Critically Ill Patients with Cancer

Dominique D. Benoit, MD, PhD[a],*, Eric A. Hoste, MD, PhD[b]

KEYWORDS

• Cancer • ICU • Acute kidney injury • Renal replacement therapy

The prognosis of cancer patients has substantially improved over the past 2 decades.[1] These improvements have been mainly achieved through the use of new or intensive chemotherapeutic regimens coupled with a better risk stratification of patients due to advances in radiology, immunohistology, and cytogenetics, and through the advances in supportive care. Unfortunately, this has also led to an increased occurrence of potential life-threatening complications requiring treatment in the intensive care unit (ICU).[2]

Acute kidney injury (AKI) is a common and dreaded complication in this population. Cancer patients who are admitted to the ICU with or because of AKI, or who develop AKI during their ICU stay typically have worse outcomes, especially in the presence of multiple organ failure.[2–6] Until recently, it remained a matter of controversy whether these patients would benefit from advanced life-supportive therapy[2,7–10] including renal replacement therapy (RRT).[11] Several studies in different settings worldwide have now shown that the presence of an underlying cancer alone can no longer be considered a contraindication to start RRT[12–15] or to refer such patients to the ICU for advanced life-supportive therapy,[15–36] even after the recent administration[37] or for the urgent initiation of systemic chemotherapy.[38,39] Moreover, whereas survival of cancer patients who require RRT in the presence of multiple organ failure was exceptional until about a decade ago,[4–6,9,10,21,22] this is no longer so today,[12–15,23,25] especially in the setting of septic shock.[12,20,27] A notable exception remains the critically ill allogeneic bone marrow or peripheral stem cell transplantation recipient,[40,41] although even in this setting some improvement in outcome has been achieved.[42]

AKI may also have serious implications for critically ill cancer survivors. Duration of mechanical ventilation is longer in cancer patients with AKI than in those without AKI.[43]

[a] Department of Intensive Care Medicine, Medical Unit, 12K12IB, Ghent University Hospital, De Pintelaan 185, 9000 Gent, Belgium
[b] Department of Intensive Care Medicine, Surgical Unit, 1K12IC, Ghent University Hospital, De Pintelaan 185, 9000 Gent, Belgium
* Corresponding author.
E-mail address: dominique.benoit@ugent.be (D.D. Benoit).

Crit Care Clin 26 (2010) 151–179
doi:10.1016/j.ccc.2009.09.002
0749-0704/09/$ – see front matter © 2010 Elsevier Inc. All rights reserved.
criticalcare.theclinics.com

Impairment in the functional status resulting from protracted ICU and hospital stay together with an incomplete or delayed recovery in renal function may compromise the optimal administration of potentially life-saving chemotherapy, thereby further affecting the long-term prognosis of these patients.[3,14,15] Thus, early identification of patients at risk of AKI followed by, when possible, preventive measures or early interventions will be of critical importance to try to reduce the associated mortality, morbidity, and economic burden in these patients.

Preventive measures aiming to improve the outcome of critically ill cancer patients developing AKI are, however, largely cause-specific. Most often, AKI results from several nephrotoxic insults in cancer patients, although a main cause is often identifiable in daily practice.[3,6,12–15] AKI may occur as a direct (ie, malignant invasion of the kidney, urinary tract obstruction) or indirect (ie, thrombotic thrombocytopenic purpura/hemolytic uremic syndrome, hypercalcemia) consequence of the cancer itself, its treatment (ie, drug induced nephropathy, tumor lysis syndrome), or associated complications (ie, septic shock, cardiac failure). Unfortunately, sepsis is by far the most common main cause of AKI in cancer patients,[3,6,12–15] and AKI in this setting is much less easy to prevent and to treat than AKI resulting from tumor lysis syndrome (TLS) and contrast- or drug-induced AKI.

The aim of this article is to provide a comprehensive overview of AKI in adult critically ill cancer patients. First, the definitions of AKI are expanded. The authors subsequently focus on the incidence, mortality, and morbidity of AKI in critically ill cancer patients, and compare these issues with the general ICU population with AKI. Third, an overview is given of the main causes of AKI in critically cancer patients and how to prevent or treat them. Finally, the authors focus on the difficult exercise of ICU and referral to treatment triage decision making in the individual critically ill cancer patient. Given the limited data available, critically ill allogeneic hematopoietic stem cell recipients with AKI are only briefly commented on throughout this article. The reader is referred to a recent review that focuses on this population in the non-ICU setting.[44]

DEFINITION AND EARLY IDENTIFICATION OF ACUTE KIDNEY INJURY

A major limitation to the correct interpretation of data on the epidemiology of AKI is the use of different definitions for AKI. At least 35 different definitions for AKI are used in the medical literature,[45,46] ranging from minor derangement of kidney function to severe AKI, such as AKI defined by the need for treatment with RRT. Comparison of incidence and outcome data of studies on AKI are hampered by this abundance of definitions. The RIFLE classification (Risk of renal dysfunction, Injury to the kidney, Failure of kidney function, Loss of kidney function, End-stage kidney disease) for AKI is a consensus definition that was developed by experts in AKI.[45] This definition was later slightly modified and renamed into the AKI diagnostic and staging system by the Acute Kidney Injury Network (AKIN), a collaboration between the major world societies on nephrology and intensive care medicine.[47] The RIFLE classification was welcomed by the AKI society, as can be concluded from the fact that, since its publication, over 30 studies including more than 300,000 patients have been published in which this classification was used. In addition, in recent years almost all studies on AKI have used the RIFLE classification.[46]

The RIFLE classification defines AKI according to an increase of serum creatinine or a decrease of in urine output into 3 increasing severity stages: RIFLE-*R*isk, -*I*njury, and -*F*ailure, or AKI stages 1 to 3 (**Fig. 1**). Patients meet the diagnostic criteria for AKI when they meet the criteria for RIFLE-Risk or stage 1 AKI within a 48-hour period. At present, there remains limited clinical experience regarding the minor modifications in the AKI

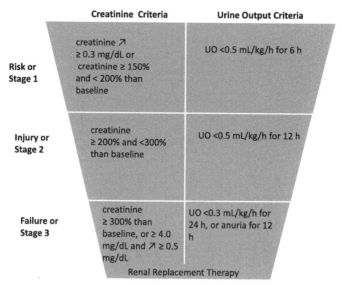

Fig. 1. Classification of AKI. The RIFLE and AKI staging system. UO, urine output. (*Adapted from* Bellomo R, Ronco C, Kellum JA, et al. Acute renal failure—definition, outcome measures, animal models, fluid therapy and information technology needs: the Second International Consensus Conference of the Acute Dialysis Quality Initiative (ADQI) Group. Crit Care 2004;8(4):R204–12; with permission. Also available on the Acute Dialysis Quality Initiative Web site, http://www.ccm.upmc.edu/adqi/ADQI2/ADQI2g1.pdf.)

staging system, but the initial reports demonstrate that it calibrates well with the RIFLE classification.[48]

The RIFLE is a very sensitive classification, yet clinically relevant, as patients meeting the RIFLE criteria demonstrate poorer outcome. Even after adjusting for other covariates for mortality the odds ratio (OR) for in-hospital mortality for RIFLE-Risk, -Injury, -Failure were 1.5, 2, and 3, respectively.[46]

Because of the many variable definitions for AKI that have been used over time in the literature, this article essentially focuses on AKI patients treated with RRT.

EPIDEMIOLOGY OF ACUTE KIDNEY INJURY IN CRITICALLY ILL CANCER PATIENTS

The incidence and hospital mortality associated with RRT in the general critically ill cancer population and the most important subgroups are depicted in detail in **Tables 1** and **2**, respectively. These tables include studies from 1990 onwards, focusing exclusively on cancer patients admitted to the ICU with life-threatening complications and for whom sufficient data were available.[5,6,9,12–39] Studies mainly focusing on postsurgical cancer patients were not considered. The studies comparing outcomes between AKI patients with and without comorbidities under which cancer patients were included are discussed here.[49–52]

Incidence

Critically ill cancer patients have a higher incidence of AKI treated with RRT than critically ill patients without cancer.[12,14,32,49–51] It is important to bear in mind that the differences in occurrence rate between these 2 populations are probably underestimated in all these studies because of selection and treatment bias due to the higher

Table 1
Incidence or short-term (ICU, 28-day, or hospital) mortality associated with renal replacement therapy (RRT) in patients with hematologic malignancies and solid tumors admitted to the ICU[a]

	Authors, Year	No. of Patients	Admission Period	Severity of Illness	Hematologic Malignancy (%)/Allo-BM or PBSCT (%)	RRT Incidence (%)	RRT Mortality (%)
1	Brunet et al, 1990[4]	260	1983–1987	SAPS 14 MV 43%/Vasopressors NR	100%/0%	13%	73%
2	Azoulay et al, 2000[17]	120	1990–1997	SAPS II 36 MV 54%/Vasopressors 37%	0%/0%	9%	NR
3	Evison et al, 2001[5]	78	1990–1997	APACHE II 18 MV 43%/Vasopressors 47%	100%/54%	10%	75%
4	Silfvast et al, 2003[9]	30	1994–1998	APACHE II/SAPS II NR[b] MV 77%/Vasopressors NR	100%/0%	17%	80%
5	Maschmeyer et al, 2003[25]	189	1998–1999	APACHE II/SAPS II NR MV 50%/Vasopressors 50%	46%/NR[c]	26%	66%
6	Kroschinsky et al, 2002[10]	104	1995–2000	SAPS II 46 MV 52%/Vasopressors NR	100%/0%	18%	68%
7	Benoit et al, 2003[21]	124	1997–2000	APACHE II 26/SAPS II 53 MV 47%/Vasopressors 46%	100%/18%	27%	88%
8	Lamia et al, 2006[23]	92	2000–2003	SAPS II 60 MV 64%/Vasopressors 50%	100%/12%	33%	73%
9	Soares et al, 2006[28]	862	2000–2004	SAPS II 43 MV 71%/Vasopressors 54%	18%/0%	13%	NR
10	Merz et al, 2008[35]	101	2001–2005	SAPSII 48 MV 55%/Vasopressors NR	100%/<12%	11.8%	75%
11	Taccone et al, 2009[32]	473	May 2002	SAPS II NR[b] MV 64%/Vasopressors 43%	15%/NR	10%	NR

Abbreviations: allo-BM, allogeneic bone marrow; APACHE, Acute Physiology and Chronic Health Evaluation; NR, not reported; PBSCT, peripheral blood stem cell transplant; SAPS, Simplified Acute Physiology Score.
[a] Based on the most important studies published since 1990 focusing on critically ill cancer patients exclusively.
[b] APACHE II and/or SAPS II not available for the general study population.
[c] Not specified whether autologous or allogeneic hematopoietic transplantation.

number of decisions to forgo life-sustaining treatments in cancer patients both at the ward level and in the ICUs,[53] especially in centers that have less experience in the treatment of these complex patients. In a study from the authors' center, 55 of the 222 (22.5%) patients with hematologic malignancies admitted to the medical ICU between 1997 and 2002 received RRT compared with 248 of the 4293 (5.8%) patients without hematologic malignancy (P<.001).[12] Darmon and colleagues[14] reported similar incidences; 94 of the 538 (17.4%) hematologic and solid tumor patients admitted to the ICU between January 2002 and June 2005 received RRT compared with 91 of the 1367 (6.7%) patients without cancer (P<.001). Finally, Taccone and colleagues[32] found that patients with hematologic malignancies in European ICUs were at particularly higher risk for developing AKI; 21.7% received RRT compared with 8% of the solid tumor patients and 11.4% in general ICU patients. Larger studies focusing on the impact of underlying comorbidities in the general ICU population with AKI confirm these findings. Bagshaw and colleagues[50] found that critically ill cancer patients had a higher risk for severe AKI; however, the risk was lower than in critically ill cardiac and, rather unexpectedly, lower than in critically ill stroke and chronic pulmonary disease patients, the latter suggesting treatment bias. The same investigators recently reported that patients with underlying liver disease had the highest incidence of AKI (12.1%), followed by patients with hematologic malignancies (10.5%) and metastatic cancer patients (8.2%).[49] In another large multicenter cohort study by de Mendonça and colleagues,[51] the odds ratio for the development of AKI (defined as serum creatinine >3.5 mg/dL or a urine output <500 mL/d during the ICU stay) in patients with underlying lymphoma and leukemia admitted to the ICU was 2.2 times higher than in patients without an underlying comorbidity after adjustment for confounding variables. In contrast, Merz and colleagues[35] reported no difference in incidence in RRT between patients with (12/101, 11.8%) and without underlying hematologic malignancy (299/3808, 7.8%) admitted between 2001 and 2005 in a tertiary university hospital ICU. The higher incidence of AKI and RRT in critically ill cancer patients is probably attributable to the higher susceptibility for infections,[14,20,24,27,32,35] and to the more frequent use of nephrotoxic antimicrobial and chemotherapeutic drugs in this population[6,12–15] although, of interest, the authors' group found that previous chemotherapy within the 3 weeks before ICU admission did not have an impact on the incidence of RRT in 186 hematologic cancer patients admitted with severe sepsis and septic shock.[37]

Depending on the definition of AKI and the case-mix in the study population, between 13% and 42% of the cancer patients admitted to the ICU have AKI and 8.0% to 59.6% receive RRT during their ICU stay (see **Tables 1 and 2**). The reported incidences are usually higher in critically ill patients with hematologic malignancies, particularly in those suffering from multiple myeloma, and in the subgroups of cancer patients with septic shock. The incidence of RRT varies from 8% to 13% in solid tumor patients[17,29,31] to 10% to 34% in patients with hematologic malignancies.[4,5,9,10,21,23,32,33,35] In a large cohort including 975 critically ill predominantly solid tumor patients admitted to a cancer center in Brazil, Soares and colleagues[15] reported an incidence in RRT of 10%. In a cohort including 1753 patients with hematologic malignancies admitted because of acute respiratory failure to 1 of 28 participating medical ICUs in Paris (France) between 1997 and 2004, 595 (33.9%) had AKI and 287 (16.3%) received RRT.[33] The incidence further increased to 32% to 44% in multiple myeloma patients[18,26] and up to 25% to 60% in series including septic shock patients exclusively,[24,27] whereas it was reported to be 15% to 25% in sepsis patients[20,37] and 16% to 34% in patients who received mechanical ventilation.[16,22,43] The incidence of RRT in patients requiring urgent systemic chemotherapy because of

Table 2
Incidence and short-term (ICU, 28-day, or hospital) mortality associated with renal replacement therapy (RRT) in the most important subgroups of patients with hematologic malignancies and solid tumors admitted to the ICU[a]

Authors,Year	No. of Patients	Admission Period	Severity of Illness	Hematologic Malignancy (%)/Allo-BM or PBSCT (%)	RRT Incidence (%)	RRT Mortality (%)
A. Subgroup of cancer patients with acute respiratory failure and/or who received (invasive and noninvasive) mechanical ventilation in the ICU						
1 Azoulay et al, 2001[16]	237	1990–1998	SAPS II 58 MV 100%/Vasopressors 50%	71%/0%	23%	NR
2 Depuydt et al, 2004[22]	166	1997–2002	SAPS II NR[b] MV 100%/Vasopressors 58%	100%/17%	34%	91%
3 Azoulay et al, 2004[19]	203	1997–2002	APACHE II NR/SAPS II NR MV 73%/Vasopressors 53%	91%/10%	9%	NR
4 Cornet et al, 2005[36]	58	1995–2002	APACHE II NR/SAPS II NR MV 100%/Vasopressors 62%	100%/9%	16%	55%
5 Vieira et al, 2007[43]	140	2003	APACHE II NR[b] MV 100%/Vasopressors	15%/0%	16%	NR
6 Lecuyer et al, 2008[33]	1753	1997–2004	SAPS II 53 MV 83%/Vasopressors 49%	100%/9%	16%	NR
B. Subgroup of cancer patients with sepsis, severe sepsis or septic shock admitted to the ICU						
1 Larché et al, 2003[24]	88	1995–2000	SAPS II 66 MV 77%/vasopressor 100%	92%/0%	25%	NR
2 Benoit et al, 2005[20]	172	2000–2003	APACHE II 26 MV 66%/Vasopressors 46%	100%/14%	20%	74%
3 Pène et al, 2008[27]	238	1998–2005	SAPS II NR[b] MV 85%/Vasopressors 100%	55%/14%	51%	80%
4 Vandijck et al, 2008[37]	186	2000–2006	APACHE II 26 MV 65%/Vasopressors 58%	100%/14%	22%	NR
C. Subgroup of cancer patients who received RRT in the ICU						
1 Lanore et al, 1991[6]	43	1983–1989	SAPS 13 MV 47%/Vasopressors 50%	100%/12%	NR	72%

2 Berghmans et al, 2004[13]	32	1997–2002	APACHE II 31 MV 47%/Vasopressors 50%	50%/28%	NR	53%
3 Benoit et al, 2005[12]	49	1997–2002	APACHE II 30 MV 88%/Vasopressors 86%	100%/12%	23%[c]	84%
4 Soares et al, 2006[15]	98	2000–2004	APACHE II 23/SAPS II 60 MV 90%/Vasopressors 84%	37%/0%	10%[c]	70%
5 Darmon et al, 2007[14]	55	2002–2005	SAPS II 53 MV 64%/Vasopressors 51%	78%/0%	17%[c]	51%
D. Subgroups with specific malignancies admitted to the ICU						
1 Azoulay et al, 1999[18]	75	1992–1998	SAPS II 52 MV 73%/Vasopressors 67%	Multiple myeloma	32%	NR
2 Peigne et al, 2009[26]	196	1990–2006	SAPS II 57 MV 51%/Vasopressors 46%	Multiple myeloma	39%	NR
3 Soares et al, 2007[31]	121	2000–2005	SAPS II 50 MV 83%/Vasopressors 58%	Head and neck cancer	10%	NR
4 Soares et al, 2007[29]	143	2000–2006	SAPS II 47 MV 70%/Vasopressors 57%	Lung cancer	8%	NR
E. Subgroup of cancer patients who received chemotherapy in the ICU in an urgent setting						
1 Darmon et al, 2005[39]	100	1997–2003	SAPS II 39 MV 54%/Vasopressors 42%	88%/0%	30%	60%
2 Benoit et al, 2006[38]	37	1997–2005	APACHE II 24 MV 35%/Vasopressors 32%	100%/0%	24%	44%
F. Subgroup of cancer patients admitted ≥21 days in the ICU						
1 Soares et al, 2008[34]	163	2000–2005	SAPS II 46 MV 91%/Vasopressors 60%	15%/0%	13%	56%

a Based on the most important studies published since 1990 focusing on specific subgroups of critically ill cancer patients exclusively.
b APACHE II and/or SAPS II not available for the general study population.
c Incidence calculated by dividing the number of patients admitted in the study cohort and the total number of critically ill cancer patients admitted during the study period.

cancer-related organ failure is 25% to 30%.[38,39] Of note, the incidence of RRT has increased over the past few decades, indicating an increasing referral rate of severely ill cancer patients to the ICU as well as in the subsequent initiation of RRT, at least in specialized centers.[26,27]

Outcome and Prognostic Indicators

Crude mortality rates in critically ill patients with AKI are systematically higher in those with cancer than in those without.[12,49–52,54] Among the 222 consecutive critically ill patients who received RRT in the medical ICU between 1997 and 2002 at the authors' center, those with hematologic malignancies had higher crude ICU (79.5% vs 55.7%, $P = .002$) and in-hospital (83.7% vs 66.1%, $P = .016$) mortality rates, and lower 6-month survival estimates (14% vs 28%, $P = .018$) compared with those without hematological malignancies.[12] However, the presence of a hematologic malignancy was no longer associated with a lower chance in 6-month survival after adjustment for the duration of hospitalization before ICU admission, a surrogate marker of comorbidity and functional status, or the severity of illness on ICU admission. Bagshaw and colleagues[50] similarly reported a 1-year survival of 15.8% in 38 patients with cancer compared with 40.1% in 202 patients without cancer ($P = .005$) in a cohort with severe AKI; however, the presence of cancer was not associated with a higher risk of death in the multivariate analysis. Darmon and colleagues[14] compared outcomes between critically ill patients who received RTT with and without underlying cancer. Both groups had similar hospital and 6-month mortality rates of 51.1% versus 42.9% ($P = .3$) and 65% versus 63.1% ($P = .99$), respectively, and the presence of cancer was again not associated with a higher risk of death after adjusting for confounders. Although in contrast with 2 other multicenter cohort studies,[51,52] these recent studies clearly indicate that the difference in mortality between cancer and noncancer patients is not as marked as commonly perceived once severity of illness is taken into account, and that the presence of underlying cancer alone is not sufficient enough to withhold RRT.

Similar to that for the general ICU population,[49–52,55] short and subsequent long-term outcome in critically ill cancer patients will essentially depend on the severity of AKI[15] and the number and severity of associated organ failures,[4–6,9,12–35,37–39] as well as on their reversibility.[20–24,35] Soares and colleagues[15] reported a 6-month mortality rate in critically ill cancer patients with AKI of 33% without associated organ failure and of 65%, 80%, and 93% in those with 1, 2, and 3 or more associated organ failures, respectively. The performance status and associated comorbidities have an additional adverse impact on both short-term and long-term outcome in cancer patients.[15,28–31,56] Age[28] and cancer characteristics by itself,[21,57] with the exception of extensive metastatic or uncontrolled recurrent disease in solid tumor patients,[28,29,31] have only a minor impact on the 6-month mortality in critically ill cancer patients. However, these factors are usually more informative about the short- and long-term prognosis in mechanically ventilated patients[22,24,30] and in patients with AKI.[15] Furthermore, outcomes have been found to be worse in patients who experience further deterioration in renal function despite advanced life support in the ICU.[14,15] In one study,[14] worsening in renal function was independently associated with an increased mortality (20% excess in absolute risk of death in univariate analysis, $P = .08$), whereas in another study[15] none of the patients who required RRT beyond day 4 survived. Finally, although never fully investigated, the main cause of AKI may also play an important role. Sepsis-induced AKI is often associated with protracted multiple organ dysfunction whereas this will be less or only rarely the case in AKI caused by nephrotoxic drugs or TLS, the latter especially since the introduction of recombinant urate oxidase. Not surprisingly, studies including a high percentage of

TLS patients report a lower overall mortality[6,14] compared with studies including a low percentage of these patients.[12,15] For instance, in a study before the urate oxidase era, only 3 out of the 11 (27%) cancer patients who received RRT for TLS-associated AKI died.[6] Preemptive or even prophylactic use of RRT to prevent further renal injury secondary to acute nephrocalcinosis may additionally explain the lower observed mortality in these patients.[3] Causes for which no effective treatment exists will carry a grim prognosis regardless of whether RRT is initiated. This situation explains the higher fatality rate observed in series including[12] or focusing on critically ill[40,41,58] or non–critically ill allogeneic hematopoietic stem cell recipients with AKI, wherein AKI is often associated with sinusoidal obstruction syndrome (formerly called hepatic veno-occlusive disease).[3,44]

Soares and colleagues[15] found that age older than 60 years, poor performance status, uncontrolled cancer, and 2 or more organ failures associated with AKI were independently associated with 6-month mortality. The 6-month survival rates in patients with no or 1, and 2 to 3 risk factors were 62% and 16%, respectively, whereas none of the 30 patients with more than 3 risk factors survived for longer than 80 days. These figures, however, are usually poorer in series including exclusively patients with hematologic malignancies who received RRT. RRT in the context of mechanical ventilation or multiple organ failure has usually been associated with a hospital mortality of 85% to 95% in critically ill cancer patients,[4–6,12,22,23] particularly in the older series[4,6] and in series including[5,12,22,23] or focusing on the hematopoietic transplant recipients.[40,41,58] At present, the authors believe that this no longer holds true for sepsis-related multiple organ failure outside the hematopoietic transplant setting, at least if induced by a documented or clinically suspected bacterial infection.[2,12,20–22,37] Whereas in an older series by Lanore and colleagues[6] only 1 of the 25 patients (4%) with sepsis-related AKI survived to hospital discharge, the authors recently reported that 7 of the 27 (26%) patients with documented or clinically suspected bacterial infection survived to hospital discharge, and 6 patients were still alive at 6 months.[12] Similar survival rates were recently reported by Pène and colleagues[27] in septic shock patients requiring RRT; 6 out of the 34 (17.6%) patients survived to hospital discharge in the period 1998 to 2001, and 18 out of the 88 (20.6%) patients survived in the period 2002 to 2005. These figures approach the survival rates that are reported in the general ICU population with septic shock requiring RRT.[50,55] In contrast, only 1 out of the 22 patients with other complications survived to hospital discharge in the authors' own series ($P = .056$).[12] In these patients, AKI was related to cardiogenic shock, fungal or viral infection, cardiopulmonary resuscitation, and post bone marrow transplant–related complications such as sinusoidal obstruction syndrome, thrombotic thrombocytopenic purpura/hemolytic uremic syndrome (TTP/HUS), and graft-versus-host disease, all complications for which less or no effective treatment exists.[12,20–22,25,37] In conclusion, although this finding certainly requires confirmation, the authors think that particularly the subgroup of patients with documented or clinically suspected bacterial sepsis should benefit from RRT in the setting of multiple organ failure.

Initiating RRT in patients referred to the ICU for urgent chemotherapy because of cancer-induced organ failure would have been considered as futile by most physicians a few years ago. Two large centers, independently from each other, have recently shown that it is feasible and justifiable to administer chemotherapy to critically ill patients with predominantly hematologic malignancies, at least at first presentation of the disease.[38,39] Although clearly these patients were highly selected, meaningful long-term survival was observed despite the concomitant need for other advanced life-supportive therapy (mechanical ventilation, vasopressors) during their ICU stay.

Although impaired functional status and incomplete recovery in renal function may jeopardize optimal administration of chemotherapy and subsequent long-term outcome, to date there are no studies that have specifically focused on the morbidity of critically ill cancer patients with AKI. Previous studies comparing cancer and non-cancer patients who received RRT in the ICU found no difference in length of stay between these groups.[12,14] Soares and colleagues[15] observed a complete and partial recovery in renal function in cancer patients of 82% and 12% respectively, and only 6% required chronic dialysis. Darmon and colleagues[14] found that 10 (21% of the hospital survivors) and 6 (22% of 6-month survivors) patients, respectively, fulfilled the criteria of end-stage kidney disease according to the RIFLE criteria. This finding is in contrast to that of Berghmans and colleagues,[13] who observed a complete and partial recovery of the renal function in only 34% and 25%, respectively.

CAUSES OF ACUTE RENAL FAILURE IN CRITICALLY ILL CANCER PATIENTS

AKI usually results from a combination of nephrotoxic insults in critically ill cancer patients, although a main insult is often identifiable in daily practice.[6,12,13,15] AKI may occur as a direct or indirect consequence of the cancer itself, its treatment, or associated complications. The most common causes of acute renal failure in cancer patients admitted to the ICU are listed in **Table 3**.[6,12–15] Sepsis was the most common cause of AKI followed by nephrotoxic drugs. Dependent on the center, diagnostic criteria and whether it was considered as a main or concomitant cause, TLS, and cancer-related diffuse intravascular coagulopathy (DIC) were responsible for approximately 3% to 40% of the AKI cases, followed by urinary tract obstruction in 5% to 16%, and multiple myeloma kidney in 2% to 11%. AKI related to posttransplant complication, such as sinusoidal obstruction syndrome, was present in about 10% of the patients in 2 centers.[12,13] The underlying cancer rarely may cause AKI by direct invasion of the kidney. Early recognition and subsequent initiation of chemotherapy in patients with chemosensitive malignancies may result in a prompt recovery of the renal function in this setting.[38,39] Since the widespread introduction of bisphosphonates with the intention to relieve skeletal pain and reduce skeletal-related complications in multiple myeloma and metastatic breast cancer,[59] referral to the ICU due to hypercalcemic-induced AKI has become relatively infrequent. Hypercalcemia-related AKI usually resolves with aggressive rehydration, and intraventricular administration of pamidronate (40–80 mg) or zoledronic acid (2–4 mg) within 48 to 72 hours. RRT should be considered as a last-resort treatment.

SEPSIS

As in general ICU patients,[49,51,52,55] sepsis and, more particularly, severe sepsis and septic shock, is the most common main contributing factor to the development of AKI in critically ill cancer patients. Patients with hematologic malignancies, who often experience longer duration of neutropenia compared with solid tumor patients, are at particularly high risk of bacterial and, less frequently, fungal sepsis.[2,19–21,25,32,37,60] In a multicenter study comparing outcomes of cancer patients admitted in European ICUs, 37.7% and 21.7% of the patients with hematologic malignancies were admitted with severe sepsis and septic shock, respectively, compared with 15.8% and 7.7% of the solid tumor patients and 17.3% and 7.4% of the patients without cancer.[32] Sepsis was responsible for 49.5% of the ICU admission in patients with hematologic malignancies compared with only 12.6% in patients without hematologic malignancies in the study by Merz and colleagues.[35] Although neutropenic patients certainly are more

Table 3	
Common causes of acute kidney injury in cancer patients admitted to the ICU[a]	
Indirectly Related to the Underlying Malignancy	**Incidence**
Hypoperfusion/Shock[6,12–15]	44%–84%
Sepsis[6,12–15]	58%–65%
Cardiac failure/Cardiogenic shock[12]	16%
Hemorrhagic shock[12]	2%
Nephrotoxic drugs[6,13–15]	16%–44%
Antimicrobial agents[b]	
Vancomycin[14]	25%
Aminoglycoside[14]	23%
Deoxycholate amphotericin B[14]	9%
Radiographic contrast agents[14,15]	4%–16%
Chemotherapeutic agents[14,15]	2%–3%
Methotrexate[6,14]	2%
Cisplatinum[14]	1%
Other (NSAID, ACE)[14]	2%–3%
Post-allogeneic BMT/HSCT[6,12,13]	9%–12%
Sinusoidal obstruction syndrome	8%
Hemolytic-uremic syndrome	5%
Directly Related to the Underlying Cancer	
Tumor lysis syndrome[6,14,15]	3%–42%
DIC/TMA[14,c]	30%
Urinary tract obstruction[14,15]	5%–16%
Multiple myeloma kidney[14,15]	2%–11%
Hypercalcemia[6]	5%
Other/unknown[15]	5%

Abbreviations: ACE, angiotensin-converting enzyme inhibitor; BMT, bone marrow transplant; DIC, diffuse intravascular coagulopathy; HSCT, hematopoietic stem cell transplant; NSAID, nonsteroidal ant-inflammatory drugs; TMA, thrombotic microangiopathy.
[a] This listing is based on 5 cohorts including exclusively critically ill cancer patients with acute kidney injury, 1 published in 1991[6] and 4 after 2003.[12–15]
[b] Total percentage is not listed because potential combinations were not provided in the initial publication.
[c] TMA may also be indirectly related to the underlying cancer.

susceptible to infection, it is however no longer evident that such patients do worse once admitted to the ICU,[2,19,20,24,27,30,35,37,60] even in the presence of AKI.[12,14,15] Whether this should be attributed to the shorter duration of neutropenic episodes since the widespread use of granulocyte colony stimulating factors (G-CSF) in patients with hematological malignancies in the early 2000s remains unclear.[2,37]

Outcome of septic shock cancer patients has improved over the past decade,[24,27] at least in patients who do not evolve to AKI.[27] Larché and colleagues[24] reported a reduction in 30-day mortality from 79% to 55.5% ($P = .01$) between the period 1995 to 1997 and 1998 to 2000 in septic shock cancer patients, resulting in a fivefold lower odds of death in the subsequent multivariate analysis. This finding was recently confirmed by Pène and colleagues,[27] who observed a decrease in hospital mortality in cancer patients with septic shock from 78.9% in the period 1998 to 2001 to 63.5% in the period 2002 to 2005 (*P*<.01). The most obvious improvement was observed in patients who did not require RRT; mortality was 78.6% in the first period versus 35.0% in the later period (*P*<.001), whereas mortality was about 80% in patients requiring RRT irrespective of the admission period. Similar mortality rates of about 30% in the absence of pulmonary infiltrates, increasing up to 65% in the presence of pulmonary infiltrates or mechanical ventilation and 70% to 80% in case of multiple organ failure or combined mechanical ventilation and RRT requirement, were reported by the authors' group[12,20,22] and others,[5] irrespective of the recent administration of previous systemic chemotherapy.[37] This improvement in outcome can be attributed to the better selection of patients with respect to the underlying cancer status and subsequent long-term survival, and to the advances in the treatment of sepsis and in ICU support in general.[2,8,16,18,24,27,37] Another underestimated factor that may have contributed to this improvement may be the more rapid referral of unstable patients to the ICU over the years, related to better communication and collaboration between critical care physicians and hemato-oncologists.[2,37,38] This factor may also partially explain the systematically lower reported mortality rates in dedicated ICUs with a high annual case volume,[12,20,24,27,37] compared with less dedicated general ICUs with lower annual case volume of hematologic patients with sepsis[9,32] and acute respiratory failure.[33] Rapid referral to the ICU might be of upmost importance in septic patients refractory to initial volume resuscitation[2,24,27,37] who are at particular risk for AKI. Close monitoring combined with aggressive resuscitation aiming to preserve adequate perfusion of vital organs[2,20,37,61] and early initiation of noninvasive mechanical ventilation in the absence of severe hemodynamic instability[16,19,22,62] may prevent further deterioration in organ (and renal) function, and the subsequent requirement for advanced life-sustaining measures such as RRT and invasive mechanical ventilation. Although data concerning the impact on renal function is lacking, both of these interventions have been shown to reduce mortality.[61,62] Cancer patients who fail to respond to these advanced resuscitation attempts in the ICU have a particularly grim prognosis.[14–16,19,22] Future studies should aim to evaluate the impact of case volume, early ICU referral, and resuscitation modalities on the incidence of AKI and mortality in cancer patients with sepsis.

Besides systemic vasodilatation and the resultant decrease in effective circulating volume that may be counteracted by the above interventions, inflammation, endothelial damage, and formation of thrombi in the microcirculation may further predispose septic patients to the development of AKI, multiple organ failure, and ultimately increased mortality.[63] Sepsis should essentially be considered as a procoagulant state that may lead to consumptive coagulopathy and microthrombosis.[63,64] Correlations have been found between the dynamic evolution of DIC parameters during the first day of ICU admission, and progression from single to multiple organ failure and subsequent death in patients with severe sepsis.[64] DIC has also been associated with glomerular microthrombi and AKI.[65] Several compounds that target this procoagulant inflammatory state have been investigated for their potential to improve outcome in sepsis. One of these agents, activated protein C, has been proven to decrease mortality in patients with severe sepsis and a high risk of death.[63] Data concerning kidney function were not reported in this trial. Activated protein C[66] and other similar compounds acting through the coagulation pathway[67] have recently been found to improve renal function in animal sepsis models. A main disadvantage of this drug, however, is the increased risk for severe hemorrhage,[63] which is already of major concern in critically ill thrombocytopenic cancer patients. In one study, only 6.8% of the cancer patients with septic shock received activated protein C.[27]

NEPHROTOXICITY RELATED TO CANCER TREATMENT AND SUPPORTIVE CARE
Antimicrobial Drugs

Several antimicrobial drugs commonly used in the supportive care of febrile cancer patients and to those with severe sepsis and septic shock may induce AKI.[14,24]

Aminoglycosides (gentamicin, tobramycin, amikacin) are commonly used in daily practice in cancer patients, although current guidelines no longer strictly recommend the use of aminoglycosides in combination with a β-lactam in febrile neutropenic patients.[68] Also, 2 large meta-analyses, one performed in immunocompetent sepsis patients[69] and another in febrile neutropenic cancer patients,[70] failed to show any survival advantage of a β-lactam/aminoglycoside combination therapy compared with β-lactam alone. Larché and colleagues[24] reported that 57% of the cancer patients admitted to the ICU because of septic shock received aminoglycosides. Darmon and colleagues[14] found that aminoglycosides were coresponsible for the development of AKI in 23% of the patients who received RRT in the ICU between 2002 and 2005. Aminoglycosides are taken up in the tubules, causing tubular and glomerular dysfunction leading to AKI, which is often nonoliguric and associated with hypokalemia, hypomagnemesia, and hypocalcemia. Absorption of aminoglycosides in the tubules is saturable. Once the tubules are completely saturated, no additional tubular absorption occurs. Thus higher concentrations of aminoglycosides do not lead to more toxicity. The nephrotoxic effects are typically time dependent, and will occur after 5 days to 1 week of therapy. Aminoglycosides have a concentration-dependent antimicrobial killing effect. There is also a postantibiotic effect; antimicrobial activity remains after the drug concentration decreases to less than the minimal inhibitory concentration. These observations have led to a once-daily dosing strategy and shorter duration of administration of aminoglycosides instead of multiple dosing, with equal efficacy and, in some studies, less nephrotoxicity.[71]

Vancomycin is often reported as a contributing factor for the development of AKI.[14] Earlier pharmacologic formulations of vancomycin in the 1950s and 1960s contained many impurities causing a brown color of the solution ("Mississippi mud"). These formulations were associated with multiple side effects such as fever, hypotension, flushing, neutropenia, ototoxicity, and nephrotoxicity. The incidence of these side effects has decreased over the years with the increasing quality of the formulation. Thus it is uncertain whether vancomycin administered as monotherapy actually causes nephrotoxicity. Vancomycin-attributed nephrotoxicity has nowadays a comparable incidence to that of other antibiotics that are not considered nephrotoxic.[72] Retrospective studies suggested that higher trough levels (>15 mg/L)[73] and higher daily dose (>4 g/d)[74] are risk factors for development of vancomycin-associated AKI. However, these trials were limited by their retrospective design, small sample size, and poor study methodology.[72] There are conflicting data regarding the effects of coadministration of vancomycin and aminoglycosides or amphotericin B and the occurrence of nephrotoxicity, with some studies suggesting a 3- to 7-fold increased risk.[72]

The major side effect of amphotericin B is its extreme nephrotoxicity. Amphotericin B increases cell membrane permeability of the tubules and causes intrarenal vasoconstriction, leading to polyuria, hypokalemia, hypomagnesemia, tubular acidosis, and AKI. Nephrotoxicity of amphotericin is dose- and time-dependent. Of note, a continuous infusion of amphotericin over 24 hours was associated with less nephrotoxicity when compared with an infusion duration of 4 hours.[75] Liposomal formulations of amphotericin do not contain the nephrotoxic vehicle deoxycholate, which was used in older preparations to bring amphotericin into solution. These formulations are considerably less nephrotoxic, while their efficacy remains.[76] Newer antifungals such as caspofungin and voriconazole combine comparable or even superior antifungal effect and decreased nephrotoxicity, and have replaced amphotericin as a first-line antifungal therapy in many clinical situations.[76]

Contrast Nephropathy

Intravascular administration of iodinated contrast agents may lead to contrast-induced AKI. The most important risk factors for contrast-induced AKI are chronic kidney disease, concomitant administration of other nephrotoxins, and diabetes.[77,78] It is unclear whether multiple myeloma by itself is a risk factor for contrast-induced AKI.[79] Furthermore, intra-arterial administration of contrast, large volumes of contrast, and administration of contrast agents with an osmolality that is significantly higher than serum, such as with high-osmolar (2000 mosmol/kg H_2O) or hypoosmolar (600–800 mosmol/kg H_2O) contrast media are associated with an increased incidence of contrast induced AKI.[77,78] Preventive measures for contrast-induced AKI should be undertaken in patients with an estimated glomerular filtration rate of less than 60 mL/min. These measures include discontinuation of other nephrotoxic drugs if possible, prehydration with either normal saline or isotonic sodium bicarbonate,[80,81] use of iso-osmolar contrast agents in at-risk patients (ie, patients with diabetes or cardiovascular disease), and limiting the total volume of contrast agent administered. Administration of N-acetylcysteine is controversial, with several studies and meta-analyses demonstrating protective effects while others are unable to confirm this finding. Unfortunately, studies on the effects of N-acetylcysteine are underpowered and heterogeneous, compromising valid meta-analysis.[82] In addition, there is controversy as to whether N-acetylcysteine actually prevents nephrotoxicity, or if it merely influences serum creatinine concentration by mechanisms other than kidney function.[83] Finally, hemofiltration may reduce the incidence of contrast-induced AKI and associated in-hospital mortality in high-risk patients,[84] although the observed beneficial effects in these open trials can also be attributed to ICU admission and the resultant increase in care and monitoring.

Toxicity Specifically Related to the Cancer Treatment

Among the chemotherapeutic agents commonly associated with AKI in critically ill cancer patients are cisplatin and methotrexate (see **Table 3**).

Cisplatin, cisplatinum, or *cis*-diamminedichloroplatinum(II) (CDDP), a DNA-alkylating agent, is one of the most extensively studied nephrotoxic chemotherapeutic agents. Cisplatin is widely used to treat various types of cancers including sarcomas, small cell lung cancer, ovarian cancer, and germ cell tumors, and is used in second- or third-line regimens for relapsing high-grade lymphomas. Carboplatin and oxaliplatin are derivates of cisplatin and have fewer side effects. Cisplatin causes direct tubular toxicity leading to salt-wasting nephropathy with hyponatremia, hypomagnemesia, and mostly mild AKI. The nephrotoxicity is dose dependent.[85] The dose of cisplatin should not exceed 120 mg/m², and a cumulative dose of more than 850 mg is associated with a significant increased risk for a reduction in kidney function over a 5-year follow-up period. Preventive measures for cisplatin nephrotoxicity are isotonic saline infusions and amifostine (910 mg/m²).[86]

Methotrexate is an antimetabolite and antifolate drug frequently used in the treatment of acute lymphoblastic leukemia, high-grade non-Hodgkin lymphoma (especially the Burkitt type), and sarcomas. Methotrexate can cause AKI by crystallization and precipitation in the tubules. AKI in turn may enhance general methotrexate toxicity and further cause or aggravate hepatitis, neutropenia, mucositis, and neurologic impairment.[87] If not detected early, multiple organ dysfunction may develop, either directly induced by the drug itself or indirectly by bacterial translocation through the gastrointestinal mucosa. Mucositis is severe in these circumstances. Precipitation of methotrexate can be prevented by enhancing the urine output and alkalinization of the urine to a pH greater than 7.5. Also, leucovorin (folinic acid) administration, 50 mg 4 times per day should be started 24 hours after administration of methotrexate as rescue to reduce multiple organ toxicity. Other nephrotoxic drugs, as well as drugs that may inhibit folate metabolism (trimethoprim-sulfamethoxazole) or decrease albumin binding (aspirin) should be interrupted. Pleural effusions and ascites should be drained because methotrexate accumulates in these compartments, thereby contributing to delayed excretion.[88] This situation is particularly relevant in critically ill patients with capillary leak. Toxic drug levels (15 μmol/L at 24 h, 1.5 μmol/L at 48 h, and 0.5 μmol/L at 72 h) should be treated with high doses of leucovorin. Methotrexate is albumin bound, and therefore hemodialysis is not an optimal therapy to remove the drug in cases of severe toxicity. Hemoperfusion and high-flux hemodialysis have been used as alternatives. Finally, carboxypeptidase-C2 in combination with high-dose leucovorin may be beneficial for patients with methotrexate-induced renal dysfunction and significantly elevated plasma methotrexate concentrations. This bacterial enzyme decreases methotrexate concentrations by a median of 98.7% (range 84%–99.5%) within 15 minutes by converting it into an inactive metabolite.[89]

TUMOR LYSIS SYNDROME

TLS is a metabolic disorder that results from the massive destruction of malignant cells and the subsequent abrupt release of intracellular anions (phosphate), cations (potassium), metabolic products of proteins, and nucleic acids (uric acid) into the extracellular space and the bloodstream.[90–92] This rapid release may overwhelm the body's homeostatic mechanism to process and excrete these materials and result in the life-threatening clinical spectrum of TLS, which is characterized by AKI, seizures, arrhythmias, and finally sudden death.[3,90–92] Uric acid, catabolized from purine nucleic acids through hypoxanthine and xanthine by xanthine oxidase, is a key player in the pathogenesis of TLS. Hyperuricemia in combination with volume depletion, which is often present in cancer patients, will lead to the formation of uric acid crystals in the renal tubules thereby obstructing the urine flow. Hyperphosphatemia may further aggravate this process through the precipitation of calcium phosphate crystals once the solubility product of calcium and phosphate is reached. This acute nephrocalcinosis, together with calcium phosphate deposition in other tissues, may result in severe hypocalcemia which is, however, rarely symptomatic in daily practice.[91,92] Hyperkalemia, resulting from the kidney's inability to clear the massive load of intracellular potassium released by lysed tumor cells and occasionally secondary to excess iatrogenic administration of potassium during induction therapy, may be further exacerbated by the development of AKI.[90] Patients with preexisting acute or chronic renal insufficiency are predisposed to the development of TLS and are more vulnerable to its effect.[91]

Although this syndrome may develop in virtually every hematologic or solid malignancy with a large tumor burden, high proliferative rate, or a high sensitivity to chemotherapy, life-threatening TLS requiring ICU admission is generally limited in daily practice to patients with high-grade non-Hodgkin lymphoma, acute lymphoblastic leukemia and, to a lesser extent, acute myelogenous leukemia. There remains a paucity of data available concerning the overall incidence of TLS and specifically in the critically ill cancer population. Soares and colleagues[15] found that TLS was the main cause of AKI in 10 (3%) of 309 critically ill predominantly solid tumor patients. In an older series including exclusively critically ill hematologic malignancy patients who received RRT,[6] TLS was considered the main cause of AKI in 25%. Darmon and colleagues[14] more recently found TLS to be a concomitant cause in 40% of critically ill mainly hematologic malignancy patients. The proportion of laboratory-defined versus clinically apparent TLS was not reported in the latter study.

Recognition of patients at risk and the timely initiation of preventive prophylactic strategies to prevent or reduce the severity of the clinical manifestations are essential in TLS. The cornerstone of this strategy is to reduce hyperuricemia. This reduction can be achieved by increasing the renal clearance (appropriate hydration) and inhibiting the formation of uric acid (allopurinol), or more recently, by converting uric acid to a more soluble form to facilitate its excretion (intravenous recombinant form of urate oxidase, rasburicase).[91] The reader is referred to the "Oncologic Emergencies" section of this issue for a more detailed discussion of the therapeutic approach of TLS. RRT is indicated when resolution of TLS is unlikely despite the administration of rasburicase, in the case of life-threatening electrolyte disorders, or the presence of volume overload.[3,90–92] RRT may also prevent further insults to the kidney due to further deposition of uric acid crystals and acute nephrocalcinosis through extracorporeal removal of urate and phosphate. Darmon and colleagues[92] have proposed that RRT should be initiated if hyperphosphatemia persists for more than 4 to 6 hours after the initiation of saline infusion. Because of potential rebound effect after dialysis, extended daily dialysis or isolated sequential dialysis followed by continuous hemofiltration should be the standard of care in TLS patients requiring RRT.[92]

CANCER-RELATED MICROANGIOPATHY
Diffuse Intravascular Coagulation

DIC is observed relatively frequently in cancer patients outside the setting of sepsis.[93] The reported incidence is approximately 7% in solid tumor patients,[94] increasing up to 10% to 15% in case of metastatic disease,[93] to 15% to 20% in patients presenting with acute lymphoblastic leukemia, and to more than 90% in those with acute promyelocytic leukemia.[93,94] Darmon and colleagues[14] reported that DIC was present in 26% of the cancer patients admitted to the ICU with AKI. Cancer-related DIC has in general a less fulminant clinical presentation than sepsis or trauma-related DIC.[93] The predominant clinical manifestations are usually hemorrhage, particularly in leukemia patients at least at presentation of their disease,[93,95] and venous thromboembolism.[93,94] Both will, however, only rarely cause AKI or multiple organ failure, except indirectly in the case of severe hemorrhage and massive pulmonary emboli, respectively. Organ failure(s) directly resulting from major, or minor but more diffuse, arterial thrombosis or microangiopathy has typically been associated with (mucin-producing) adenocarcinomas of the stomach, pancreas, ovary, breast, and lung,[96–103] and to a lesser extent of the prostate[103] and cervix.[104] The exact mechanism of this uncommon more aggressive thromboembolic diathesis, often designated as Trousseau syndrome, remains unclear. Formation of platelet-rich microthrombi resulting from the interaction between mucin secreted into the bloodstream and P-and L-selectins, respectively, together with the exposure of tissue factor–rich tumor cell surface or the release of tissue factor–rich microvesicles by the tumor-inducing fibrin formation and platelet aggregation by thrombin production are thought to be essential.[101] Although more frequently diagnosed in patients with metastatic disease, cases have been reported in patients with localized or occult malignancy.[97,101] The clinical picture is heterogeneous and may vary from stroke,[100,104] migratory thrombophlebitis,[96,97,99,101] bilateral acral cyanosis, or even limb gangrene[103] to the more catastrophic picture of purpura fulminans or multiple organ failure.[98,102] AKI may result from cortical necrosis in this setting.[98] In exceptional cases surgery with resultant manipulation of the tumor may precipitate the syndrome.[98] In the case of thromboembolic events at multiple sites, systemic embolization secondary to underlying concomitant nonbacterial thrombotic (marantic) endocarditis should be excluded[105] because it may be a part of this syndrome.[96,97,99,101,105] In this particular setting, arterial embolization most frequently involves the spleen, kidney, brain, and heart, respectively. Premortem diagnosis is rare.[105] Although overt DIC usually rapidly resolves after the initiation of cancer treatment,[102,103] cancer patients with DIC have a poorer prognosis than those without.[94] Control and, if possible, elimination of the underlying causative malignancy should be achieved as soon as possible, and unfractionated heparin is the preferred treatment in the case of thrombotic diathesis.[96,97,99,101] Catastrophic Trousseau syndrome presenting with multiple organ failure is usually rapidly fatal.[98,102]

Thrombotic Thrombocytopenic Purpura/Hemolytic Uremic Syndrome

Differentiating DIC from TTP/HUS is not always straightforward, especially in myelosuppressed cancer patients, and both syndromes are probably often misdiagnosed in daily practice and the literature[3,106]; this is also suggested by both syndromes having essentially been associated with the same tumor types. In contrast to DIC, routine laboratory coagulation parameters are usually unaffected in TTP/HUS, and the presence of schistocytes on peripheral blood examination is mandatory for the diagnosis. Repeated assessments should be performed in patients with a high clinical suspicion of TTP/HUS and absence of schistocytes on the initial blood examination.

About 3% to 15% of patients with TTP/HUS have an underlying cancer.[107–109] Darmon and colleagues[14] found that TTP/HUS was present in 3% of the cancer patients admitted with AKI to the ICU. An underlying malignancy should be suspected in TTP/HUS patients refractory to plasma exchange or with a discrepantly high lactate dehydrogenase (LDH) on presentation.[107] TTP/HUS may be associated with the cancer itself or its treatments. Similar to cancer-related DIC, TTP/HUS has most often been associated with advanced adenocarcinoma of the breast,[106,107,110–113] stomach, colon, pancreas, and prostate.[106,107,110–113] Extensive bone marrow infiltration with or without secondary myelofibrosis is often present on bone marrow puncture/biopsy.[107,110–112] Chemotherapeutic agents used to treat these malignancies, as well as other tumors, have also frequently been implicated. Mitomycin was the first widely reported chemotherapeutic agent implicated in the development of HUS/TTP in the literature in the mid 1980s.[106,113–115] Since then an expansive number of agents, solely or in combination, have been added to the list.[114] Regimens containing 5-fluorouracil,[106,113] cisplatin and, more recently, gemcitabine have frequently been implicated.[114] The incidence of TTP/HUS in cancer patients receiving gemcitabine, a nucleoside analogue that was initially introduced for the treatment of unresectable pancreatic carcinoma in 1996 and subsequently expanded to the treatment of non–small lung carcinoma, lymphoma, breast cancer and, more recently, advanced ovarian carcinoma, has been estimated at between 0.015% and 1.4%.[114,116] About 33% to 55% of these patients will require RRT.[114] Finally, TTP/HUS has been observed in the hematopoietic essentially myeloablative allogeneic stem cell transplantation population. The reported incidence varies widely, in part due to different diagnostic criteria.[44] Direct endothelial injury from calcineurin inhibitors, high-dose chemotherapy, and total body irradiation are thought to be responsible.[44] These factors have also been associated with the sinusoidal obstruction syndrome and graft-versus-host disease, conditions that are often present concomitantly with TTP/HUS.[117]

Compared with idiopathic TTP/HUS, the outcome of cancer-related and post-hematopoietic stem cell related TTP/HUS is dismal.[44,106,107,110–115,117] Both conditions are not or only poorly responsive to plasmapheresis, most likely because ADAMST13 deficiency does not play a key role in their pathogenesis. Moreover, many patients died because of the underlying disseminated malignancy and other concomitant severe post-hematopoietic stem cell transplant related complications, respectively. As with patients with catastrophic cancer-related DIC, advanced life-supportive therapy in the ICU should be for restrictive use. An exception is clearly cancer patients in complete remission or with stable disease who consequently are most likely to experience chemotherapy-related TTP/HUS.[106,114] Cessation of the implicated drug(s) together with a trial of plasma exchange and, if required, RRT are the primary treatment modalities. In general, renal function improves with the discontinuation of the drug and the subsequent remission of TTP/HUS, but often does not return to baseline.[114]

ACUTE KIDNEY INJURY SECONDARY TO URETERAL OBSTRUCTION

Ureteral obstruction is the fifth most common main or concomitant cause of AKI in cancer patients admitted to the ICU.[14,15] Ureteral obstruction carries an ominous prognosis, as it is usually observed in the context of extensive metastatic solid tumors often poorly responsive to chemotherapy. Median survival is only 3 to 7 months.[118–120] Ureteral obstruction may result from a direct intrinsic or extrinsic compression of the ureters by a pelvic (bladder, prostate, cervix, ovaries) or abdominal (colorectal) tumor, extrinsic compression from the retroperitoneal cavity (sarcoma), or metastatic lymph nodes (metastasis of essentially abdominal and pelvic tumors but also of the breast or lung and non-Hodgkin lymphoma).[118–120] Cancer patients presenting with AKI secondary to ureteral obstruction usually present with vague and nonspecific symptoms,[119] and AKI is often a coincidental laboratory finding in this setting. Therefore, physicians should always exclude post-renal obstruction as a concomitant cause of AKI in cancer patients with sepsis, especially in the setting of a discrepancy between the degree of AKI and sepsis (hemodynamic instability and the routine DIC laboratory parameters), and in patients with known or suspected extensive malignancy. Abdominal ultrasonography is the investigation of choice for the detection of ureteral obstruction, and can easily be performed at the bedside in the ICU.

In the case of non-Hodgkin lymphoma, corticosteroids with or without concomitant chemo- or radiotherapy will often result in ureteral decompression within a couple of days, at least at first presentation of the disease. Long-term survival may be achieved in these patients, in contrast to the extensive solid tumor patient, in whom percutaneous nephrostomy or stenting will often be mandatory in cases of hydronephrosis and AKI. Given the usually palliative context and that these procedures may further affect the quality of life of these already frail patients (ie, tube movement and dislodgment, incomplete resolution of the obstruction and the subsequent need of reinterventions, urinary tract infections), it will be important to address all these issues with the patient and the relatives.[119] Percutaneous nephrostomy is preferred over retrograde ureteral stenting in cases of gross invasion of a bladder, and prostatic or cervical cancer on cytoscopy.[118,119] The success rate of retrograde ureteral stenting is higher in colorectal and breast cancer patients.[118] Patients should be monitored for postobstructive polyuria and electrolyte derangements. Recovery of the renal function depends on the degree and duration of the obstruction and whether the obstruction is uni- or bilateral.

MULTIPLE MYELOMA KIDNEY

AKI is a common feature of multiple myeloma and often provides a clue to the diagnosis of this disease, particularly in the presence of a high serum total protein concentration in routine laboratory investigations. Only 52% of the multiple myeloma patients have normal renal function on presentation[121,122] and, depending on the definition, about 20% to 46% of de novo multiple myeloma patients present with AKI.[122–124] Multiple myeloma represents about 3% of cancer patients[30] and 10% to 21% of patients with hematologic malignancy admitted to the ICU, respectively.[10,16,20,21,23] About 32% to 44% of the critically ill multiple myeloma patients receive RRT during their ICU stay.[18,26] AKI seems to be correlated with a high tumor mass, because it is most often observed in patients with a high light chain urine protein excretion,[123,125,126] high serum LDH, multiple bone lesions, or extensive marrow plasmocytosis.[123] Reversibility of AKI is more informative about the long-term prognosis than the response to chemotherapy in multiple myeloma patients.[121,124]

Similar to TLS and methotrexate nephropathy that causes AKI secondary to the intrarenal crystallization of uric acid and the drug or its metabolites, respectively, multiple myeloma causes intrarenal tubular obstruction through the formation of light chain casts. Free light chains, which are by-products of intact immunoglobulin synthesis, are normally rapidly removed from the circulation by renal clearance. However, in multiple myeloma patients serum concentrations of these molecules may be several thousand times higher than normal.[126] These casts develop after excessively filtered monoclonal light chains bind to the Tamm-Horsfall glycoprotein, which is secreted by the thick ascending limb of the loop of Henle.[127] Light-chain nephropathy has been traditionally considered the most common cause of AKI in multiple myeloma patients,[121,125,126] and substantial efforts have already been undertaken to try to lower serum light chain concentrations and subsequently improve renal function in these patients. For many years, plasma exchange in combination with chemotherapy was considered the standard of care in cast nephropathy, at least in some centers.[121] However, a recent randomized controlled trial failed to show an outcome benefit of plasma exchange in multiple myeloma with AKI treated with conventional chemotherapy.[125] Irreversible tubular damage due to a time delay in diagnosing multiple myeloma and insufficient removal of monoclonal free light chains by plasma exchange were thought to be responsible. Studies assessing the value of extended high cutoff hemodialysis, which is much more efficient in removing free light chains than plasma exchange, are underway.[126] Another explanation for the lack of efficacy of plasma exchange is that the renal function may be altered by means other than light-chain cast nephropathy alone in multiple myeloma patients.[128] Other potential causes of AKI in this patient population, occurring solely or in combination, are light and heavy chain amyloidosis, nodular glomerulosclerosis associated with light chain and heavy chain deposition disease, acute proximal tubular damage with or without Fanconi syndrome, acute tubular interstitial nephritis, cryoglobulinemia, hyperviscosity (more often occurring in IgA and IgG3 isotypes), plasma cell infiltration, and vascular amyloisis.[128,129]

Given the complex potential multifactorial pathogenesis of the multiple myeloma kidney and because multiple myeloma and, more particularly, the production of monoclonal light and heavy chains cannot be rapidly contained by chemotherapy, critical care physicians should not expect a rapid recovery of renal function during the ICU stay even after initiation of chemotherapy. Until recently, conventional induction chemotherapy for multiple myeloma patients with AKI consisted of dexamethasone, alone or in combination with adriamycin and vincristine. This combination was preferred over oral melphalan because of a lower toxicity on the hematopoietic stem cells, which may be of major concern in patients with reduced renal function.[121] Avoiding cumulative bone marrow toxicity is of particular importance in patients who are eligible for hematopoietic stem cell transplantation.[130] Thalidomide and bortezomib recently have been introduced as induction therapy for patients eligible for hematopoietic stem cell transplantation and as salvage therapy, respectively.[121,130–132] Both drugs seem promising for the treatment of multiple myeloma-related AKI. There is limited information available concerning the impact of high-dose chemotherapy followed by autologous hematopoietic stem cell transplantation on the renal recovery in patients with multiple myeloma.[133,134]

WHO SHOULD BENEFIT FROM ADVANCED LIFE-SUPPORTIVE THERAPY, INCLUDING RENAL REPLACEMENT THERAPY?

From the aforementioned data it should be clear that the presence of an underlying cancer alone can no longer be considered a contraindication to initiate RRT in critically ill patients. Moreover, long-term survival is no longer exceptional even in multiple organ failure cancer patients requiring RRT, at least in the context of septic shock outside the allogeneic hematopoietic transplant setting.[12,27] However, these relatively good results should not be used to warrant unrealistic therapeutic perseverance or to withhold palliative care in cancer patients who are in a desperate situation. As in non-cancer patients referred to the ICU, the degree and duration of advanced life-supportive measures should be in balance with the expected long-term survival and quality of life. However, prognostication and subsequent withholding or withdrawing of treatment remains a difficult decision regarding the individual patient in daily practice. Even ICU physicians used to treating critically ill cancer patients fail to discriminate adequately between survivors and nonsurvivors.[135] Although is it clear that such a complex decision cannot simply be replaced by a rule of thumb consisting of a combination of several prognostic indicators[10,15,21] or even by a more complex scoring systems,[56,136,137] it certainly can assist physicians in their decision making.

Besides the cancer status and the subsequent expected long-term prognosis, the number of failing organs and, more particularly, their potential reversibility are important factors to take into account. As the authors have seen previously, the latter will largely depend on the availability and timely initiation of an effective treatment of the insult(s) causing multiple organ dysfunction or AKI (ie, sepsis, TLS), or on timely discontinuation (ie, drug-induced AKI including TTP/HUS) or removal of the causative agent (ie, uric acid in TLS, light-chain nephropathy) by RRT, plasma exchange, or other means. In patients who progress to multiple organ failure or AKI despite these measures, the underlying cancer status will become more important in the decision making because protracted ICU stay and chronic critical illness may compromise future administration of chemotherapy. Unavailability of an effective treatment will be associated with a uniformly poor prognosis in the context of multiple organ failure (ie, adenocarcinoma-related TTP/HUS and catastrophic DIC, sinusoidal obstruction syndrome in the hematopoietic transplant setting) irrespective of whether RRT or other advanced life-supportive measures are initiated. ICU referral should in this setting only be on a very selective basis. Of course, the quality of life as perceived by the patient and above all the preferences of the patient or their relatives should also be taken into account. Providing appropriate care to these complex patients is only possible after honest communication has taken place regarding the most likely scenarios with the relatives,[138,139] and preferably, if allowed by her or his acute illness at that moment, with the patient.[11,140–143] To achieve this goal close collaboration between the ICU team, hemato-oncologist, and nephrologist are mandatory. In case of doubt a trial of 3-day ICU admission may be considered.[144]

SUMMARY

Critically ill cancer patients have a higher incidence of AKI treated with RRT than critically ill patients without cancer. AKI may occur as a direct or indirect consequence of the cancer itself, its treatment, or associated complications. The presence of an underlying cancer alone can no longer be considered a contraindication to initiate RRT in critically ill patients. Moreover, recent studies have shown that long-term survival is no longer exceptional in multiple organ failure cancer patients requiring RRT, at least in the context of septic shock outside the allogeneic hematopoietic transplant setting. However, these relatively good results should not be used to justify unrealistic therapeutic perseverance or to withhold palliative care in cancer patients who are in a desperate situation. Similar to that for any other critically ill patient, the decision to initiate advanced life-supportive therapy as well as its duration should be in proportion with the patient's expected long-term prognosis and quality of life. Close collaboration between critical care physicians, hemato-oncologists, and nephrologists in cases of AKI, and timely communication of realistic expectations to the relatives and, if possible, to the patient before admission to the ICU and during ICU stay is therefore essential.

ACKNOWLEDGMENTS

The authors would like to thank Pieter Depuydt, MD, PhD and Jean-Patrick Harvey, MD, respectively staff member and resident in training at the Department of Intensive Care of Ghent University Hospital Medical Unit, for reviewing the manuscript and for their useful comments.

REFERENCES

1. Brenner H. Long-term survival rates of cancer patients achieved by the end of the 20th century: a period analysis. Lancet 2002;360(9340):1131–5.
2. Benoit DD, Depuydt PO, Decruyenaere JM. Should we remain reluctant to admit critically ill cancer patients to the intensive care unit? In: Vincent J-L, editor. Yearbook of intensive care and emergency medicine. Berlin/Heidelberg/New York: Springer-Verlag; 2009. p. 845–55.
3. Darmon M, Ciroldi M, Thiery G, et al. Clinical review: specific aspects of acute renal failure in cancer patients. Crit Care 2006;10(2):211.
4. Brunet F, Lanore JJ, Dhainaut JF, et al. Is intensive care justified for patients with haematological malignancies? Intensive Care Med 1990;16(5):291–7.
5. Evison J, Rickenbacher P, Ritz R, et al. Intensive care unit admission in patients with haematological disease: incidence, outcome and prognostic factors. Swiss Med Wkly 2001;131(47–48):681–6.
6. Lanore JJ, Brunet F, Pochard F, et al. Hemodialysis for acute renal failure in patients with hematologic malignancies. Crit Care Med 1991;19(3):346–51.
7. Azoulay E, Afessa B. The intensive care support of patients with malignancy: do everything that can be done. Intensive Care Med 2006;32(1):3–5.

8. Pène F, Soares M. Can we still refuse ICU admission of patients with hematological malignancies? Intensive Care Med 2008;34(5):790–2.
9. Silfvast T, Pettila V, Ihalainen A, et al. Multiple organ failure and outcome of critically ill patients with haematological malignancy. Acta Anaesthesiol Scand 2003;47(3):301–6.
10. Kroschinsky F, Weise M, Illmer T, et al. Outcome and prognostic features of intensive care unit treatment in patients with hematological malignancies. Intensive Care Med 2002;28(9):1294–300.
11. Groeger JS, Aurora RN. Intensive care, mechanical ventilation, dialysis, and cardiopulmonary resuscitation. Implications for the patient with cancer. Crit Care Clin 2001;17(3):791–803, x.
12. Benoit DD, Hoste EA, Depuydt PO, et al. Outcome in critically ill medical patients treated with renal replacement therapy for acute renal failure: comparison between patients with and those without haematological malignancies. Nephrol Dial Transplant 2005;20(3):552–8.
13. Berghmans T, Meert AP, Markiewicz E, et al. Continuous venovenous haemofiltration in cancer patients with renal failure: a single-centre experience. Support Care Cancer 2004;12(5):306–11.
14. Darmon M, Thiery G, Ciroldi M, et al. Should dialysis be offered to cancer patients with acute kidney injury? Intensive Care Med 2007;33(5):765–72.
15. Soares M, Salluh JI, Carvalho MS, et al. Prognosis of critically ill patients with cancer and acute renal dysfunction. J Clin Oncol 2006;24(24):4003–10.
16. Azoulay E, Alberti C, Bornstain C, et al. Improved survival in cancer patients requiring mechanical ventilatory support: impact of noninvasive mechanical ventilatory support. Crit Care Med 2001;29(3):519–25.
17. Azoulay E, Moreau D, Alberti C, et al. Predictors of short-term mortality in critically ill patients with solid malignancies. Intensive Care Med 2000;26(12):1817–23.
18. Azoulay E, Recher C, Alberti C, et al. Changing use of intensive care for hematological patients: the example of multiple myeloma. Intensive Care Med 1999; 25(12):1395–401.
19. Azoulay E, Thiery G, Chevret S, et al. The prognosis of acute respiratory failure in critically ill cancer patients. Medicine (Baltimore) 2004;83(6):360–70.
20. Benoit DD, Depuydt PO, Peleman RA, et al. Documented and clinically suspected bacterial infection precipitating intensive care unit admission in patients with hematological malignancies: impact on outcome. Intensive Care Med 2005; 31(7):934–42.
21. Benoit DD, Vandewoude KH, Decruyenaere JM, et al. Outcome and early prognostic indicators in patients with a hematologic malignancy admitted to the intensive care unit for a life-threatening complication. Crit Care Med 2003; 31(1):104–12.
22. Depuydt PO, Benoit DD, Vandewoude KH, et al. Outcome in noninvasively and invasively ventilated hematologic patients with acute respiratory failure. Chest 2004;126(4):1299–306.
23. Lamia B, Hellot MF, Girault C, et al. Changes in severity and organ failure scores as prognostic factors in onco-hematological malignancy patients admitted to the ICU. Intensive Care Med 2006;32(10):1560–8.
24. Larchè J, Azoulay E, Fieux F, et al. Improved survival of critically ill cancer patients with septic shock. Intensive Care Med 2003;29(10):1688–95.
25. Maschmeyer G, Bertschat FL, Moesta KT, et al. Outcome analysis of 189 consecutive cancer patients referred to the intensive care unit as emergencies during a 2-year period. Eur J Cancer 2003;39(6):783–92.

26. Peigne V, Rusinova K, Karlin L, et al. Continued survival gains in recent years among critically ill myeloma patients. Intensive Care Med 2009;35(3):512–8.
27. Pène F, Percheron S, Lemiale V, et al. Temporal changes in management and outcome of septic shock in patients with malignancies in the intensive care unit. Crit Care Med 2008;36(3):690–6.
28. Soares M, Carvalho MS, Salluh JI, et al. Effect of age on survival of critically ill patients with cancer. Crit Care Med 2006;34(3):715–21.
29. Soares M, Darmon M, Salluh JI, et al. Prognosis of lung cancer patients with life-threatening complications. Chest 2007;131(3):840–6.
30. Soares M, Salluh JI, Spector N, et al. Characteristics and outcomes of cancer patients requiring mechanical ventilatory support for >24 hrs. Crit Care Med 2005;33(3):520–6.
31. Soares M, Salluh JI, Toscano L, et al. Outcomes and prognostic factors in patients with head and neck cancer and severe acute illnesses. Intensive Care Med 2007;33(11):2009–13.
32. Taccone FS, Artigas AA, Sprung CL, et al. Characteristics and outcomes of cancer patients in European ICUs. Crit Care 2009;13(1):R15.
33. Lecuyer L, Chevret S, Guidet B, et al. Case volume and mortality in haematological patients with acute respiratory failure. Eur Respir J 2008;32(3):748–54.
34. Soares M, Salluh JI, Torres VB, et al. Short- and long-term outcomes of critically ill patients with cancer and prolonged ICU length of stay. Chest 2008;134(3):520–6.
35. Merz TM, Schar P, Buhlmann M, et al. Resource use and outcome in critically ill patients with hematological malignancy: a retrospective cohort study. Crit Care 2008;12(3):R75.
36. Cornet AD, Issa AI, van de Loosdrecht AA, et al. Sequential organ failure predicts mortality of patients with a haematological malignancy needing intensive care. Eur J Haematol 2005;74(6):511–6.
37. Vandijck DM, Benoit DD, Depuydt PO, et al. Impact of recent intravenous chemotherapy on outcome in severe sepsis and septic shock patients with hematological malignancies. Intensive Care Med 2008;34(5):847–55.
38. Benoit DD, Depuydt PO, Vandewoude KH, et al. Outcome in severely ill patients with hematological malignancies who received intravenous chemotherapy in the intensive care unit. Intensive Care Med 2006;32(1):93–9.
39. Darmon M, Thiery G, Ciroldi M, et al. Intensive care in patients with newly diagnosed malignancies and a need for cancer chemotherapy. Crit Care Med 2005; 33(11):2488–93.
40. Bach PB, Schrag D, Nierman DM, et al. Identification of poor prognostic features among patients requiring mechanical ventilation after hematopoietic stem cell transplantation. Blood 2001;98(12):3234–40.
41. Letourneau I, Dorval M, Belanger R, et al. Acute renal failure in bone marrow transplant patients admitted to the intensive care unit. Nephron 2002;90(4):408–12.
42. Pène F, Aubron C, Azoulay E, et al. Outcome of critically ill allogeneic hematopoietic stem-cell transplantation recipients: a reappraisal of indications for organ failure supports. J Clin Oncol 2006;24(4):643–9.
43. Vieira JM Jr, Castro I, Curvello-Neto A, et al. Effect of acute kidney injury on weaning from mechanical ventilation in critically ill patients. Crit Care Med 2007;35(1):184–91.
44. Parikh CR, Coca SG. Acute renal failure in hematopoietic cell transplantation. Kidney Int 2006;69(3):430–5.

45. Bellomo R, Ronco C, Kellum JA, et al. Acute renal failure— definition, outcome measures, animal models, fluid therapy and information technology needs: the Second International Consensus Conference of the Acute Dialysis Quality Initiative (ADQI) Group. Crit Care 2004;8(4):R204–12.
46. Hoste EA, Schurgers M. Epidemiology of acute kidney injury: how big is the problem? Crit Care Med 2008;36(4 Suppl):S146–51.
47. Mehta RL, Kellum JA, Shah SV, et al. Acute Kidney Injury Network: report of an initiative to improve outcomes in acute kidney injury. Crit Care 2007;11(2):R31.
48. Kellum JA. Defining and classifying AKI: one set of criteria. Nephrol Dial Transplant 2008;23(5):1471–2.
49. Bagshaw SM, George C, Bellomo R. Changes in the incidence and outcome for early acute kidney injury in a cohort of Australian intensive care units. Crit Care 2007;11(3):R68.
50. Bagshaw SM, Laupland KB, Doig CJ, et al. Prognosis for long-term survival and renal recovery in critically ill patients with severe acute renal failure: a population-based study. Crit Care 2005;9(6):R700–9.
51. de Mendonça A, Vincent JL, Suter PM, et al. Acute renal failure in the ICU: risk factors and outcome evaluated by the SOFA score. Intensive Care Med 2000; 26(7):915–21.
52. Uchino S, Kellum JA, Bellomo R, et al. Acute renal failure in critically ill patients: a multinational, multicenter study. JAMA 2005;294(7):813–8.
53. Tanvetyanon T, Leighton JC. Life-sustaining treatments in patients who died of chronic congestive heart failure compared with metastatic cancer. Crit Care Med 2003;31(1):60–4.
54. Chertow GM, Christiansen CL, Cleary PD, et al. Prognostic stratification in critically ill patients with acute renal failure requiring dialysis. Arch Intern Med 1995; 155(14):1505–11.
55. Hoste EA, Lameire NH, Vanholder RC, et al. Acute renal failure in patients with sepsis in a surgical ICU: predictive factors, incidence, comorbidity, and outcome. J Am Soc Nephrol 2003;14(4):1022–30.
56. Soares M, Salluh JI, Ferreira CG, et al. Impact of two different comorbidity measures on the 6-month mortality of critically ill cancer patients. Intensive Care Med 2005;31(3):408–15.
57. Massion PB, Dive AM, Doyen C, et al. Prognosis of hematologic malignancies does not predict intensive care unit mortality. Crit Care Med 2002;30(10): 2260–70.
58. Rubenfeld GD, Crawford SW. Withdrawing life support from mechanically ventilated recipients of bone marrow transplants: a case for evidence-based guidelines. Ann Intern Med 1996;125(8):625–33.
59. Drake MT, Clarke BL, Khosla S. Bisphosphonates: mechanism of action and role in clinical practice. Mayo Clin Proc 2008;83(9):1032–45.
60. Vandijck DM, Benoit DD. Impact of recent intravenous chemotherapy on outcome in severe sepsis and septic shock patients with hematological malignancies: reply to letter by Meyer et al. Intensive Care Med 2008;34(10):1930–1.
61. Rivers E, Nguyen B, Havstad S, et al. Early goal-directed therapy in the treatment of severe sepsis and septic shock. N Engl J Med 2001;345(19):1368–77.
62. Hilbert G, Gruson D, Vargas F, et al. Noninvasive ventilation in immunosuppressed patients with pulmonary infiltrates, fever, and acute respiratory failure. N Engl J Med 2001;344(7):481–7.
63. Bernard GR, Vincent JL, Laterre PF, et al. Efficacy and safety of recombinant human activated protein C for severe sepsis. N Engl J Med 2001;344(10):699–709.

64. Dhainaut JF, Shorr AF, Macias WL, et al. Dynamic evolution of coagulopathy in the first day of severe sepsis: relationship with mortality and organ failure. Crit Care Med 2005;33(2):341–8.

65. Shimamura K, Oka K, Nakazawa M, et al. Distribution patterns of microthrombi in disseminated intravascular coagulation. Arch Pathol Lab Med 1983;107(10):543–7.

66. Gupta A, Berg DT, Gerlitz B, et al. Role of protein C in renal dysfunction after polymicrobial sepsis. J Am Soc Nephrol 2007;18(3):860–7.

67. Sharfuddin AA, Sandoval RM, Berg DT, et al. Soluble thrombomodulin protects ischemic kidneys. J Am Soc Nephrol 2009;20(3):524–34.

68. Hughes WT, Armstrong D, Bodey GP, et al. 2002 guidelines for the use of antimicrobial agents in neutropenic patients with cancer. Clin Infect Dis 2002;34(6):730–51.

69. Paul M, Benuri-Silbiger I, Soares-Weiser K, et al. Beta lactam monotherapy versus beta lactam-aminoglycoside combination therapy for sepsis in immunocompetent patients: systematic review and meta-analysis of randomised trials. BMJ 2004;328(7441):668.

70. Paul M, Soares-Weiser K, Leibovici L. Beta lactam monotherapy versus beta lactam-aminoglycoside combination therapy for fever with neutropenia: systematic review and meta-analysis. BMJ 2003;326(7399):1111.

71. Smyth AR, Tan KH. Once-daily versus multiple-daily dosing with intravenous aminoglycosides for cystic fibrosis. Cochrane Database Syst Rev 2006;3:CD002009.

72. Rybak M, Lomaestro B, Rotschafer JC, et al. Therapeutic monitoring of vancomycin in adult patients: a consensus review of the American Society of Health-System Pharmacists, the Infectious Diseases Society of America, and the Society of Infectious Diseases Pharmacists. Am J Health Syst Pharm 2009;66(1):82–98.

73. Hidayat LK, Hsu DI, Quist R, et al. High-dose vancomycin therapy for methicillin-resistant *Staphylococcus aureus* infections: efficacy and toxicity. Arch Intern Med 2006;166(19):2138–44.

74. Lodise TP, Lomaestro B, Graves J, et al. Larger vancomycin doses (at least four grams per day) are associated with an increased incidence of nephrotoxicity. Antimicrobial Agents Chemother 2008;52(4):1330–6.

75. Eriksson U, Seifert B, Schaffner A. Comparison of effects of amphotericin B deoxycholate infused over 4 or 24 hours: randomised controlled. BMJ 2001; 322(7286):579 [Clinical research ed.].

76. Blot S, Vandewoude K. Management of invasive candidiasis in critically ill patients. Drugs 2004;64(19):2159–75.

77. McCullough PA. Contrast-induced acute kidney injury. J Am Coll Cardiol 2008; 51(15):1419–28.

78. Tumlin J, Stacul F, Adam A, et al. Pathophysiology of contrast-induced nephropathy. Am J Cardiol 2006;98(6A):14K–20K.

79. McCarthy CS, Becker JA. Multiple myeloma and contrast media. Radiology 1992;183(2):519–21.

80. Merten GJ, Burgess WP, Gray LV, et al. Prevention of contrast-induced nephropathy with sodium bicarbonate: a randomized controlled trial. JAMA 2004; 291(19):2328–34.

81. Hoste EAJ, De Waele JJ, Gevaert SA, et al. Sodium bicarbonate for prevention of contrast-induced acute kidney injury: a systematic review and meta-analysis. Nephrol Dial Transplant 2009. [Epub ahead of print].

82. Vaitkus PT, Brar C. N-acetylcysteine in the prevention of contrast-induced nephropathy: publication bias perpetuated by meta-analyses. Am Heart J 2007;153(2):275–80.

83. Hoffmann U, Fischereder M, Kruger B, et al. The value of N-acetylcysteine in the prevention of radiocontrast agent-induced nephropathy seems questionable. J Am Soc Nephrol 2004;15(2):407–10.

84. Marenzi G, Lauri G, Campodonico J, et al. Comparison of two hemofiltration protocols for prevention of contrast-induced nephropathy in high-risk patients. Am J Med 2006;119(2):155–62.

85. Arany I, Safirstein RL. Cisplatin nephrotoxicity. Semin Nephrol 2003;23(5):460–4.

86. Schuchter LM, Hensley ML, Meropol NJ, et al. 2002 update of recommendations for the use of chemotherapy and radiotherapy protectants: clinical practice guidelines of the American Society of Clinical Oncology. J Clin Oncol 2002; 20(12):2895–903.

87. Widemann BC, Adamson PC. Understanding and managing methotrexate nephrotoxicity. Oncologist 2006;11(6):694–703.

88. Pauley JL, Panetta JC, Schmidt J, et al. Late-onset delayed excretion of methotrexate. Cancer Chemother Pharmacol 2004;54(2):146–52.

89. Buchen S, Ngampolo D, Melton RG, et al. Carboxypeptidase G2 rescue in patients with methotrexate intoxication and renal failure. Br J Cancer 2005; 92(3):480–7.

90. Cairo MS, Bishop M. Tumour lysis syndrome: new therapeutic strategies and classification. Br J Haematol 2004;127(1):3–11.

91. Davidson MB, Thakkar S, Hix JK, et al. Pathophysiology, clinical consequences, and treatment of tumor lysis syndrome. Am J Med 2004;116(8):546–54.

92. Darmon M, Roumier M, Azoulay E. Acute tumor lysis syndrome: diagnosis and management. In: Vincent J-L, editor. Yearbook of intensive care and emergency medicine. Berlin/Heidelberg/New York: Springer-Verlag; 2009. p. 819–27.

93. Levi M. Disseminated intravascular coagulation in cancer patients. Best Pract Res Clin Haematol 2009;22(1):129–36.

94. Sallah S, Wan JY, Nguyen NP, et al. Disseminated intravascular coagulation in solid tumors: clinical and pathologic study. Thromb Haemost 2001;86(3):828–33.

95. Stein E, McMahon B, Kwaan H, et al. The coagulopathy of acute promyelocytic leukaemia revisited. Best Pract Res Clin Haematol 2009;22(1):153–63.

96. Bell WR, Starksen NF, Tong S, et al. Trousseau's syndrome. Devastating coagulopathy in the absence of heparin. Am J Med 1985;79(4):423–30.

97. Callander N, Rapaport SI. Trousseau's syndrome. West J Med 1993;158(4): 364–71.

98. Miyashita M, Onda M, Sasajima K, et al. Multiple organ failure without sepsis following surgical treatment of advanced gastric carcinoma. Jpn J Surg 1988; 18(6):705–8.

99. Sack GH Jr, Levin J, Bell WR. Trousseau's syndrome and other manifestations of chronic disseminated coagulopathy in patients with neoplasms: clinical, pathophysiologic, and therapeutic features. Medicine (Baltimore) 1977;56(1):1–37.

100. Taccone FS, Jeangette SM, Blecic SA. First-ever stroke as initial presentation of systemic cancer. J Stroke Cerebrovasc Dis 2008;17(4):169–74.

101. Varki A. Trousseau's syndrome: multiple definitions and multiple mechanisms. Blood 2007;110(6):1723–9.

102. Voulgaris E, Pentheroudakis G, Vassou A, et al. Disseminated intravascular coagulation (DIC) and non-small cell lung cancer (NSCLC): report of a case and review of the literature. Lung Cancer 2009;64(2):247–9.

103. Langer F, Spath B, Haubold K, et al. Tissue factor procoagulant activity of plasma microparticles in patients with cancer-associated disseminated intravascular coagulation. Ann Hematol 2008;87(6):451–7.

104. Chalela JA, Raps EC, Kasner SE. Disseminated intravascular coagulation and stroke associated with cervical cancer. J Stroke Cerebrovasc Dis 1999;8(5):355–7.
105. Smeglin A, Ansari M, Skali H, et al. Marantic endocarditis and disseminated intravascular coagulation with systemic emboli in presentation of pancreatic cancer. J Clin Oncol 2008;26(8):1383–5.
106. Lesesne JB, Rothschild N, Erickson B, et al. Cancer-associated hemolytic-uremic syndrome: analysis of 85 cases from a national registry. J Clin Oncol 1989;7(6):781–9.
107. Francis KK, Kalyanam N, Terrell DR, et al. Disseminated malignancy misdiagnosed as thrombotic thrombocytopenic purpura: a report of 10 patients and a systematic review of published cases. Oncologist 2007;12(1):11–9.
108. Levandovsky M, Harvey D, Lara P, et al. Thrombotic thrombocytopenic purpura-hemolytic uremic syndrome (TTP-HUS): a 24-year clinical experience with 178 patients. J Hematol Oncol 2008;1:23.
109. Miller DP, Kaye JA, Shea K, et al. Incidence of thrombotic thrombocytopenic purpura/hemolytic uremic syndrome. Epidemiology 2004;15(2):208–15.
110. Chang JC, Naqvi T. Thrombotic thrombocytopenic purpura associated with bone marrow metastasis and secondary myelofibrosis in cancer. Oncologist 2003;8(4):375–80.
111. Spoormans I, Altintas S, Van den Brande J, et al. Purpura in a patient with disseminated breast cancer: a rapidly progressive cancer-related thrombotic thrombocytopenic purpura. Ann Oncol 2008;19(6):1204–7.
112. Werner TL, Agarwal N, Carney HM, et al. Management of cancer-associated thrombotic microangiopathy: what is the right approach? Am J Hematol 2007; 82(4):295–8.
113. Snyder HW Jr, Mittelman A, Oral A, et al. Treatment of cancer chemotherapy-associated thrombotic thrombocytopenic purpura/hemolytic uremic syndrome by protein A immunoadsorption of plasma. Cancer 1993;71(5):1882–92.
114. Zupancic M, Shah PC, Shah-Khan F. Gemcitabine-associated thrombotic thrombocytopenic purpura. Lancet Oncol 2007;8(7):634–41.
115. Cantrell JE Jr, Phillips TM, Schein PS. Carcinoma-associated hemolytic-uremic syndrome: a complication of mitomycin C chemotherapy. J Clin Oncol 1985; 3(5):723–34.
116. Muller S, Schutt P, Bojko P, et al. Hemolytic uremic syndrome following prolonged gemcitabine therapy: report of four cases from a single institution. Ann Hematol 2005;84(2):110–4.
117. Roy V, Rizvi MA, Vesely SK, et al. Thrombotic thrombocytopenic purpura-like syndromes following bone marrow transplantation: an analysis of associated conditions and clinical outcomes. Bone Marrow Transplant 2001;27(6):641–6.
118. Ganatra AM, Loughlin KR. The management of malignant ureteral obstruction treated with ureteral stents. J Urol 2005;174(6):2125–8.
119. Kouba E, Wallen EM, Pruthi RS. Management of ureteral obstruction due to advanced malignancy: optimizing therapeutic and palliative outcomes. J Urol 2008;180(2):444–50.
120. Wong LM, Cleeve LK, Milner AD, et al. Malignant ureteral obstruction: outcomes after intervention. Have things changed? J Urol 2007;178(1):178–83 [discussion: 183].
121. Gertz MA. Current therapy of myeloma induced renal failure. Leuk Lymphoma 2008;49(5):833–4.
122. Kyle RA, Gertz MA, Witzig TE, et al. Review of 1027 patients with newly diagnosed multiple myeloma. Mayo Clin Proc 2003;78(1):21–33.

123. Eleutherakis-Papaiakovou V, Bamias A, Gika D, et al. Renal failure in multiple myeloma: incidence, correlations, and prognostic significance. Leuk Lymphoma 2007;48(2):337–41.

124. Knudsen LM, Hjorth M, Hippe E. Renal failure in multiple myeloma: reversibility and impact on the prognosis. Nordic Myeloma Study Group. Eur J Haematol 2000;65(3):175–81.

125. Clark WF, Stewart AK, Rock GA, et al. Plasma exchange when myeloma presents as acute renal failure: a randomized, controlled trial. Ann Intern Med 2005;143(11):777–84.

126. Hutchison CA, Bradwell AR, Cook M, et al. Treatment of acute renal failure secondary to multiple myeloma with chemotherapy and extended high cut-off hemodialysis. Clin J Am Soc Nephrol 2009;4(4):745–54.

127. Huang ZQ, Sanders PW. Localization of a single binding site for immunoglobulin light chains on human Tamm-Horsfall glycoprotein. J Clin Invest 1997;99(4):732–6.

128. Herrera GA. Renal lesions associated with plasma cell dyscrasias: practical approach to diagnosis, new concepts, and challenges. Arch Pathol Lab Med 2009;133(2):249–67.

129. Lameire N, Van Biesen W, Vanholder R. Acute renal problems in the critically ill cancer patient. Curr Opin Crit Care 2008;14(6):635–46.

130. Kyle RA, Rajkumar SV. Multiple myeloma. N Engl J Med 2004;351(18):1860–73.

131. Tosi P, Zamagni E, Cellini C, et al. Thalidomide alone or in combination with dexamethasone in patients with advanced, relapsed or refractory multiple myeloma and renal failure. Eur J Haematol 2004;73(2):98–103.

132. Roussou M, Kastritis E, Migkou M, et al. Treatment of patients with multiple myeloma complicated by renal failure with bortezomib-based regimens. Leuk Lymphoma 2008;49(5):890–5.

133. Firkin F, Hill PA, Dwyer K, et al. Reversal of dialysis-dependent renal failure in light-chain deposition disease by autologous peripheral blood stem cell transplantation. Am J Kidney Dis 2004;44(3):551–5.

134. Lorenz EC, Gertz MA, Fervenza FC, et al. Long-term outcome of autologous stem cell transplantation in light chain deposition disease. Nephrol Dial Transplant 2008;23(6):2052–7.

135. Thiery G, Azoulay E, Darmon M, et al. Outcome of cancer patients considered for intensive care unit admission: a hospital-wide prospective study. J Clin Oncol 2005;23(19):4406–13.

136. Groeger JS, Lemeshow S, Price K, et al. Multicenter outcome study of cancer patients admitted to the intensive care unit: a probability of mortality model. J Clin Oncol 1998;16(2):761–70.

137. Groeger JS, White P Jr, Nierman DM, et al. Outcome for cancer patients requiring mechanical ventilation. J Clin Oncol 1999;17(3):991–7.

138. Apatira L, Boyd EA, Malvar G, et al. Hope, truth, and preparing for death: perspectives of surrogate decision makers. Ann Intern Med 2008;149(12):861–8.

139. Wright AA, Zhang B, Ray A, et al. Associations between end-of-life discussions, patient mental health, medical care near death, and caregiver bereavement adjustment. JAMA 2008;300(14):1665–73.

140. Steinhauser KE, Christakis NA, Clipp EC, et al. Factors considered important at the end of life by patients, family, physicians, and other care providers. JAMA 2000;284(19):2476–82.

141. Emanuel LL, Emanuel EJ, Stoeckle JD, et al. Advance directives. Stability of patients' treatment choices. Arch Intern Med 1994;154(2):209–17.

142. Emanuel EJ, Fairclough DL, Wolfe P, et al. Talking with terminally ill patients and their caregivers about death, dying, and bereavement: is it stressful? Is it helpful? Arch Intern Med 2004;164(18):1999–2004.
143. Price KJ, Kish SK. End-of-life decisions in cancer care. Crit Care Clin 2001; 17(3):805–11.
144. Lecuyer L, Chevret S, Thiery G, et al. The ICU trial: a new admission policy for cancer patients requiring mechanical ventilation. Crit Care Med 2007;35(3): 808–14.

Oncologic Emergencies

Deepti Behl, MD[a], Andrea Wahner Hendrickson, MD[a],
Timothy J. Moynihan, MD[b],*

KEYWORDS

- Hypercalcemia • Hyperviscosity • Malignant airway obstruction
- Malignant spinal cord compression

Cancer patients are at risk for several life-threatening emergencies, including metabolic, cardiologic, neurologic, and infectious events. Many of these high-risk situations can be prevented or effectively managed if promptly recognized and urgently treated. This review addresses the more commonly encountered emergencies in cancer patients.

HYPERCALCEMIA

Hypercalcemia is one of the most common oncologic emergencies. The reported incidence varies widely, and may occur in up to 30% of all cancer patients at some time in their disease course.[1]

Hypercalcemia in patients with cancer can be mediated by several different mechanisms, including humoral-related factors, such as parathyroid hormone-related peptide (PTHrP), parathyroid hormone (PTH) oversecretion, overproduction of vitamin D, or direct osteolytic effect of tumor on bone.[2]

PTHrP-mediated hypercalcemia (also termed humoral hypercalcemia of malignancy [HHM]), is by far the most common mechanism, accounting for 80% of all cases.[2] PTHrP works much like PTH, causing increased resorption of calcium from the bones and enhancing renal retention of calcium.[3] Tumors most commonly associated with PTHrP production are of squamous histology and usually arise from the lung, esophagus, head and neck, and cervix.

Ovarian, endometrial, and renal carcinoma may also produce hypercalcemia through this mechanism. Serum measurement of PTHrP is feasible, but of little to no clinical significance, so is not routinely recommended.

Tumors that overproduce PTH itself, rather than PTHrP, are rare. Only a few patients are known who have hypercalcemia because of high PTH levels.[2,4]

About 15% of cancer patients with hypercalcemia have tumors that lead to an overproduction of the active form of vitamin D. Lymphomas are particularly adept at

[a] Hematology and Oncology, Mayo Clinic College of Medicine, 200 First Street SW, Rochester, MN 55905, USA
[b] Department of Oncology, Mayo Clinic College of Medicine, 200 First Street SW, Rochester, MN 55905, USA
* Corresponding author.
E-mail address: moynihan.timothy@mayo.edu (T.J. Moynihan).

Crit Care Clin 26 (2010) 181–205
doi:10.1016/j.ccc.2009.09.004
0749-0704/09/$ – see front matter © 2010 Elsevier Inc. All rights reserved.

criticalcare.theclinics.com

secreting the active form of vitamin D, which leads to increased bone resorption and increased efficiency of intestinal absorption of calcium, leading to hypercalcemia.[5]

Cancers that have a tendency to metastasize to the bone may lead to local osteolytic cell activation and produce hypercalcemia.[6] Local production of any one of several cytokines facilitates local bone resorption. Included in these cytokines is PTHrP. Common examples of tumors producing hypercalcemia from local bone effects include breast cancer, multiple myeloma, and many lymphomas.[7] Other tumors that have a high predilection for bone metastases, such as prostate cancer, are only rarely associated with hypercalcemia, reinforcing the dependence not just on the presence of the bony metastases, but the unique characteristics and cytokine production of the tumor itself.

Clinical Presentation

The clinical manifestations of hypercalcemia are vague and nonspecific, often confused with many other comorbid conditions present in patients with advanced cancer.[8] The rate of increase of the calcium level is more important than the absolute calcium level in determining the appearance of symptoms. High levels may be well tolerated if the rate has been slow and prolonged. The most common symptoms are constipation, lethargy, abdominal pain, and polyuria. Electrocardiograph (ECG) may show a shortened QT interval and arrhythmias may occur. Acute renal failure, seizures, coma, and death may also occur if corrective measures are not taken.

Diagnosis

The best way to diagnose hypercalcemia is to obtain an ionized calcium level. Total calcium level measurement may not be as accurate, because of changes in plasma proteins, particularly albumin, which affect the level considerably. Although formulas for correction for calcium according to albumin levels are widely used, they only help in making approximations.

Although PTHrP is the most common mechanism for hypercalcemia in patients with cancer, coexistent primary hyperparathyroidism is not a rare entity and must be considered in the differential diagnosis.[2,9] PTHrP and PTH levels can be measured, but there can be no strong recommendation to check either, as most of these patients have obvious widely metastatic cancer, and the management of the patient is unlikely to be effected. In patients with minimal metastatic disease, or in tumors that are rarely associated with hypercalcemia, PTH levels are reasonable to check, especially for those with more indolent tumors, whose survival may be prolonged.

Management

Patients with clinically significant hypercalcemia are almost always intravascularly volume depleted. (**Table 1**) This, in turn, leads to a decreased glomerular filtration rate, further decreasing excretion of calcium by the kidneys. Thus, the cornerstone of the management of hypercalcemia is adequate hydration. Normal saline is immediately started, generally at rates between 200 and 300 mL/h, depending on the patient's cardiovascular status. Once adequate intravascular volume repletion has been achieved, loop diuretics should be used to facilitate calcium excretion. Thiazide diuretics should be avoided, as they worsen hypercalcemia.

One of the most useful pharmacologic agents for treatment of hypercalcemia are the bisphosphonates.[10] Pamidronate or zoledronic acid may be used, although studies show that zoledronic acid is slightly more efficacious.[11] Zoledronic acid requires a shorter infusion time, but is more expensive. Calcitonin can be used in the first 12 to 24 hours, but its effects are modest and tachyphylaxis occurs quickly.

Table 1 Treatment of hypercalcemia		
Medication	**Usual Dose**	**Points to Remember**
Normal saline	Rapid infusion 200–300 mL/h until euvolemic	Caution in patients with heart failure
Furosemide	20–40 mg IV	Only after adequate hydration
Pamidronate	60–90 mg IV	Caution if renal insufficiency present
Zoledronic acid	4 mg IV	Adjust dose for renal insufficiency
Calcitonin	4–8 IU/kg SQ or IV	Tachyphylaxis occurs quickly
Steroids	Hydrocortisone 100 mg every 6 h; or prednisone 60 mg/d by mouth	Role usually limited to lymphomas
Mithramycin/gallium nitrate		Of historical interest only

Abbreviations: IU, international units; IV, intravenous; SQ, subcutaneous.

However, it may be particularly useful in those severe cases in which the calcium level requires immediate lowering, such as in patients with seizures or arrhythmias. Because of the rapid tachyphylaxis, calcitonin should never be used as a single agent in treating hypercalcemia.

In the rare cases in which vitamin D_3 is responsible for the hypercalcemia, such as some lymphomas, steroids are useful. Agents such as mithramycin and gallium nitrate are rarely, if ever, used, as bisphosphonates tend to be effective with fewer side effects. These are largely of historical interest at this point (for a summary of the treatment of hypercalcemia, see **Table 1**).[12]

HYPONATREMIA

Hyponatremia is common in cancer patients and is defined as a serum sodium concentration of less than 136 mmol/L.[13] The most common cause is the syndrome of inappropriate secretion of antidiuretic hormone (SIADH); however, it is important to recognize that volume depletion can also be associated with hyponatremia.

Hyponatremia can be classified as mild if the sodium level is between 135 and 131 mmol/L, moderate if the level is 130 to 126 mmol/L, and severe if less than 125 mmol/L.[14] Severe hyponatremia can be life-threatening, especially if the onset is acute.

Causes of SIADH in Cancer Patients

SIADH may ensue from the tumor itself or the chemotherapy that is used to treat it. Many different tumors can actively produce antidiuretic hormone (ADH), but it is most classically associated with small cell lung cancers. Other lung tumors and duodenal, pancreatic, genitourinary, and head and neck cancers can lead to ectopic ADH production. Rare cases of SIADH have been reported with lymphomas, sarcomas, and thymomas.[14]

Certain chemotherapy drugs, notably cisplatin,[15] ifosfamide, and vincristine, can stimulate excessive ADH production or enhance its activity. These drugs are also nauseating, and nausea in itself is a potent stimulus for ADH release; the SIADH and resultant hyponatremia from these drugs can be severe.

Symptoms

Mild hyponatremia may manifest as excessive tiredness, difficulty concentrating and remembering, headache, and muscle cramps. A peculiar but uncommon symptom of hyponatremia is dysgeusia. More severe hyponatremia may manifest with diffuse neurologic symptoms including confusion, hallucinations, seizures, coma, and death.

Diagnosis

SIADH is diagnosed when a clinically euvolemic patient with normal adrenal and thyroid function has a decreased effective serum osmolality of less than 275 mOsm/kg and an increased urinary osmolality of more than 100 mOsm/kg of water. In addition, urine sodium should be greater than 40 mmol/L when the dietary sodium is not excessive.[14] Other findings may include serum uric acid less than 4 mg/dL[16] and blood urea nitrogen less than 10 mg/dL. Fractional excretion of sodium is typically greater than 1%, and that of urea greater than 55%. Levels of ADH should not be routinely checked, but are typically elevated.

Management

The definitive treatment of SIADH in the cancer patient is removal of the underlying cause. If the hyponatremia is asymptomatic, it is appropriate to ascertain the cause before management is begun. It is often possible to remove the cause in cancer patients, such as resection of a tumor or discontinuation of the offending chemotherapy drug.

In case of symptomatic hyponatremia, prompt treatment is mandated. Treatment of symptomatic hyponatremia is associated with better outcomes even when the hyponatremia is chronic.[17] If symptoms are mild, fluid restriction to about 0.5 to 1 L of free water, along with increased intake of salt and protein, is usually sufficient.

In cases of more severe symptoms, the serum sodium should be restored using 3% saline cautiously. Over-rapid correction of hyponatremia, especially if long-standing, can result in central pontine myelinosis (CPM), a debilitating neurologic condition that manifests several days after the damage is done. It is characterized by spastic quadriparesis, pseudobulbar palsy, coma, or death.[18] Therefore, it is recommended that serum sodium be corrected by no more than 8 to 10 mmol/L in 24 hours, or less than 18 mmol/L in the first 48 hours.[19] If a patient has neurologic symptoms attributable to hyponatremia, it is reasonable to increase serum sodium by 1 to 2 mmol/L/h until the neurologic condition improves, and then return to the use of normal saline. The use of furosemide-induced diuresis is now considered controversial, and it is recommended that furosemide not be used along with 3% saline.

A single case has been reported in which reinduction of hyponatremia after excessive correction of serum sodium level apparently improved a patient's outcome.[20]

CARDIAC EMERGENCIES
Superior Vena Cava Syndrome

The superior vena cava (SVC) is easily compressed by tumors arising from the lung, mediastinal structures, or lymph nodes. Malignancies are the most common cause for superior vena cava syndrome (SVCS) but, as more and more indwelling central venous access devices are used, intrinsic thrombus is becoming a significant cause for SVCS,[21,22] accounting for as many as 20% to 40% of all cases.

Etiology

The leading cause of malignancy associated with SVCS is lung cancer, accounting for as many as 60% to 85% of all cases. The most common lung cancer type that is associated with SVCS is non–small cell lung cancer (NSCLC), but that is only because NSCLC is far more common than small cell lung carcinoma (SCLC). It is estimated that 2% to 4% of all lung cancer patients will develop SVCS, but 10% of patients with SCLC will develop SVCS. The second most common cancer associated with SVCS is non-Hodgkin lymphoma, accounting for about 10% of all cases. Curiously, Hodgkin disease is rarely associated with SVCS even though it is often mediastinal in location.

Clinical presentation
SVCS causes edema in the upper body, particularly in the head and neck (**Fig. 1**). This edema may be significant enough to compromise the lumen of the larynx, causing dyspnea and stridor, and compromise of the pharyngeal lumen, causing dysphagia. There may be arm swelling and cutaneous venous dilatation as the venous return is shunted around the obstruction (**Fig. 2**). The most concerning symptoms are neurologic, such as headaches, confusion, or even coma, suggesting cerebral ischemia. Brain stem herniation and death can potentially occur.[23] However, the usual course of SVCS is that collaterals eventually develop, and symptoms tend to improve when this happens.[24]

Management
SVCS is not considered a true oncologic emergency unless neurologic symptoms are present. However, its presence is, in itself, a poor prognostic marker.[25] It is strongly recommended that, if a patient presents with SVCS without a prior tissue diagnosis of malignancy, every effort should be made to obtain biopsies and histologic diagnosis before any treatment decisions are made.[26]

If a true emergency exists, then a stent can be emergently placed in the SVC if the expertise to do so is available,[27,28] or radiation can be used. Stenting is now considered first-line treatment of SVCS from benign causes,[29] and many experts believe this can also be extrapolated to malignant causes.[30] Otherwise, therapy directed at the underlying cause should be used, and symptoms usually start improving rapidly if the tumor is responsive.

Although not a true emergency unless central nervous system (CNS) symptoms are present, the presence of SVCS at diagnosis does portend a poor prognosis in lung cancer and lymphoma, with overall median survival only 5 months.

Malignant Pericardial Effusion
Cancer patients may develop fluid accumulations in the pericardial space as a result of metastases, various treatments, or direct extension of the tumor into the space

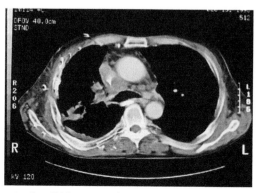

Fig. 1. CT scan demonstrating SVC compression.

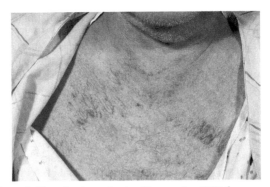

Fig. 2. Dilated collateral skin veins in patient with superior SVCS from small cell lung cancer.

(**Fig. 3**).[31] Primary malignancies of the pericardium are rare. Of these, mesothelioma is the most common, and is almost always unresectable and incurable at presentation.[32]

Most pericardial effusions are small and asymptomatic, although their presence does portend a poor prognosis, with median survival often less than 1 year.

Large effusions can be asymptomatic if they accumulate slowly, but rapidly accumulating effusions may lead to cardiac tamponade, even if small in amount.[33] It is estimated that, if an effusion occurs slowly, the pericardium may accommodate as much as 2 L of fluid without life-threatening compromise of ventricular filling.[34]

Signs and symptoms

The classic Beck triad of distended neck veins, silent precordium, and hypotension in cardiac tamponade is rarely seen in malignancy, as, more often, the fluid accumulation tends to be subacute rather than acute. Patients typically complain of shortness of breath, chest discomfort, and fatigue. Clinical examination reveals distant heart sounds, a narrow pulse pressure, and pulsus paradoxus.[35,36] An electrocardiogram (ECG) tends to show low-voltage complexes with nonspecific ST-T changes. Electrical alternans may be seen in patients with a large pericardial effusion, but this is not diagnostic for cardiac tamponade physiology (**Fig. 4**).[33]

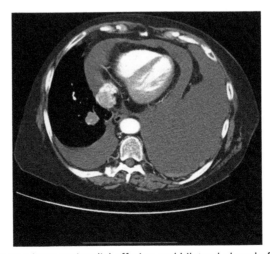

Fig. 3. CT scan showing large pericardial effusion and bilateral pleural effusions.

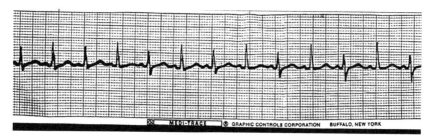

Fig. 4. ECG demonstrating electrical alternans in patient with pericardial tamponade.

Management

Echocardiography is useful in making the diagnosis of both effusions and demonstrating the physiology of tamponade, and also guides the drainage of the fluid to relieve symptoms.[37,38] There is probably no advantage to draining asymptomatic effusions, even if they are large.[39] A catheter may be left in place for a few days after drainage has been performed.

In the case of chemosensitive tumors, systemic chemotherapy may be useful. Intrapericardial installation of chemotherapy agents such as bleomycin,[40] carboplatin,[41] or mitomycin-C[42] has been studied in Japan and found to be safe. A recent study, also in Japan, found that overall survival is probably unchanged by such maneuvers.[43]

Surgical procedures, such as a subxiphoid pericardiostomy and percutaneous balloon pericardiotomy, are sometimes undertaken. These are low-morbidity procedures and usually can be accomplished under local anesthesia.[44] Subxiphoid pericardiostomy may be more appropriate for stable patients.[45] Video-assisted thoracoscopic (VATS) pericardial window is another safe and highly effective surgical alternative.[46]

Tumor Lysis Syndrome

Tumor lysis syndrome (TLS) results from rapid cell breakdown with the release of large amounts of nucleic acids, phosphorous, and potassium into the circulation. Although most commonly seen after administration of chemotherapy for highly sensitive tumors such as leukemias and lymphomas, spontaneous TLS has been reported to occur in a wide variety of tumors, most commonly those with a rapid growth pattern, the classic example being Burkitt lymphoma.

Nucleic acids are rapidly broken down into uric acid, which is not water soluble. Precipitation of uric acid crystals can occur in many organs, including the kidneys (causing renal failure), the cardiac conduction system (causing arrhythmias), and the joint spaces (causing an acute flare of gout). **Fig. 5** illustrates how nucleic acids are catabolized. Allopurinol inhibits the enzyme xanthine oxidase, thus decreasing uric acid production, whereas rasburicase is a recombinant form of the enzyme urate oxidase, which is not found in humans, and leads to the further degradation of uric acid into water-soluble allantoin. It is Food and Drug Administration (FDA)-approved for use in the pediatric population at high risk for the development of tumor lysis, and has also demonstrated efficacy in the adult population.[47–50] Risk factors for the development of TLS include intravascular volume depletion, rapidly growing malignancy, renal insufficiency, large tumor burden, and hyperuricacidemia.

Severe hyperphosphatemia can lead to renal failure by precipitation in the renal tubules of calcium phosphate crystals. This compound can deposit in the heart, causing arrhythmias. Acute, severe hyperkalemia can also produce life-threatening arrhythmia.

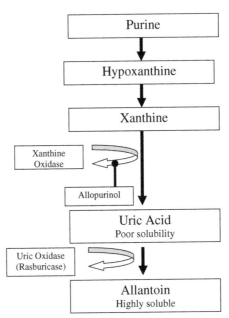

Fig. 5. Metabolism of uric acid with sites of action of allopurinol and xanthene oxidase.

TLS is defined by laboratory and clinical criteria. The Cairo-Bishop definition and grading is well accepted and recognizes laboratory and clinical parameters (**Box 1**).

Signs and Symptoms
The signs and symptoms relate to the underlying electrolyte and metabolic abnormalities, and are not specific for this syndrome.

Management
TLS is best managed proactively, anticipating its occurrence and taking measures to avoid it. The most important measure is to ensure adequate hydration. The aim is to ensure a urine output of 100 mL/m² if there is no cardiac limitation. Alkalinization of the urine is believed to be beneficial, but may be harmful if only allopurinol is being used, because xanthine is even less water soluble in an alkaline environment, and may precipitate within the renal tubules.[51] Once adequate hydration is assured, loop diuretics may be used to increase urine output, if needed.

Allopurinol is routinely instituted in moderate-risk situations 2 to 3 days before starting chemotherapy, but in high-risk situations, or situations in which allopurinol may be of limited benefit (such as high uric acid at baseline, or high uric acid despite allopurinol use), it is recommended that allopurinol be omitted and the patient started on rasburicase instead[52] (**Table 2**). Allopurinol causes buildup of xanthine and hypoxanthine, compounds that are poorly water soluble, heightening the risk of renal failure in these situations. Rasburicase, facilitates the break down of uric acid into allantoin, which is easily excreted in urine. Although rasburicase is approved only in pediatric patients by the FDA in the United States, there is adult experience with its use in France.[53] An expert panel considered that the rationale and recommendations discussed earlier are equally applicable in adults.[52] **Table 3** shows general guidelines for starting allopurinol and rasburicase.

Box 1
TLS laboratory definition using Cairo-Bishop classification

Laboratory TLS

Uric acid more than or equal to 8 mg/dL ($\geq$476 μmol/L) or 25% increase from baseline

Potassium more than or equal to 6.0 mEq/L ($\geq$6 mmol/L) or 25% increase from baseline

Phosphorus more than or equal to 6.5 mg/dL ($\geq$2.1 mmol/L) or 25% increase from baseline

Calcium less than or equal to 7 mg/dL ($\leq$1.75 mmol/L) or 25% decrease from baseline

Clinical TLS

Creatinine more than or equal to 1.5 times upper limit of normal

Cardiac arrhythmia or sudden death

Seizure

Note: Two or more laboratory changes within 3 days before, or 7 days after, cytotoxic therapy.
Data from Cairo MS, Bishop M. Tumour lysis syndrome: new therapeutic strategies and classification. Br J Haematol 2004;127(1):3–11.

Hyperphosphatemia is managed by placing the patient on a phosphorous-restricted diet, using oral phosphate binders, and, in extreme cases, dialysis.

Hyperkalemia is managed by using calcium gluconate, insulin and dextrose, and sodium polystyrene sulfonate, in addition to adequate hydration and diuresis as already mentioned. The accompanying table outlines the management of electrolyte abnormalities in TLS (**Table 4**).

MALIGNANT SPINAL CORD COMPRESSION

Malignant spinal cord compression (MSCC) is a devastating neurologic complication that occurs in approximately 1 in 12,700 cancer patients in the United States each

Table 2
Risk stratification forTLS

Type of Cancer	Risk		
	High	Intermediate	Low
NHL	Burkitt, lymphoblastic, B-ALL	DLBCL	Indolent NHL
ALL	WBC $\geq$ 100,000	WBC 50,000–100,000	WBC $\leq$50,000
AML	WBC $\geq$50,000 monoblastic	WBC 10,000–50,000	WBC $\leq$10,000
CLL		WBC 10,000–100,000 Tx w/fludarabine	WBC $\leq$10,000
Other hematologic malignancies (including CML and multiple myeloma) and solid tumors		Rapid proliferation with expected rapid response to therapy	Remainder of patients

Abbreviations: ALL, acute lymphoblastic leukemia; AML, acute myeloid leukemia; B-ALL, Burkitt acute lymphoblastic leukemia; CML, chronic myeloid leukemia; DLBCL, diffuse large B-cell lymphoma; NHL, non-Hodgkin lymphoma; CLL, chronic lymphocytic leukemia; Tx, treatment.

Table 3 Treatment recommendations for TLS	
Agent	**Recommendation**
Allopurinol	Dosing: 100 mg/m^2/dose every 8 h (10 mg/kg/d divided every 8 h) PO (maximum, 800 mg/d) or 200–400 mg/m^2/d in 1–3 divided doses; IV (maximum, 600 mg/d)
	Reduce dose by 50% or more in renal failure
	Reduce 6-mercaptopurine or azathioprine doses by 65%–75% with concomitant allopurinol
	May need to adjust doses of dicumarol, thiazide diuretics, chlorpropamide, cyclosporine, or allopurinol when they are used concomitantly with allopurinol
Rasburicase	Contraindicated in glucose-6-phosphate dehydrogenase–deficient patients, and in patients with a known history of anaphylaxis or hypersensitivity reactions, hemolytic reactions, or methemoglobinemia reactions to rasburicase or any of the excipients
	Administration: 0.05–0.2 mg/kg IV over 30 min
	Uric acid levels should be monitored regularly and used as a guide to modulate dosing; to measure uric acid levels place blood sample immediately on ice to avoid continual pharmacologic ex vivo enzymatic degradation
	10% incidence of antibody formation

year.[54] MSCC most commonly occurs when the malignancy metastasizes to the spine, with subsequent erosion into the epidural space causing compression of the spinal cord. Rarely, tumors will metastasize directly to the epidural or intradural tissue. Although all tumor types have the potential to cause MSCC, breast, prostate, and lung each account for approximately 15% to 20% of the cases, with non-Hodgkin lymphoma, renal cell carcinoma, and myeloma each causing 5% to 10% of cases.[12,54]

Pathophysiology

MSCC most commonly occurs when metastatic tumor reaches the vertebral bodies via hematogenous spread with secondary erosion into the epidural space, thus causing compression of the spinal cord. In approximately 15% of cases it occurs when a paravertebral lesion spreads into the spinal canal through an intervertebral foramen and directly compresses the spinal cord. This mechanism is most commonly seen in neuroblastomas and lymphomas.[55] Metastatic lesions can also cause MSCC via destruction of vertebral cortical bone leading to vertebral collapse with displacement of bone fragments into the epidural space. In rare cases, metastases occur directly to the spinal cord and meninges.[55–57] The damage to the spinal cord occurs via direct compression causing demyelination, axonal damage, and secondary vascular compromise. Animal models implicate vascular damage as the most prominent and destructive of the 2 mechanisms. Acute compression causes occlusion of epidural venous plexus, compromising the blood-spinal cord barrier, resulting in inflammation and vasogenic edema. At this stage, the damage can often be reversed by corticosteroids. When the arterial blood flow is impaired due to compression, spinal cord ischemia, infarction, and irreversible damage result.[58,59]

Clinical Presentation

The most common clinical presentation is back pain, which occurs in approximately 90% of cases. A prior diagnosis of malignancy is known in most cases, although in

Table 4
Treatment of metabolic abnormalities associated with TLS

Problem	Intervention	Dosages	Comments
Renal insufficiency and hypovolemia	IV fluids	Normal saline, 3 L/m^2 daily (200 mL/kg daily)	Use with caution if history of CHF
	Dialysis	—	Patients with oliguric renal failure not responding to IV fluids or patients with CHF
Hyperuricemia	Allopurinol	100 mg/m^2 per dose orally every 8 h (10 mg/kg/d divided in 3 doses) or 200–400 mg/m^2/d IV in divided doses every 8–12 h; commonly used dosages include 600 mg initially followed by 300 mg/d	Reduce dose in renal failure; multiple drug interactions (6-mercaptopurine and azathioprine); IV allopurinol should be used only in patients unable to take oral medications
	Rasburicase	0.05–0.2 mg/kg IV	Contraindicated in G6PD deficiency; transfer blood samples on ice to the laboratory; risk of sensitization and allergic reactions; expensive
Hyperphosphatemia (phosphate level> 6.5 mg/mL [>2.1 mmol/L])	Minimize phosphate intake	—	Low phosphorus diet; phosphorus-free IV fluids
	Phosphate binders (aluminum hydroxide)	50–150 mg/kg daily orally	May interfere with drug absorption
	Dialysis	—	If no response to medical therapy
Hyperkalemia	Insulin (regular)	10 units IV	—
	Dextrose (50%)	50–100 mL IV	—
	Calcium gluconate (10%)	10–20 mL (100–200 mg) IV	Do not give with bicarbonate; use if arrhythmias or ECG changes; can repeat as needed
	Sodium bicarbonate	45 mEq IV (1 ampule of 7.5% NaHCO$_3$)	Use if acidosis; can repeat in 30 min
	Sodium polystyrene sulfonate (Kayexalate)	15–30 g every 6 h orally (can be used rectally)	Can be given with sorbitol
	Albuterol	Inhaled 2.5 mg	For severe hyperkalemia
	Dialysis	—	Severe hyperkalemia not responsive to other measures; renal failure; volume overload
Hypocalcemia	Calcium gluconate (10%)	5–20 mL (50–200 mg) IV	Only if symptomatic; repeat as necessary; use with caution in patients with severe hyperphosphatemia

Abbreviation: CHF, congestive heart failure.

5% to 15% of cases MSCC is the initial presentation of malignancy.[60] The nature of the pain can vary with local, radicular, or referred pain. Referred pain is common with cervical compression, often presenting as subscapular pain; thoracic compression as lumbrosacral or hip pain; and lumbrosacral compression presenting as thoracic pain.[61] The most common location for MSCC is in the thoracic spine, followed by the lumbrosacral region and, lastly, cervical spine. Multiple levels are involved in almost half of all patients. Breast and lung cancer tend to metastasize more frequently to the thoracic spine, whereas colon and pelvic carcinomas tend to develop metastatic lesions in the lumbosacral spine.[54] Other presenting symptoms include motor weakness, sensory impairment, and autonomic dysfunction. In cauda equina syndrome, patients will present with decreased sensation over the buttocks, posterior-superior thighs, and perineal region. Cauda equina syndrome may present as urinary retention, and overflow incontinence (90% sensitivity, 95% specificity).[54,61]

The severity of MSCC can be scored according to several grading systems, including the Frankel grading system, which classifies each patient into 1 of the following 5 categories: (A) complete paraplegia, (B) only sensory function, (C) nonambulation, (D) ambulation, and (E) no neurologic symptoms or signs. The Barthel index also includes assessment of bowel and bladder function.[54,62] These can be useful in assessing severity and response to therapy.

Diagnosis

The gold standard for the diagnosis of MSCC is magnetic resonance imaging (MRI) with a sensitivity of 93%, specificity of 97%, and overall accuracy of 95% (Fig. 6).[56,63] Plain radiographs are not adequate in making the diagnosis, and have a false-negative rate of 10% to 17% and so should not be used to rule out compression. Plain films will also not detect paraspinous masses that have entered the intervertebral foramen if there is no bone erosion.[56,60] If MRI is contraindicated or not available, computed tomography myelography can be used.[12,57] There is no clinical model to rule out MSCC in cancer patients with back pain, and, therefore, all new onset back pain should prompt an immediate assessment and consideration for an MRI in this patient population. Lack of neurologic deficits is ideal and should not inhibit further investigation, but may alter the urgency of the evaluation. For those patients with back pain only, and a normal neurologic examination, emergent imaging of the spinal axis is not mandatory, but should be completed in the next 48 to 72 hours. Those with neurologic deficits need emergent evaluation before nerve damage becomes permanent. Finding unsuspected lesions is not uncommon, and up to one-third of patients have more than 1 site of compression, therefore imaging of the entire spine is required.[56]

Treatment

Corticosteroids are first-line treatment of most patients with MSCC. Steroids reduce the vasogenic edema and inflammation, and seem to have a tumoricidal effect on leukemias, lymphomas, and, occasionally, breast cancer.[56] Because the most important prognostic indicator for ambulatory outcome is the pretreatment motor function, immediate initiation of therapy is of utmost importance. Although the use of high-dose dexamethasone to promote posttreatment ambulation is a grade A recommendation from an evidence-based guideline, the optimal dose of dexamethasone is still unclear and debated because of the significant side effects of high-dose steroids. Several studies have been conducted to determine the optimal dose of dexamethasone to balance outcome with adverse effects. Two studies revealed an 11% to 14% frequency of serious side effects including a fatal ulcer, rectal bleeding and bowel

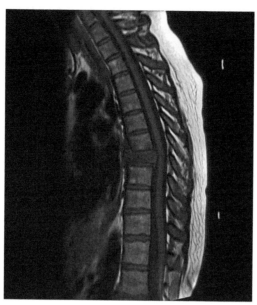

Fig. 6. Breast cancer presenting as spinal cord compression in 48-year-old woman with a strong family history of breast cancer. This case is unusual as the initial manifestation of breast cancer and in that only one level of spinal axis is involved.

perforations when doses as high as 96 mg intravenous (IV) were given. When the dose was decreased to 16 mg/d there were no serious side effects, and no detectable difference in ambulatory rates, between the groups.[64,65] Another study by Vecht and colleagues compared an initial IV dose of 10 mg to the high dose of 100 mg. There was no difference in treatment arms in terms of pain reduction, ambulation, or bowel function, although the sample size was small and not adequately powered to determine equivalence.[64–66] There is no current consensus on the best dose, but dexamethasone is typically given at 10 to 16 mg IV bolus followed by 4 to 6 mg every 4 hours, with a taper during, or immediately after, completion of radiation.[12,54,56] Due to the severity of loss of ambulation, one option that is still used is giving higher doses in patients who present with paraplegia or rapidly progressive symptoms.[56]

Radiation therapy plays a critical role in the treatment of MSCC. Although there is no consensus in dosing schedules, the therapy port usually extends 1 or 2 vertebral bodies above and below the site of compression, and is often given at 30 Gy in 10 fractions. Radiation given at greater than 30 Gy has not been shown to improve outcomes, but treatment regimens can range in duration, thus changing the dose per fraction.[54,58,67,68] In the past, radiation therapy and steroids have been the standard of care for MSCC; however, the role of surgery is becoming increasingly evident. In 2005, Patchell and colleagues[69] reported the first phase III randomized clinical trial comparing the role of decompressive surgery and radiation to that of radiation alone. Patients were given 100 mg of dexamethasone followed by 24 mg every 6 hours, and then treated with radiation therapy (30 Gy in 10 fractions) alone or surgery (generally within 24 hours) followed by the same course of radiation within 2 weeks of surgery. The study was discontinued after enrollment of 100 of the 200 planned patients because predetermined stopping criteria were met. The percentage of ambulatory patients was significantly higher in the group treated with surgery plus radiation

(84% vs 57%), as was their duration of ambulation (median 122 days vs 13 days) and median survival (126 days vs 100 days). It is difficult to extrapolate these data to all MSCC patients, as there were strict inclusion criteria. However, in patients who fulfill the criteria as outlined by Patchell and noted in **Box 2**, decompressive surgery for maximal tumor resection and stabilization followed by radiotherapy should be considered.[57,69]

BRAIN METASTASES AND INCREASED INTRACRANIAL PRESSURE

Brain metastases represent the most common type of intracranial tumor and are a common complication in cancer patients. The incidence of metastases varies by tumor type, with lung cancer being the most common, followed by breast and melanoma. Lung and melanoma tend to present as multiple brain lesions, whereas breast, colon, and renal tumors more commonly produce solitary lesions.[70,71] These lesions in the brain can lead to neurologic deficits, seizures, and increased intracranial pressure (ICP). Untreated patients have an average median survival of about 4 weeks. Prognosis is dependent on Karnofsky performance status, presence of systemic disease, and primary tumor.[70]

Pathophysiology

Most brain metastases are secondary to hematogenous spread from the primary tumor. Accordingly, as 90% of cerebral blood flow occurs in the supratentorial region, most metastatic lesions occur in the supratentorial region. Within the brain, the lesions tend to occur at the borders of the territories of the major arteries (watershed areas) and at the gray-white matter junction. The most common cause of increased ICP is cerebral edema. Vasogenic edema occurs when the blood-brain barrier is disrupted by the tumor. Tumors can also induce increased ICP from hydrocephalus due to

---

Box 2
Patchell criteria for decompressive surgery

Inclusion criteria

At least 18 years of age

Tissue-proven diagnosis of cancer (not of CNS or spinal column origin)

MRI evidence of MSCC (displacement of the spinal cord by an epidural mass)

At least 1 neurologic sign or symptom (including pain)

Not paraplegic for more than 48 hours

MSCC restricted to 1 area (can include several contiguous spinal or vertebral segments)

Expected survival of at least 3 months

General medical status acceptable for surgery

Exclusion criteria

Multiple discrete lesions

Radiosensitive tumors (lymphomas, leukemia, multiple myeloma, and germ cell tumors)

Mass with compression of only the cauda equina or spinal roots

Preexisting neurologic problems not directly related to MSCC

Prior radiotherapy that would exclude them from receiving study dose

increased cerebrospinal fluid (CSF) volume in the ventricular space, because normal flow or absorption is obstructed by the tumor itself.[72]

Clinical Presentation

Approximately 75% of patients with brain metastases have neurologic symptoms at the time these lesions are detected. Symptoms vary significantly and depend on the location of the lesions or lesions. The most common presenting feature is subacute onset of headache, which occurs in roughly 50% of cases, but can also present with focal neurologic deficits, seizures including status epilepticus, neurocognitive changes or any combination of these features. Generally, these symptoms arise over days to weeks, but can appear acutely if there is hemorrhage into the lesion, which occurs more frequently with melanoma, choriocarcinoma, and renal and thyroid carcinoma.[70,73] Metastatic lesions become an oncologic emergency in cases of increased ICP and status epilepticus. Patients with increased ICP classically present with headache, nausea, and vomiting. The headaches tend to be more severe in the mornings and when supine. Other symptoms include weakness, ataxia, seizures, and mental status changes. If papilledema is detected on physical examination, this almost always indicates ICP. The triad of signs referred to as the Cushing response (hypertension with wide pulse pressure, bradycardia, and an irregular respiratory rate) is a late effect and needs to be addressed immediately.

Diagnosis

Contrast-enhanced MRI is the most sensitive and specific diagnostic tool available. Computerized tomography (CT) can be used if MRI is not available or contraindicated, but it is less sensitive, especially if the tumor is small or located in the posterior fossa. However, CT is the preferred scanning technique in an acute situation when hemorrhage or hydrocephalus is suspected.[12,70,72]

Treatment

The first line treatment of patients with increased ICP is dexamethasone. Corticosteroids seem to restore leaky capillary permeability, reduce peritumoral edema, and reduce local brain compression, which can relieve the symptoms. The effect of steroids is usually seen within 24 hours, but the full effect is not seen for several days, and changes on imaging may not appear for a week. There is no consensus on dose, but this usually ranges from 10 to 24 mg IV bolus, followed by 4 mg every 6 hours.[12,70] In severe cases, mannitol and hyperventilation are used. Mannitol can be administered as IV boluses or as continuous infusion to decrease cerebral edema. Intubation and controlled hyperventilation lead to a rapid decrease in cerebral edema. The effect of mannitol and hyperventilation are transient and not definitive therapy. These should be reserved for critical cases in patients with rapidly declining clinical states.[71] More definitive treatment modalities include whole-brain radiation therapy (WBRT), surgery, or stereotactic radiosurgery. Whole-brain radiation is the classic treatment of patients with multiple brain metastases or with a tumor too large for surgery or stereotactic radiosurgery. WBRT generally improves median survival to 3 to 6 months, compared with 1 to 2 months with supportive care alone.[70,71] Surgical debulking can also be performed, depending on tumor location, and is the most rapid way to alleviate increased ICP. Stereotactic radiosurgery can be used in selected cases. Chemotherapy can be used in highly chemosensitive tumors such as germ cell, lymphoma, or small cell carcinomas, or in cases in which radiation therapy is not an option.

Seizures occur in about one-quarter of patients with intracranial metastases, and these patients require anticonvulsant therapy. In cases of status epilepticus, treatment usually consists of lorazepam, phenytoin, or fosphenytoin.[12,70] In the past, patients with brain metastases were treated prophylactically with antiepileptic medications, but this is no longer recommended as a meta-analysis. Sirven and colleagues[74] revealed that prophylactic treatment does not reduce the frequency of first seizures in this patient population. These medications also have significant side effects, including bone marrow suppression, and interactions with chemotherapeutic and targeted agents, as many are metabolized via P450, and most of these antiepileptic medications induce the cytochrome P450 system.[70]

HYPERVISCOSITY SYNDROME DUE TO DYSPROTEINEMIA (MONOCLONAL GAMMOPATHY)

Hyperviscosity syndrome (HVS) refers to the clinical consequences of increased blood viscosity. These can occur secondary to a variety of malignancies including monoclonal gammopathies, such as Waldenstrom macroglobulinemia (WM), multiple myeloma, and acute leukemias. This section of the review focuses on hyperviscosity secondary to dysproteinemia. The most common cause of HVS due to dysproteinemia is WM, which occurs in up to 30% of these patients.[75]

Pathophysiology

HVS occurs as a result of increased viscosity of the blood, and leads to adverse effects on tissue perfusion. In normal blood, the most important determinant of blood viscosity is the hematocrit, with serum protein concentration playing a lesser role. In normal physiologic conditions, fibrinogen is the key component in protein concentration in blood because of its large molecular size, shape, and charge. In cases of HVS, excessive amounts of circulating immunoglobulins (Igs) are produced. IgM is the most likely culprit, as it is the largest Ig (molecular weight [MW] 1,000,000). These proteins are mainly intravascular and, as the concentration increases, they form aggregates and bind water via their carbohydrate contents. This process increases the osmotic pressure and increases the resistance to blood flow. Igs are also cationic and lower the repellant forces between anionic red blood cells, which can lead to rouleaux formation and reduction in the malleability they need to travel through the microvasculature. Eventually, this leads to impaired transit of blood cells, microvascular congestion, decreased tissue perfusion, and tissue damage. Although this is predominately via IgM, it can occur with IgA molecules, as they tend to polymerize and aggregate. It can also occur with the IgG3 subclass, as these undergo a concentration-dependent aggregation.[75,76]

There is no concise relationship between serum viscosity (SV) and clinical symptoms. The normal range for SV is 1.2 to 2.8 centipoise (cP). In general, patients will not become symptomatic with a SV less than 3, although more recent studies have shown retinal changes in levels as low as 2.1 cP.[77] In WM patients, about one-third of those with an SV greater than 4 will not have symptoms. High-risk patients have a serum IgM level greater than 4 g/L, although IgM levels of 3 g/L can produce symptoms in some patients.[12,75]

Clinical Presentation

The signs and symptoms of HVS vary and are nonspecific in nature. The classic triad of symptoms includes neurologic abnormalities, visual changes, and bleeding, although all 3 need not be present to make the diagnosis.[75] Neurologic manifestations include headache, altered mental status, vertigo, ataxia, or paresthesias.

Hyponatremia and hypercalcemia are often present. The hyponatremia seen on laboratory studies is pseudohyponatremia due to an artifact from the hyperproteinemia.[78] Visual changes are secondary to vascular changes, which play a major role in HVS. These vascular changes can be detected early on at lower SV in the periphery of the retina, which then progresses to central retinal hemorrhages and vascular dilatation as the viscosity increases.[78,79] The classic fundoscopic examination, which should be performed in all patients with suspected HVS, reveals dilated, engorged veins that look like sausage links; a condition known as fundus paraproteinaemicus. If untreated, this will progress to complete retinal vein occlusion, and flame-shaped hemorrhages. The retinal vein changes can lead to blurry vision, decreased visual acuity, and eventually blindness if not treated.[75,80] Mucosal bleeding is another common clinical manifestation of HVS. The proteins coat the platelets and hinder their clot formation ability. Bleeding can be seen in the gastrointestinal tract, gingival, uterus, or cause epistaxis. Purpura can also be seen on physical examination.[75]

Other clinical consequences of HVS include congestive heart failure, ischemic acute tubular necrosis, pulmonary edema, with multiorgan system failure and death if treatment is not promptly initiated.[12,75]

Diagnosis

There is no single diagnostic test to assess for HVS. Physical examination and history are important, as are laboratory studies, including electrolyte panel, SV, peripheral blood smear, and quantitative Ig levels. The diagnostic workup will need to rule out other causes of the presenting symptoms, and will vary depending on presentation.

Treatment

The mainstay of therapy is plasmapheresis. Plasmapheresis is the fastest, most effective method to reduce plasma viscosity. It is especially rapid in IgM-related cases, as most IgM is intravascular. In cases of IgA- or IgG-related HVS, it may take several sessions to achieve the same result as seen in 1 treatment with IgM-related HVS. If plasmapheresis is not readily available, phlebotomy of 100 to 200 mL of whole blood has been used to reduce acute symptoms. Normal saline, given until repletion of intravascular volume, followed by loop diuretics, is another means to reduce hypercalcemia and SV.[81] Ultimately, the underlying dysproteinemia needs to be addressed as these therapies do not control the underlying disease. The definitive treatment varies according to diagnosis, but often involves chemotherapeutic agents such as alkylating agents or nucleoside analogs.[12,78] Until SV is reduced and capillary perfusion improved, red-cell transfusions should be avoided unless critical, as this can increase SV, thus worsening HVS.

HYPERLEUKOCYTOSIS AND LEUKOSTASIS

Although most leukemias present with more subtle features, up to 30% of adult acute myelogenous leukemias can present with hyperleukocytosis, putting patients at risk for leukostasis. Hyperleukocytosis has been conventionally defined as an initial white blood cell (WBC) count greater than 100,000/μL. Hyperleukocytosis is more common in acute leukemias, especially in acute lymphoblastic leukemia (ALL) with 11q23 rearrangement, and acute monocytic leukemia (AML) subtypes M3v, M4, and M5. Hyperleukocytosis portends a poor prognosis, with higher risk of early mortality, especially in ALL. The WBC count is the most important prognostic factor in ALL; patients who present with a WBC greater than 50,000/μL have a particularly poor prognosis, and few children with hyperleukocytosis become long-term survivors.[82–84]

Pathophysiology

Initial studies suggested that the increase in circulating leukocytes caused sludging of the leukemic blasts on the microvasculature secondary to increased whole blood viscosity. There is increasing evidence that interactions between the vascular endothelial cells and leukemic blasts enhance the aggregation of blasts. There is also differential expression of adhesion molecules on the lymphoblast cells and myeloblast, which has been implicated in the higher incidence of leukostasis in AML versus ALL.[84,85]

Clinical Presentation

The presentation of leukostasis due to leukemias is similar to the HVS seen with dysproteinemia. In general, the presenting symptoms are related to the respiratory system and CNS. Pulmonary symptoms can range from exertional dyspnea to severe respiratory distress. Arterial blood gases should be interpreted with caution, as pseudohypoxia, as detected with low arterial oxygen tension, may be secondary to rapid consumption of plasma oxygen from the increased leukocytes. Chest radiograph findings can vary from normal to diffuse infiltrates. Neurologic manifestations span the spectrum from mild confusion to somnolence. Intracranial hemorrhage also occurs and can present with focal neurologic deficits. Other symptoms include retinal hemorrhage, retinal vein thrombosis, myocardial infarction, limb ischemia, renal vein thrombosis, and disseminated intravascular coagulation. Fever is also common and high. Although infection is found in only a few cases, it does need to be ruled out, as this syndrome can mimic sepsis syndromes.[12,83,84]

Diagnosis

As with HVS, there is no specific diagnostic test. Laboratory evaluation should include evaluation for thrombocytopenia, coagulopathy, and TLS.

Treatment

Leukoreduction can be achieved quickly with leukapheresis. Although there are no evidence-based guidelines for initiation of leukapheresis, it is usually initiated at a blast count greater than 100,000/μL, or the presence of symptoms regardless of blast count. In ALL, leukapheresis is usually not done unless symptoms develop or the white count becomes greater than 200,000/μL. Supportive measures that should be initiated include hydration with IV fluids with careful monitoring of fluid balance, as these patients are at risk for cardiopulmonary complications. TLS should be prevented with the use of allopurinol or recombinant urate oxidase. Transfusions should be avoided unless absolutely necessary, as this may increase blood viscosity and can exacerbate the syndrome. Induction chemotherapy should be initiated immediately.[83,84] Single-fraction radiation to the cranium for cerebral leukostasis, or to the lungs for pulmonary leukostasis causing hypoxia, have been used as temporizing measures in select patients, although this is controversial and there are no controlled studies that confirm benefit.[12]

AIRWAY OBSTRUCTION

Malignant airway obstruction can arise from locally advanced tumors that arise from the region of the tracheobronchial tree or from lesions metastatic to the mediastinum or major airways. Primary bronchogenic carcinomas are estimated to be the most common cause of malignant airway obstructions, and it is estimated that up to 30% of patients with primary lung tumors will, at some point in their course, develop airway obstruction.[86] In patients with primary bronchogenic cancers, airway obstruction does not seem to adversely effect overall survival, with median survival of 8.2 versus 8.4 months respectively for patients with and without airway obstruction.[87] However, prompt recognition and treatment can lead to a markedly improved quality of life, with up to 95% of patients reporting a decrease in dyspnea with prompt treatment.[88]

Causes

Primary lung cancers are the most common cause of malignant airway obstruction, but other local tumors, such as thyroid, esophageal, primary mediastinal (including thymic, lymphoma, and germ cell), and rare tumors such as pulmonary carcinoid or adenocystic, can also cause obstruction. Metastatic lesion directly to the bronchial tree, lymph nodes, or mediastinal structures include lung, breast, thyroid, colon, sarcoma, and melanoma, although virtually any cancer can cause obstruction.

Presentation

Symptoms at presentation include stridor, dyspnea, hemoptysis, and cough. These symptoms are nonspecific and are often mistaken for more common conditions, such as an exacerbation of chronic obstructive pulmonary disease (COPD), asthma, infections, bronchitis, or heart disease. The rate of development of symptoms is often dependent on the tumor and its aggressiveness. Patients with slow-growing tumors may have a prolonged course of symptoms, with a sudden exacerbation due to local accumulation of secretions or bleeding.

Physical Examination Findings

Physical examination findings may include similarly nonspecific findings such as stridor, wheezing, or loss of breath sounds. Regional lymphadenopathy may help to point to the cause and identify tissue for diagnostic evaluation.

Evaluation

Chest radiographs are nonsensitive and nonspecific, but may show tracheal narrowing. CT scanning is more sensitive and more likely to show bronchial narrowing (**Fig. 7**). Axial and coronal views can often delineate the anatomy, and may provide significant help for the pulmonologist in evaluation and bronchoscopy. CT can also define the mediastinal anatomy and help guide evaluation for primary and metastatic lesions.

Bronchoscopy offers the advantage of allowing the anatomy to be directly visualized, allowing treatment of an obstruction, and obtaining tissue for diagnosis. Care must be taken in evaluating what type of procedure to perform, as bronchoscopy can increase the risk for completion of obstruction, and anesthesia may further limit gas exchange. The choice between rigid versus flexible bronchoscopy will depend on the anatomy, the experience of the physician, and the treatment options locally available.

Spirometry can demonstrate presence of central airway obstruction, but, in the emergent setting, is less likely to be useful compared with bronchoscopy and CT scanning. Flow-volume loops may demonstrate a classic pattern suggestive of major airway obstruction.

Treatment

The primary and most urgent goal of treatment is to establish a patent airway to allow for proper gas exchange. Bronchoscopy done with a rigid scope allows for rapid opening of the airway and can often simultaneously obtain tissue diagnosis for those

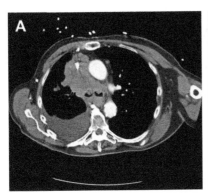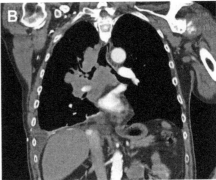

Fig. 7. Axial (*A*) and coronal (*B*) views of bilateral mainstem bronchi with intrinsic tumor masses causing obstruction from NSCLC.

cases that present de novo. Rigid bronchoscopy also allows for placement of metallic, self-expanding stents that are particularly useful for cases of extrinsic airway compression or control of bleeding. Flexible bronchoscopy can also be used to place certain stents, remove secretions or tumor, and obtaining tissue for diagnosis. Airway dilatation (bronchoplasty) can be completed, but the effect of this on malignant airway compression tends to be transient, and some other form of more definitive tumor control should follow, such as radiation or chemotherapy.

Stents

Several different types of stents are available for use in airway obstruction.[89] The most common stents are those made from silicone, metal, or a hybrid of the two. Stents are the treatment of choice to relieve acute airway obstruction in patients with extrinsic tumor compression[90] or with tracheoesophageal fistulas.[91] Although there is no evidence of a survival advantage for patients treated with stenting, 95% of patients do report relief of symptoms[88] after stent placement. Complications from stenting occur in up to 15% of patients, and include tumor ingrowth, stent migration (less common with metallic stents[92]), retained secretions, development of excessive granulation tissue, and, rarely, perforations.[93,94]

Laser

Neodymium-doped yttrium aluminum garnet (Nd:YAG) or CO_2 lasers can be used to open the airway in patients with malignant intrinsic airway obstruction.[95] A recent review[96] of the effectiveness of laser therapy showed a 76% decrease in dyspnea and 94% rate of hemoptysis control, with no procedure-related mortality. Similar to bronchoplasty, the effects are temporary and need to be combined with other antitumor therapies to maintain patent airways. Complications include perforation of the bronchial wall, combustion of the endotracheal tube or fiber-optic bronchoscope, hypoxemia, and respiratory failure.

Photodynamic Therapy

Photodynamic therapy is available at a limited number of centers. It uses the IV injection of light-sensitive molecules, then local activation of the material by exposure to light of a certain wavelength. Patients must avoid all sunlight exposure for up to 6 weeks following the procedure, as all tissues are exposed to the light-sensitizing porphyrin. This technique is of limited value in acute airway obstruction because of its slow therapeutic effect.

Radiation Therapy

For tumors that are sensitive, whether airway obstruction is due to intrinsic tumor or extrinsic compression, radiation therapy can be an effective treatment. When airway obstruction is severe and acute, some more rapid intervention to establish airway and gas exchange is warranted, which may be then be supplemented by addition of radiation. External beam therapy is the most commonly applied modality, but, in regions that have previously undergone radiation therapy, local brachytherapy may be applicable.[97,98]

Chemotherapy

Tumors that are sensitive to chemotherapy, such as lymphomas, SCLCs, and germ cell tumors, may also respond rapidly to systemic chemotherapy. If gas exchange is sufficient to maintain the patient while administering chemotherapy, this is a reasonable treatment. For patients with critical airway compression, a more immediate form of therapy to alleviate the obstruction is called for, which can then be supplemented by subsequent chemotherapy.

REFERENCES

1. Abeloff MD. Hypercalcemia. Abeloff's clinical oncology. 4th edition. Philadelphia: Churchill Livingston; 2004.
2. Stewart AF. Clinical practice. Hypercalcemia associated with cancer. N Engl J Med 2005;352(4):373–9.
3. Horwitz MJ, Tedesco MB, Sereika SM, et al. Direct comparison of sustained infusion of human parathyroid hormone-related protein-(1-36) [hPTHrP-(1-36)] versus hPTH-(1-34) on serum calcium, plasma 1,25-dihydroxyvitamin D concentrations, and fractional calcium excretion in healthy human volunteers. J Clin Endocrinol Metab 2003;88(4):1603–9.
4. Nussbaum SR, Gaz RD, Arnold A. Hypercalcemia and ectopic secretion of parathyroid hormone by an ovarian carcinoma with rearrangement of the gene for parathyroid hormone. N Engl J Med 1990;323(19):1324–8.
5. Seymour JF, Gagel RF. Calcitriol: the major humoral mediator of hypercalcemia in Hodgkin's disease and non-Hodgkin's lymphomas. Blood 1993;82(5):1383–94.
6. Horwitz M, Stewart AF. Hypercalcemia associated with malignancy. In: Favus MJ, editor. Primer on the metabolic bone diseases and disorders of mineral metabolism. 6th edition. Washington, DC: American Society for Bone and Mineral Research; 2006. p. 195–9.
7. Roodman GD. Mechanisms of bone lesions in multiple myeloma and lymphoma. Cancer 1997;80(Suppl 8):1557–63.
8. Deftos LJ. Hypercalcemia in malignant and inflammatory diseases. Endocrinol Metab Clin North Am 2002;31(1):141–58.
9. Hutchesson AC, Bundred NJ, Ratcliffe WA. Survival in hypercalcaemic patients with cancer and co-existing primary hyperparathyroidism. Postgrad Med J 1995;71(831):28–31.
10. Body JJ. Hypercalcemia of malignancy. Semin Nephrol 2004;24(1):48–54.
11. Major P, Lortholary A, Hon J, et al. Zoledronic acid is superior to pamidronate in the treatment of hypercalcemia of malignancy: a pooled analysis of two randomized, controlled clinical trials. J Clin Oncol 2001;19(2):558–67.

12. Halfdanarson TR, Hogan WJ, Moynihan TJ. Oncologic emergencies: diagnosis and treatment. Mayo Clin Proc 2006;81(6):835–48.
13. Adrogue HJ, Madias NE. Hyponatremia. N Engl J Med 2000;342(21):1581–9.
14. Ellison DH, Berl T. Clinical practice. The syndrome of inappropriate antidiuresis. N Engl J Med 2007;356(20):2064–72.
15. Bressler RB, Huston DP. Water intoxication following moderate-dose intravenous cyclophosphamide. Arch Intern Med 1985;145(3):548–9.
16. Beck LH. Hypouricemia in the syndrome of inappropriate secretion of antidiuretic hormone. N Engl J Med 1979;301(10):528–30.
17. Ayus JC, Arieff AI. Chronic hyponatremic encephalopathy in postmenopausal women: association of therapies with morbidity and mortality. JAMA 1999; 281(24):2299–304.
18. Laureno R, Karp BI. Myelinolysis after correction of hyponatremia. Ann Intern Med 1997;126(1):57–62.
19. Verbalis JG, Goldsmith SR, Greenberg A, et al. Hyponatremia treatment guidelines 2007: expert panel recommendations. Am J Med 2007;120(11 Suppl 1): S1–21.
20. Soupart A, Ngassa M, Decaux G. Therapeutic relowering of the serum sodium in a patient after excessive correction of hyponatremia. Clin Nephrol 1999;51(6): 383–6.
21. Bertrand M, Presant CA, Klein L, et al. Iatrogenic superior vena cava syndrome. A new entity. Cancer 1984;54(2):376–8.
22. Otten TR, Stein PD, Patel KC, et al. Thromboembolic disease involving the superior vena cava and brachiocephalic veins. Chest 2003;123(3):809–12.
23. Abner A. Approach to the patient who presents with superior vena cava obstruction. Chest 1993;103(Suppl 4):394S–7S.
24. Wilson LD, Detterbeck FC, Yahalom J. Clinical practice. Superior vena cava syndrome with malignant causes. N Engl J Med 2007;356(18):1862–9.
25. Arinc S, Gonlugur U, Devran O, et al. Prognostic factors in patients with small cell lung carcinoma. Med Oncol 2009. [Epub ahead of print].
26. Urban T, Lebeau B, Chastang C, et al. Superior vena cava syndrome in small-cell lung cancer. Arch Intern Med 1993;153(3):384–7.
27. Nguyen NP, Borok TL, Welsh J, et al. Safety and effectiveness of vascular endoprosthesis for malignant superior vena cava syndrome. Thorax 2009;64(2):174–8.
28. Lanciego C, Chacon JL, Julian A, et al. Stenting as first option for endovascular treatment of malignant superior vena cava syndrome. AJR Am J Roentgenol 2001;177(3):585–93.
29. Rizvi AZ, Kalra M, Bjarnason H, et al. Benign superior vena cava syndrome: stenting is now the first line of treatment. J Vasc Surg 2008;47(2):372–80.
30. Cheng S. Superior vena cava syndrome: a contemporary review of a historic disease. Cardiol Rev 2009;17(1):16–23.
31. DeCamp MM Jr, Mentzer SJ, Swanson SJ, et al. Malignant effusive disease of the pleura and pericardium. Chest 1997;112(Suppl 4):291S–5S.
32. Warren WH. Malignancies involving the pericardium. Semin Thorac Cardiovasc Surg 2000;12(2):119–29.
33. Spodick DH. Acute cardiac tamponade. N Engl J Med 2003;349(7):684–90.
34. Reddy PS, Curtiss EI, O'Toole JD, et al. Cardiac tamponade: hemodynamic observations in man. Circulation 1978;58(2):265–72.
35. Shabetai R. Pericardial and cardiac pressure. Circulation 1988;77(1):1–5.
36. Swami A, Spodick DH. Pulsus paradoxus in cardiac tamponade: a pathophysiologic continuum. Clin Cardiol 2003;26(5):215–7.

37. Tsang TS, Oh JK, Seward JB. Diagnosis and management of cardiac tamponade in the era of echocardiography. Clin Cardiol 1999;22(7):446–52.
38. Tsang TS, Seward JB. Management of pericardial effusion: safety over novelty. Am J Cardiol 1999;83(4):640.
39. Merce J, Sagrista-Sauleda J, Permanyer-Miralda G, et al. Should pericardial drainage be performed routinely in patients who have a large pericardial effusion without tamponade? Am J Med 1998;105(2):106–9.
40. Maruyama R, Yokoyama H, Seto T, et al. Catheter drainage followed by the instillation of bleomycin to manage malignant pericardial effusion in non-small cell lung cancer: a multi-institutional phase II trial. J Thorac Oncol 2007;2(1):65–8.
41. Moriya T, Takiguchi Y, Tabeta H, et al. Controlling malignant pericardial effusion by intrapericardial carboplatin administration in patients with primary non-small-cell lung cancer. Br J Cancer 2000;83(7):858–62.
42. Kaira K, Takise A, Kobayashi G, et al. Management of malignant pericardial effusion with instillation of mitomycin C in non-small cell lung cancer. Jpn J Clin Oncol 2005;35(2):57–60.
43. Kunitoh H, Tamura T, Shibata T, et al. A randomised trial of intrapericardial bleomycin for malignant pericardial effusion with lung cancer (JCOG9811). Br J Cancer 2009;100(3):464–9.
44. Vaitkus PT, Herrmann HC, LeWinter MM. Treatment of malignant pericardial effusion. JAMA 1994;272(1):59–64.
45. Allen KB, Faber LP, Warren WH, et al. Pericardial effusion: subxiphoid pericardiostomy versus percutaneous catheter drainage. Ann Thorac Surg 1999;67(2):437–40.
46. Georghiou GP, Stamler A, Sharoni E, et al. Video-assisted thoracoscopic pericardial window for diagnosis and management of pericardial effusions. Ann Thorac Surg 2005;80(2):607–10.
47. Pui CH. Rasburicase: a potent uricolytic agent. Expert Opin Pharmacother 2002;3(4):433–42.
48. Pui CH, Mahmoud HH, Wiley JM, et al. Recombinant urate oxidase for the prophylaxis or treatment of hyperuricemia in patients with leukemia or lymphoma. J Clin Oncol 2001;19(3):697–704.
49. Jeha S, Kantarjian H, Irwin D, et al. Efficacy and safety of rasburicase, a recombinant urate oxidase (Elitek), in the management of malignancy-associated hyperuricemia in pediatric and adult patients: final results of a multicenter compassionate use trial. Leukemia 2005;19(1):34–8.
50. Jeha S, Pui CH. Recombinant urate oxidase (rasburicase) in the prophylaxis and treatment of tumor lysis syndrome. Contrib Nephrol 2005;147:69–79.
51. Cairo MS, Bishop M. Tumour lysis syndrome: new therapeutic strategies and classification. Br J Haematol 2004;127(1):3–11.
52. Coiffier B, Altman A, Pui CH, et al. Guidelines for the management of pediatric and adult tumor lysis syndrome: an evidence-based review. J Clin Oncol 2008;26(16):2767–78.
53. Coiffier B, Mounier N, Bologna S, et al. Efficacy and safety of rasburicase (recombinant urate oxidase) for the prevention and treatment of hyperuricemia during induction chemotherapy of aggressive non-Hodgkin's lymphoma: results of the GRAAL1 (Groupe d'Etude des Lymphomes de l'Adulte Trial on Rasburicase Activity in Adult Lymphoma) study. J Clin Oncol 2003;21(23):4402–6.
54. Abrahm JL, Banffy MB, Harris MB. Spinal cord compression in patients with advanced metastatic cancer: "all I care about is walking and living my life". JAMA 2008;299(8):937–46.

55. Gilbert RW, Kim JH, Posner JB. Epidural spinal cord compression from metastatic tumor: diagnosis and treatment. Ann Neurol 1978;3:40–51.
56. Cole JS, Patchell RA. Metastatic epidural spinal cord compression. Lancet Neurol 2008;7:459–66.
57. Kwok Y, Tibbs PA, Patchell RA. Clinical approach to metastatic epidural spinal cord compression. Hematol Oncol Clin North Am 2006;20:1297–305.
58. Ushio Y, Posner R, Posner JB, et al. Experimental spinal cord compression by epidural neoplasms. Neurology 1977;27:422–9.
59. Kato A, Ushio Y, Hayakawa T, et al. Circulatory disturbance of the spinal cord with the epidural neoplasm in rats. J Neurosurg 1985;63:260–5.
60. Schiff D. Spinal cord compression. Neurol Clin 2003;21(1):67–86.
61. Deyo RA, Rainville J, Kent DL. What can the history and physical examination tell us about low back pain? JAMA 1992;268(6):760–5.
62. Makris A, Kunkler IH. The Barthel index in assessing the response to palliative radiotherapy in malignant spinal cord compression: a prospective audit. Clin Oncol 1995;7(2):82–6.
63. Li KC, Poon PY. Sensitivity and specificity of MRI in detecting malignant spinal cord compression and in distinguishing malignant from benign compression fractures of the vertebrae. Magn Reson Imaging 1988;6(5):547–56.
64. Heimdal K, Hirschberg H, Slettebo H, et al. High incidence of serious side effects of high dose dexamethasone treatment in patients with epidural spinal cord compression. J Neurooncol 1992;12(2):141–4.
65. Sorensen S, Helweg-Larsen S, Mouridsen H, et al. Effect of high dose dexamethasone in carcinomatous metastatic spinal cord compression treated with radiotherapy: a randomised trial. Eur J Cancer 1994;30A(1):22–7.
66. Vecht CJ, Haaxma-Reiche H, van Putten WL, et al. Initial bolus of conventional versus high dose dexamethasone in metastatic spinal cord compression. Neurology 1989;39:1255–7.
67. Rades D, Karstens JH, Hoskin PJ, et al. Escalation of radiation dose beyond 30 Gy in 10 fractions for metastatic spinal cord compression. Int J Radiat Oncol Biol Phys 2007;67(2):525–31.
68. Loblaw DA, Smith K, Lockwood G, et al. The Princess Margaret Hospital experience of malignant spinal cord compression [abstract]. Proc Am Soc Clin Oncol 2003;22:119.
69. Patchell RA, Tibbs PA, Regine WF, et al. Direct decompressive surgical resection in the treatment of spinal cord compression caused by metastatic cancer: a randomised trial. Lancet 2005;366:643–8.
70. Tosoni A, Ermani M, Brandes A. The pathogenesis and treatment of brain metastases: a comprehensive review. Crit Rev Oncol Hematol 2004;55:199–215.
71. Peacock KH, Lesser GJ. Current therapeutic approaches in patients with brain metastases. Curr Treat Options Oncol 2006;7:479–89.
72. Lee ELT, Armstrong T. Increased intracranial pressure. Clin J Oncol Nurs 2008; 12(1):37–41.
73. Barker F. Surgical and radiosurgical management of brain metastases. Surg Clin North Am 2005;85:329–45.
74. Sirven JI, Wingerchuk DM, Drazkowski JF, et al. Seizure prophylaxis in patients with brain tumors: a meta-analysis. Mayo Clin Proc 2004;79(12):1489–94.
75. Mullen EC, Wang M. Recognizing hyperviscosity syndrome in patients with Waldenstrom macroglobulinemia. Clin J Oncol Nurs 2007;11(1):87–95.
76. Buxbaum J. Hyperviscosity syndrome in dysproteinemias. Am J Med Sci 1972; 264:123–6.

77. Menke MN, Feke GT, McMeel JW, et al. Effect of plasmapheresis on hyperviscosity-related retinopathy and retinal hemodynamics in patients with Waldenström's macroglobulinemia. Invest Ophthalmol Vis Sci 2008;49(3):1157–60.
78. Vitolo U, Ferreri A, Montoto S. Lymphoplasmacytic lymphoma-Waldenström's macroglobulinemia. Crit Rev Oncol Hematol 2008;67:172–85.
79. Menke MN, Feke GT, McMeel JW, et al. Hyperviscosity-related retinopathy in Waldenström macroglobulinemia. Arch Ophthalmol 2006;124:1601–6.
80. Chiang CC, Begley S, Henderson SO. Central retinal occlusion due to hyperviscosity syndrome. J Emerg Med 2000;18:23–6.
81. Zarkovic M, Kwaan HC. Correction of hyperviscosity by apheresis. Semin Thromb Hemost 2003;29:535–42.
82. Inaba H, Fan Y, Pounds S, et al. Clinical and biologic features and treatment outcome of children with newly diagnosed acute myeloid leukemia and hyperleukocytosis. Cancer 2008;113(3):522–9.
83. Majhail NS, Lichtin AE. Acute leukemia with a very high leukocyte count: confronting a medical emergency. Cleve Clin J Med 2004;71(8):633–7.
84. Porcu P, Cripe LD, Ng EW, et al. Hyperleukocytic leukemias and leukostasis: a review of pathophysiology, clinical presentation and management. Leuk Lymphoma 2000;39(1-2):1–18.
85. Porcu P, Farag S, Marcucci G, et al. Leukocytoreduction for acute leukemia. Ther Apher 2002;6:15–23.
86. Noppen M, Meysman M, D'Haese J, et al. Interventional bronchoscopy: 5-year experience at the Academic Hospital of the Vrije Universiteit Brussel (AZ-VUB). Acta Clin Belg 1997;52(6):371–80.
87. Chhajed PN, Baty F, Pless M, et al. Outcome of treated advanced non-small cell lung cancer with and without central airway obstruction. Chest 2006;130(6):1803–7.
88. Wood DE, Liu YH, Vallieres E, et al. Airway stenting for malignant and benign tracheobronchial stenosis. Ann Thorac Surg 2003;76(1):167–72 [discussion: 173–4].
89. Chin CS, Litle V, Yun J, et al. Airway stents. Ann Thorac Surg 2008;85(2):S792–6.
90. Wood D. Airway stenting. Chest Surg Clin N Am 2003;13(2):211–29.
91. Freitag L, Tekolf E, Steveling H, et al. Management of malignant esophagotracheal fistulas with airway stenting and double stenting. Chest 1996;110(5):1155–60.
92. Dumon JF, Cavaliere S, Diaz-Jiminez JP. Seven-year experience with the Dumon prosthesis. J Bronchol 1996;31:6–10.
93. Lemaire A, Burfeind WR, Toloza E, et al. Outcomes of tracheobronchial stents in patients with malignant airway disease. Ann Thorac Surg 2005;80(2):434–7 [discussion: 437–8].
94. Makris D, Marquette CH. Tracheobronchial stenting and central airway replacement. Curr Opin Pulm Med 2007;13(4):278–83.
95. Cavaliere S, Venuta F, Foccoli P, et al. Endoscopic treatment of malignant airway obstructions in 2,008 patients. Chest 1996;110(6):1536–42.
96. Han CC, Prasetyo D, Wright GM. Endobronchial palliation using Nd:YAG laser is associated with improved survival when combined with multimodal adjuvant treatments. J Thorac Oncol 2007;2(1):59–64.
97. Chella A, Ambrogi MC, Ribechini A, et al. Combined Nd-YAG laser/HDR brachytherapy versus Nd-YAG laser only in malignant central airway involvement: a prospective randomized study. Lung Cancer 2000;27(3):169–75.
98. Suh JH, Dass KK, Pagliaccio L, et al. Endobronchial radiation therapy with or without neodymium yttrium aluminum garnet laser resection for managing malignant airway obstruction. Cancer 1994;73(10):2583–8.

Acute Care Nurse Practitioners in Oncologic Critical Care: The Memorial Sloan-Kettering Cancer Center Experience

Rhonda D'Agostino, ACNP-BC[a,b,*], Neil A. Halpern, MD[c,d]

KEYWORDS

- Acute care nurse practitioner • Nurse practitioner
- Intensive care • Critical care
- Oncologic intensive care • Physician alternative

Reductions in the number of residency positions, restrictions on residency work hours, expansion of an aging population, and requirements to meet the Leapfrog critical care medicine (CCM) criteria have highlighted a deficit in CCM physician staffing.[1–7] Nurse practitioners (NPs) and physician assistants (PAs) are being used to fill the intensivist void in the intensive care unit (ICU).[4,8–11]

NP and PA programs were originally developed in the 1960s to provide outpatient primary care and pediatric services.[10] Subsequently, in the early 1990s, the role of these nonphysician or midlevel providers was expanded to include inpatient care in the ICU and non-ICU settings.[12] The predominance of the medical literature shows that the NP and PA groups have had a positive impact on patient care and outcomes, throughput, implementation of care guidelines, and cost control in each environment

[a] Department of Anesthesiology and Critical Care Medicine, Memorial Sloan-Kettering Cancer Center, 1275 York Avenue C1179, New York, NY 10065, USA
[b] Critical Care Nurse Practitioner Program, Memorial Sloan-Kettering Cancer Center, 1275 York Avenue C1179, New York, NY 10065, USA
[c] Critical Care Medicine Service, Department of Anesthesiology and Critical Care Medicine, Memorial Sloan-Kettering Cancer Center, 1275 York Avenue C1179, New York, NY 10065, USA
[d] Weill Cornell Medical College, 525 East 68th Street, New York, NY 10065, USA
* Corresponding author. Department of Anesthesiology and Critical Care Medicine, Memorial Sloan-Kettering Cancer Center, 1275 York Avenue C1179, New York, NY 10065.
E-mail address: bruynr@mskcc.org (R. D'Agostino).

Crit Care Clin 26 (2010) 207–217
doi:10.1016/j.ccc.2009.09.003
0749-0704/09/$ – see front matter © 2010 Elsevier Inc. All rights reserved.

criticalcare.theclinics.com

where they have practiced, including the ICU.[4,13,14] There is no consensus, however, on how to incorporate the NPs or PAs into the multidisciplinary CCM team or on how to provide the enhanced training that these groups require to provide care in the ICU.[4,15]

In this article, we describe the development and function of our CCM NP program in the 20-bed, closed, mixed medical-surgical adult ICU of the Memorial Sloan-Kettering Cancer Center, a 435-bed, tertiary care oncology center in New York City. Currently, CCM NPs, in addition to house staff trainees and CCM fellows, provide full-time comprehensive ICU patient care as well as consultative and rapid response team (RRT) services outside the ICU (**Box 1**). The NPs function as "physician alternatives" in collaboration and under the direction of the CCM attending physician group.[12]

Box 1
CCM NP responsibilities

Patient care

Obtaining histories

Performing physical examinations

Participating in daily clinical rounds

Ordering and interpreting diagnostic tests

Prescribing and adjusting medications

Performing/supervising invasive procedures

Managing mechanical ventilation

Documenting procedures and progress notes

Assessing patients for changes in clinical status

Stabilizing new ICU admissions

Formulating plans of care with CCM attending

Participating in multidisciplinary rounds

Coordinating services with other teams

Communicating with patients and families

Consultative and RRT

Providing critical care consultation and follow-up

First responders for the institution's RRT

Participate as a team member in medical codes

Coordinate ICU admissions and discharges

Teaching

Provide support and education to clinical nursing staff

Precept students (NP and medical)

Data control, quality improvement, and research

Maintain and update the CCM census database

Record patient data on daily CCM care bundles

Perform and participate in quality or performance improvement activities and clinical research

CONCEPTION, DESIGN, AND IMPLEMENTATION OF THE CCM NP PROGRAM

Historically, our ICU patients were cared for by anesthesiology and internal medicine house staff with CCM fellow and attending supervision. During the planning steps for our ICU expansion from 12 to 20 beds it became apparent that additional house staff or physician alternatives would be required. However, additional house staff were not available or necessarily wanted, thus the physician alternative model with NPs and PAs was explored. We recruited both NPs and PAs but elected the NP, rather than the PA, approach for 3 reasons. First, the NP program was far larger and more developed in our hospital. Second, we thought that NPs who had already worked in the critical care setting as registered nurses (RNs) would not only be more experienced than PAs but would also be easier to train and more attuned to the nuances of CCM practice. Third, the NPs were willing to work nights and weekends, whereas the PAs were not so inclined.

As we considered governance paradigms, it was evident that the existing nursing organizational structure in our institution where NPs report directly to nursing leadership would be incompatible with our goals of a direct expansion of the CCM physician team.[16–18] We felt that the fostering of a close and direct collaborative relationship between the CCM physicians and NPs would be inhibited by the existence of separate and potentially conflicting obligations to the nursing department. In addition, we felt that nurse managers, although well experienced in addressing staff nurse issues, were not suited to develop the educational programs for the new NPs or to evaluate their medical decision-making skills.[8,16] Therefore, we devised a joint governance model where the Department of Anesthesiology and Critical Care Medicine would direct the education, training, clinical supervision, scheduling, and discipline of the new CCM NPs, and the Department of Nursing would govern financing, administrative supervision, and credentialing (**Fig. 1**).

RECRUITMENT

In the fall of 2006, recruitment efforts commenced with the goal of establishing an NP-staffed CCM team (11 NPs) by April 2007 when the new and larger ICU would open.

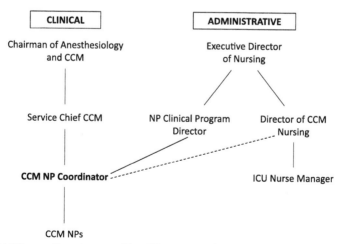

Fig. 1. CCM NP reporting structure. The CCM NP Coordinator directly reports to the Service Chief of CCM and the NP Clinical Program Director. The NP Coordinator also collaborates with the Department of Nursing through the Director of CCM Nursing. The CCM NP Coordinator functions within the nursing governance at the same level of a nurse manager.

Prior critical care (ICU, PACU, ED, Step-down) experience as either an RN or an NP was considered a prerequisite for employment as well as (**Fig. 2**) a master's degree in nursing, specialty certification from a national NP certifying body (ANCC, American Nurse Credentialing Center; AANP, American Academy of Nurse Practitioners; and AACN, American Association of Critical Care Nurses), and New York State licensure. Although there are many NP educational tracks (acute care, adult primary care, psychology/mental health, family, gerontological, pediatric, and neonatal), we sought NPs who were ACNP (acute care nurse practitioner) trained because of their concentrated exposure to didactic and clinical critical care medicine.[4,11,14,19,20]

We looked for a pioneering mindset among the applicants that would indicate a willingness to take a chance on a job opportunity within an uncharted role and practice environment. Candidates who were self-directed, resourceful, and ambitious or who had demonstrated leadership qualities were hired. We recognized that this new program would have growing pains, and therefore, would need hardy, resilient individuals equal to the task. Interviews were conducted by 2 CCM attendings and the NP Clinical Program Director. Despite pessimism about the feasibility of finding 11 qualified candidates even within 1 year, 10 NPs were hired within 6 months. This indicated to us that there was a pool of NPs eager to step forward into CCM. Subsequently, an additional 10 NPs were hired and a program coordinator selected, as further responsibilities were placed on the CCM team and the house staff complement continued to diminish.

TRAINING

The new NPs underwent a custom designed 3-month CCM formal educational training program (**Box 2**). Daytime and evening lectures were conducted by a CCM attending to accommodate all NP shifts. On rounds, the CCM attendings focused on developing NPs' case presentation skills and helped them learn to organize and prioritize the care

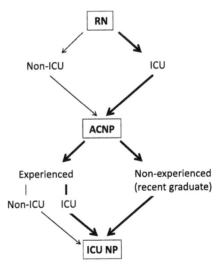

Fig. 2. Different career tracks starting from RN to NP. Our preference (*bold arrows*) is ACNPs with prior ICU nursing experience. Alternatively, if the applicant had NP experience we preferred NPs with ICU experience; however there are few such candidates.

Box 2
CCM NP training course curriculum

Admissions and discharges

    Admission process

    Distinguishing medical and surgical problems and needs

    Order writing by protocol

    Discharge process

    Critical care medicine consults

Clinical

    Chest radiograph interpretation

    ECG interpretation

    Ventilator management

    Noninvasive positive pressure ventilation

    Fluid resuscitation

    Antibiotics selection

    Multiorgan failure

    Continuous renal replacement therapy

    Shock states and vasopressors

    Prophylactic regimens

    Acute coronary syndromes and arrhythmias

    Sedation regimens

    Delirium management

    Common ICU emergencies

    Postoperative care and common surgical procedures

Devices

    Venous and arterial catheters

    Airways

    Chest tubes and drainage systems

    What to do when devices fail

CCM information systems

    Data-tracking program

    Hand-offs between teams and shifts

    Care bundles: ventilator-associated pneumonia, central venous catheter

CCM template notes

    Consultation/RRT notes

    Daily progress notes

    Procedure notes

of patients with complex and multiple active medical and/or surgical problems. Mannequins (**Fig. 3**) were acquired to teach insertion techniques for central venous and arterial cannulation. When proficient in the simulation classroom, the NPs were directly supervised in catheter insertion by CCM fellows and attendings. Airway skills and ventilator management were likewise taught using mannequins (**Fig. 4**) and through biweekly hands-on ventilator workshops. The CCM NPs were sent to the operating rooms to enhance their intubation experience in real life. While in the operating suites, the NPs were also assigned to observe designated types of surgical procedures typical of ICU admissions and to recognize the potential postoperative problems associated with them. Being in the operating rooms had the added benefit of developing collegial relationships with the anesthesiology and surgical teams. Advanced training modules in imaging (ultrasonography and computed tomography) and electrocardiogram (ECG) interpretation were offered to experienced NPs. Multiple educational approaches were used for this intensive NP training regimen. These included the traditional didactic lecture format, interactive small group sessions and role-playing, and advanced media tools, such as the SMART board (SMART Technologies ULC, Calgary, Alberta, Canada). A multimedia critical care web site with various self-directed learning options was developed. The web site includes podcasts of daytime lectures, a repository of required reading articles, and links to other educational web sites.

All NPs took the Fundamental Critical Care Support (FCCS) course offered by the Society of Critical Care Medicine. This course teaches basic critical care principles for the non-intensivist health care provider. NPs also attended formal simulation training in a local simulation center with a focus on code management, emergency airway skills and team building.

DIVISION OF LABOR

The CCM service functions daily with 3 teams: house staff, NP, and consultative/RRT (**Fig. 5**). No distinctions are made between house staff and NP ICU admitting teams when triaging ICU admissions, although our original intent was to select patients with

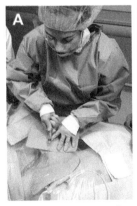 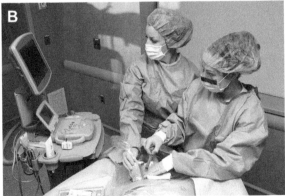

Fig. 3. Central venous catheter (CVC) insertion. (*A*) Using a mannequin and full sterile preparation, NPs learn to insert a CVC. Arterial catheter insertion is similarly taught. The mannequin has different color fluids in its vessels and arterial pulsation to differentiate between central venous and arterial structures. (*B*) Once the NP is comfortable with the technical aspects of catheter insertion, they are taught how to use ultrasonographic guidance.

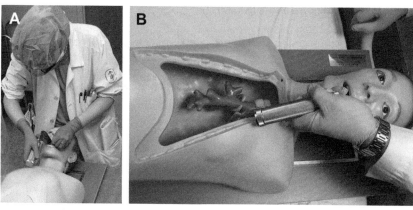

Fig. 4. Airway (*A*) Intubation training on an airway mannequin. (*B*) Direct observation of the airway tree and lungs for manually insufflating air after correct ET placement.

lower acuity for placement on the NP service.[12–15] We strove to maintain an equal census between the 2 admitting teams. Hence, the CCM NP service is usually responsible for 10 beds, and each NP manages 3 to 4 patients. Because the house staff allocation continued to decrease, NPs were integrated into the house staff team to supplement coverage. The CCM NP role inside the ICU includes presenting in morning and evening rounds, managing complex critical patients, performing and supervising procedures (arterial and central venous catheters, intubation, and thoracentesis), and meeting with families (see **Box 1**). NPs also staff the CCM consultative/RRT service around-the-clock in conjunction with a CCM fellow. The consultative/RRT service evaluates new consults for ICU admission, follows up ICU discharges and rejections, and handles ventilator management outside the ICU. The NPs of this service serve as "first-responders" to RRT and code calls, determine in consultation with the CCM fellow if the RRT call must be elevated to a CCM consultation, and work with cardiology in handling acute coronary syndrome cases.

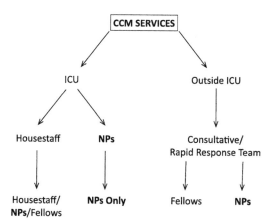

Fig. 5. Pathways of the CCM service. The CCM service cares for patients inside the ICU (house staff and NP teams) and outside the ICU. The house staff team is staffed with anesthesiology interns, NPs, and a CCM fellow. Fellows periodically rotate on the NP team. The consultative and RRT work is divided between the CCM fellows and NPs. A CCM attending directs each of the 3 teams.

REPORTING STRUCTURE AND MANAGEMENT

The NP team is managed by an NP Coordinator who reports directly to the CCM Service Chief (see **Fig. 1**). The NP coordinator is at similar rank to nurse managers, attends nursing administrative meetings and serves as a liaison between the CCM NP group and the Department of Nursing via a direct reporting relationship with the hospital's NP Clinical Program Director. Similar to physicians with administrative duties in our hospital, the NP Coordinator continues to have clinical responsibilities.

TRANSITIONING

Our NPs faced personal challenges when transitioning from previous roles as bedside nurses or nurse practitioners to CCM NPs.[21,22] Day to day activities including formal rounds presentations, rapid review and assimilation of extensive medical records, and performing procedures were "foreign" to the incoming NPs. Additionally, the change from being a facilitator of care to becoming an independent CCM provider and thinker fostered insecurities with their clinical practice, role development, and autonomy. Similarly, the shift from being primarily a source of comfort and support at family meetings to becoming an active clinical contributor was a major role adjustment.

There was also occasional resistance from the bedside nursing staff to comply with NP orders. Our nursing and physician teams were not accustomed to dealing with CCM NPs. The CCM physicians were also concerned about the NPs' knowledge and clinical capabilities and were uncertain about the NPs skill set in dealing with patients and family members and addressing end of life care.[19,23–28] Fortunately, with extensive training and time, as well as increasing familiarity and trust, these issues have largely resolved.

For the NP transition to be successful, the CCM program must recognize that the CCM NPs are not doctors. NP schooling is much shorter and less comprehensive than physician education and training. NP approaches to critical thinking and problem solving are also different then those of doctors. Thus, the onus is upon the CCM program to create the environment and educational curriculum for the NPs to thrive.

COMMUNICATION

Excellent communication skills are crucial for working successfully in the ICU environment. The CCM NP must deal with diverse circumstances, including coordination of care between multiple teams, speaking with the families of ICU patients, and addressing EOL issues.[29]

CCM NPs in their coordinator of care-roles[30] in the ICU constantly interact with admitting and consultative services. When all parties are in agreement with the diagnosis and care plan, this task is straightforward; however, when conflicts in diagnosis or management emerge, interactions may become frustrating and difficult. Disagreements between the ICU and admitting services may be legitimate and develop because of differences in opinion. Alternatively, disputes may be secondary to uncommunicated deviations from the agreed-upon care plan, loss of order writing control by the primary team within the "closed" ICU environment, and disappointment in unanticipated complications and poor outcomes. Regardless of the cause, it is essential that the CCM NPs maintain decorum and equilibrium in navigating these situations and foster a unified health care team approach to treatment, patients, and their families.

The physician-patient relationship may be even more important for oncology patients than other patients because of the insidious nature of cancer and the fear associated with cancer and its therapies. Thus, patients with cancer and their families usually develop a bond with their primary oncologists or oncologic surgeons. This relationship becomes even more pronounced when the patient suddenly and unexpectedly becomes critically ill. Thus, CCM practitioners, including NPs, are challenged to quickly develop a close connection with the family members.

In the oncologic setting in particular, families and providers may feel compelled to "keep going" even when the cause seems futile. This circumstance occurs especially if the patient is young and has received aggressive care in hope of a cancer cure or extension of life. Training the CCM NPs to recognize denial on the part of the clinician or family and to interact in complicated family dynamics requires extensive preparation and most of all, experience. The NPs must learn to deal with unrealistic expectations on the part of family members and admitting physicians.[31,32] Sometimes, even having EOL discussions may be discouraged by the admitting teams or the families,[33] thus presenting an ethical quandary to the CCM NPs who may feel that an inappropriately high level of care is being rendered.

We provide the NPs with enhanced communication training through their mandatory attendance in a formalized communication skill workshop managed by the Department of Psychiatry where EOL discussion skills are developed and refined. NPs participate in videotaped simulation sessions with professional actors playing family members or other physicians. These interactions are then analyzed, and constructive suggestions are offered for a host of common EOL scenarios that range from giving bad news, to initiating and completing EOL discussions, and arranging palliative care and withdrawal of life-supportive therapy.

EMOTIONAL SUPPORT

Working in an oncologic ICU may be more emotionally draining than working in a standard ICU setting. Cancer mortality among the young is common. NPs are also faced with moral distress in recognizing that health care proxies often do not uphold advanced directives limiting care.[32] Thus, it is critical that the ICU and hospital provide psychological support to the NPs to prevent burn out.

FUTURE DIRECTIONS

We are now exploring billing for NP services (procedures and RRT calls) that are not currently billed by the CCM attendings. We are also developing a job description for charge NPs for each shift with responsibilities for oversight and direction of the junior NPs, scheduling, and advancing cohesiveness of the team. Finally, we are looking to create a post-NP CCM fellowship training program.[4]

SUMMARY

Relatively little information exists about NP practice models in the adult ICU, let alone in an oncologic ICU setting. Our collaborative physician-NP practice model governed primarily through critical care, provides a well-trained, highly functional NP team. The growth and transformation of this program has brought to light the challenges that may well be faced by other institutions seeking to cultivate their own CCM NP teams. It is our hope that this descriptive article of the development of our CCM NP group will allow others pursuing the same path to benefit from our experience.

ACKNOWLEDGMENTS

The authors would like to thank Kate Tayban, ACNP-BC; Camille Lineberry, ACNP-BC; Deborah Stein, ACNP-BC; Lauren Scoma, ACNP-BC and Nina Raoof, MD for their contributions to this manuscript.

REFERENCES

1. Fischer JE. Continuity of care: a casualty of the 80-hour work week. Acad Med 2004;79:381.
2. Ewart GW, Marcus L, Gaba MM, et al. The critical care medicine crisis: a call for federal action: a white paper from the critical care professional societies. Chest 2004;125:1518.
3. Kelley MA, Angus D, Chalfin DB, et al. The critical care crisis in the United States: a report from the profession. Chest 2004;125:1514.
4. Kleinpell RM, Ely EW, Grabenkort R. Nurse practitioners and physician assistants in the intensive care unit: an evidence-based review. Crit Care Med 2008;36: 2888.
5. Weinstein DF. Duty hours for resident physicians—tough choices for teaching hospitals. N Engl J Med 2002;347:1275.
6. Cajulis CB, Fitzpatrick JJ. Levels of autonomy of nurse practitioners in an acute care setting. J Am Acad Nurse Pract 2007;19:500.
7. The Leapfrog Group. ICU Physician Staffing (IPS). Available at: www.leapfroggroup.org. Accessed May 24, 2009.
8. Bahouth M, Esposito-Herr MB, Babineau TJ. The expanding role of the nurse practitioner in an academic medical center and its impact on graduate medical education. J Surg Educ 2007;64:282.
9. Gordon CR, Axelrad A, Alexander JB, et al. Care of critically ill surgical patients using the 80-hour Accreditation Council of Graduate Medical Education workweek guidelines: a survey of current strategies. Am Surg 2006;72:497.
10. Silver HK, Ford LC, Stearly SG. A program to increase health care for children: the pediatric nurse practitioner program. Pediatrics 1967;39:756.
11. Kleinpell RM. Acute care nurse practitioner practice: results of a 5-year longitudinal study. Am J Crit Care 2005;14:211.
12. Snyder JV, Sirio CA, Angus DC, et al. Trial of nurse practitioners in intensive care. New Horiz 1994;2:296.
13. Hoffman LA, Tasota FJ, Scharfenberg C, et al. Management of patients in the intensive care unit: comparison via work sampling analysis of an acute care nurse practitioner and physicians in training. Am J Crit Care 2003;12:436.
14. Hoffman LA, Tasota FJ, Zullo TG, et al. Outcomes of care managed by an acute care nurse practitioner/attending physician team in a subacute medical intensive care unit. Am J Crit Care 2005;14:121.
15. Brilli RJ, Spevetz A, Branson RD, et al. Critical care delivery in the intensive care unit: defining clinical roles and the best practice model. Crit Care Med 2007;29: 2001.
16. Almost J, Laschinger HK. Workplace empowerment, collaborative work relationships, and job strain in nurse practitioners. J Am Acad Nurse Pract 2002;14:408.
17. Parrinello KM. Advanced practice nursing: an administrative perspective. Crit Care Nurs Clin North Am 1995;7:9.
18. Roschkov S, Rebeyka D, Comeau A, et al. Cardiovascular nurse practitioner practice: results of a Canada-wide survey. Can J Cardiovasc Nurs 2007;17:27.

19. Cummings GG, Fraser K, Tarlier DS. Implementing advanced nurse practitioner roles in acute care: an evaluation of organizational change. J Nurs Adm 2003; 33:139.
20. Howie-Esquivel J, Fontaine DK. The evolving role of the acute care nurse practitioner in critical care. Curr Opin Crit Care 2006;12:609.
21. Bahouth MN, Esposito-Herr MB. Orientation program for hospital-based nurse practitioners. AACN Adv Crit Care 2009;20:82.
22. Kelly N, Mathews M. The transition to first position as nurse practitioner. J Nurs Educ 2001;40:156–63.
23. Vazirani S, Hays RD, Shapiro MF, et al. Effect of a multidisciplinary intervention on communication and collaboration among physicians and nurses. Am J Crit Care 2005;14:71.
24. Reay T, Golden-Biddle K, Germann K. Challenges and leadership strategies for managers of nurse practitioners. J Nurs Manag 2003;11:396.
25. Jensen L, Scherr K. Impact of the nurse practitioner role in cardiothoracic surgery. Dynamics 2004;15:14.
26. Howie JN, Erickson M. Acute care nurse practitioners: creating and implementing a model of care for an inpatient general medical service. Am J Crit Care 2002;11: 448.
27. Richmond TS, Becker D. Creating an advanced practice nurse-friendly culture: a marathon, not a sprint. AACN Clin Issues 2005;16:58.
28. Molitor-Kirsch S, Thompson L, Milonovich L. The changing face of critical care medicine: nurse practitioners in the pediatric intensive care unit. AACN Clin Issues 2005;16:172.
29. Halpern NA, Raoof ND, Voigt LP, et al. Challenging family dialogues within the intensive care unit: an intensivist's perspective. J Hosp Med 2008;3:354.
30. Sidani S, Doran D, Porter H, et al. Processes of care: comparison between nurse practitioners and physician residents in acute care. Nurs Leadersh (Tor Ont) 2006;19:69.
31. Rydvall A, Lynoe N. Withholding and withdrawing life-sustaining treatment: a comparative study of the ethical reasoning of physicians and the general public. Crit Care 2008;12:R13.
32. Rohan E, Bausch J. Climbing Everest: oncology work as an expedition in caring. J Psychosoc Oncol 2009;27:84.
33. Pieracci FM, Ullery BW, Eachempati SR, et al. Prospective analysis of life-sustaining therapy discussions in the surgical intensive care unit: a housestaff perspective. J Am Coll Surg 2008;207:468.

End-of-Life Issues in Critically Ill Cancer Patients

Susan Gaeta, MD*, Kristen J. Price, MD

KEYWORDS

- End-of-life • Intensive care unit • Cancer
- Advance directives • Management

"To cure sometimes, to relieve often, to comfort always"
15th Century French proverb

Over the past decade, the probability of surviving an admission to the ICU for a cancer patient has improved. This trend can be attributed to three factors. First, improvement in the treatment of solid tumors and hematological malignancies has led to a 20% overall decrease in mortality from 1978 to 1998. Second, earlier admission to the ICU has resulted in better survival rates. Third, there has been some improvement in selecting patients likely to benefit from ICU admission.[1]

Despite the above factors, some critically ill cancer patients will die during a hospital admission that includes an ICU admission. A review of an epidemiologic study demonstrated that one in five patients will die during a hospitalization that included an ICU admission.[2] This number includes all patients, not just cancer patients, and does not necessarily indicate a death in the ICU. One may conclude that this percentage may be higher or lower depending on the type of ICU—medical, surgical, open or closed, rural or urban, and their respective admission criteria for cancer patients. Most of the deaths in the ICU will follow withholding or withdrawing of life support.[3] Before discussing end-of-life issues in critically ill cancer patients it is beneficial to review those factors or barriers that may lead to a greater probability of death in a critically ill cancer patient admitted to the ICU.

ADMISSION CRITERIA TO ICU AND TRANSITIONING TO PALLIATION AFTER A TRIAL OF AGGRESSIVE SUPPORT

The first factor to consider is the criteria used in determining admission of a cancer patient to an ICU. The criteria may vary depending on the type of hospital: community,

Department of Critical Care Medicine, University of Texas MD Anderson Cancer Center, 1515 Holcombe Boulevard, Box # 0112, Houston, TX 77030, USA
* Corresponding author.
E-mail address: sgaeta@mdanderson.org (S. Gaeta).

Crit Care Clin 26 (2010) 219–227
doi:10.1016/j.ccc.2009.10.002
0749-0704/09/$ – see front matter © 2010 Elsevier Inc. All rights reserved.

tertiary, or a comprehensive cancer center. In general, most physicians will admit cancer patients to the ICU if their condition is medically reversible, but will not admit cancer patients with only palliative care treatment options. However, a great deal of variation exists between these two admission options. This variation can, in part, be explained by the uncertainty of the reversibility of the condition. Thus, some cancer patients are admitted to the ICU with the intent to give a trial of aggressive support.

The timing of the transition from cure to palliation after a trial of aggressive support is seemingly straightforward; however, this decision is delayed at times for different reasons. Depending on the type of ICU administrative model—closed, semi-closed, or open—the intensivist's role may be that of a consultant to the primary oncologist and he or she may not be willing to discuss end-of-life issues. In a survey of oncologists attending a meeting of the American Society of Clinical Oncology, 18% of the respondents stated that they would have a discussion about do-not-resuscitate (DNR) orders "a few days or few hours before the patient's death."[4] Based on these findings, approximately one in five oncologists potentially may not discuss DNR status until after the patient has had a cardiac arrest or has been on life support for some time. On the other hand, when the ICU is a closed unit with the intensivist serving as the primary attending, he or she may feel that it is not his or her role to discuss end-of-life issues. Also changing from one intensivist to another affects the timing of the decision because of varying viewpoints and approaches between intensivists.

USE OF ADVANCE DIRECTIVES IN CRITICALLY ILL CANCER PATIENTS

Confounding the decision of when to transition from intensive care to palliation is the lack of patients' advance directives as to when to limit or withhold aggressive support. The Patient Self Determination Act (PSDA) signed into law on November 5, 1990, and effective December 1, 1991, was to have addressed the increased use of advance directives. The law was in response to the US Supreme Court case *Cruzan v Director, Missouri Department of Health and Human Services*.[5] In brief, Ms Cruzan was a 26-year-old who was rendered comatose after a motor vehicle accident in 1983. In 1986, after not recovering and remaining in a persistent vegetated state, her parents asked that artificial nutrition be stopped. However, the Missouri State Hospital insisted that a court order was needed to stop enteral feeding. The trial court ruled to stop enteral feeding, but the Missouri Supreme Court reversed the lower court's ruling. Subsequently, in 1990, the US Supreme Court reviewed the Missouri Supreme Court ruling and upheld the ruling in regard to incompetent patients, but also added that competent patients would be allowed to refuse unwanted medical treatment. Furthermore, in incompetent patients, like Nancy Cruzan, the US Supreme Court allowed individual states to determine requirements for surrogate decision making regarding withdrawal of life-sustaining therapy. In response to this ruling, Senator Danforth of Missouri sponsored the PSDA.[6]

The purpose of the PSDA was to give patients the right to make decisions regarding their medical care, including the right to accept or refuse treatment, and to make an advance directive. The law also requires that health care facilities and agencies discuss advance health care directives with patients when they are admitted.[5]

Soon after the PSDA went into effect, research was conducted to evaluate its impact on completion of advance directives and decision making with regards to end-of-life decisions. The studies on the impact of PSDA on decision making for the most part have demonstrated negative results. The most widely known of these studies is the Study to Understand Prognosis and Preferences for Outcomes and Risk of Treatments (SUPPORT) which demonstrated that the intervention did not facilitate informed end-of-life decision making. The SUPPORT study was a multicenter study looking at whether advance directives assist in decision making with regard to end-of-life decisions in the general population. The study was conducted at five US teaching hospitals and included a total of 9,105 patients. This study was conducted in two phases: an observational phase and an interventional phase. The interventional phase was a randomization of 4,804 patients to a treatment or control group. The patients in the treatment group were intervened via the "presence of a trained nurse facilitator to provide detailed prognostic information to the patients and medical staff, to work with patients and families to elicit and document patient preferences, and to facilitate communication between patients and physicians." No difference was noted between the two groups with regard to any of the five major measured outcomes: incidence and timing of DNR orders; patient-physician agreement on preferences for cardiopulmonary resuscitation (CPR); days in an ICU, in a coma, or ventilated before death; presence of pain; and hospital resource use.[6]

In SUPPORT, the maximum number of cancer patients that were enrolled was 16.9%. This low percentage of enrollment of cancer would make one wonder if, in a larger cohort of cancer patients, advance directives would have an effect on decision making with regard to end-of-life decisions when admitted to an ICU.

Kish and colleagues[7] conducted a prospective study as part of a Multicenter Outcomes Study of Critically Ill Cancer Patients on consecutive admissions to the medical ICU from July 1994 to March 1996 at a tertiary cancer center. The study objectives were to determine the incidence of critically ill cancer patients admitted to the ICU with advance directives and the characteristics of those patients and their hospital outcomes. Only 27% of the 872 patients admitted to the ICU had advance directives. The demographics of the patients who had advance directives tended to be Caucasian and older. The study concluded that advance directives are infrequently established in critically ill cancer patients and that, since the majority of the patients tended to be Caucasian, cultural differences might need to be taken into consideration when discussing end-of-life decisions in the ICU. Additionally, they found that patients with hematological malignancies and those with relapse and progressive disease tended to have more advance directives. There was an association between advance directives and actual mortality. Upon review of the data, using logistic regression, severity of illness was the most important predictor of mortality in comparison to type of malignancy, disease status, and presence of an advance directive.

Wallace and colleagues,[8] using the data from the study by Kish and colleagues,[7] examined matched pairs with the same characteristics except for the presence of advance directives, then analyzed their cases to determine if the presence of an advance directive at the time of ICU admission influenced the decision to initiate life-support therapy. The investigators showed that the presence of an advance directive was not statistically significant to affect the decision of initiating life-supporting therapy. However, the presence of the advance directive was helpful in making decisions regarding resuscitation status, withdrawal of support, and discharge from the ICU. These patients had more DNR orders written and shorter length of stay in the ICU.[8]

The majority of studies that have been conducted to determine if advance directives facilitate end-of-life decisions have shown that they have a negative effect both in cancer and noncancer patients. However, a retrospective study by Hammes and colleagues evaluated a program titled *Respecting Your Choices*, an intervention focused on advance care planning as an "ongoing process" rather than an event to produce a product such as an advance directive. In addition, the program facilitated discussions about values and preferences instead of completing a document. "The study demonstrated that 85% of the individuals had advance directives and 95% of these were available in the medical record." Furthermore, the advance directives were completed long in advance of death (median time was 1.2 years).[6] The focus on patient's values and preferences, a dynamic process based on the current patient's status, is probably the reason why the Hammes program is successful.

CONVENING MULTIDISCIPLINARY FAMILY MEETINGS

Once the decision has been made to transition to comfort care it is important that a family meeting be convened that includes members from the multidisciplinary team. Ideally, this is not the first family meeting to be convened since the patient's admission to the ICU. Mularski and colleagues[9] recommend that discussions be held with the patient and the patient's family to discuss goals of ICU care, advance planning, and identification of a surrogate decision maker before transfer to the ICU. In another study focusing on an intensive communication intervention, Lilly and colleagues[10] recommended that a family meeting be convened within 72 hours of admission to the ICU. The purpose of the meeting is to discuss the facts, options for treatments, the patient's perspective on death and dying, and to agree on the care plan and on the criteria that would determine success or failure of the care plan. Furthermore, having frequent family meetings during an ICU admission—as opposed to having only one to discuss end-of-life issues—may provide an opportunity to build trust between the intensivist and the patient's family.[6]

The presence of the multidisciplinary team at the family meeting is recommended to provide emotional support to patient's family, and the team can gain insight into their values and beliefs. This multidisciplinary team makeup may include individuals from the social work, chaplaincy, ethics, and palliative care departments. Also helpful is to have both the primary attending and intensivist present at the family meeting. It is important that before convening the family meeting, the various health care providers meet to discuss the patient's disease, prognosis, and treatment options and resolve any disagreements before the family meeting. If disagreements still persist, avoid debating these issues in front of patient's family since it may lead to family members becoming confused and frustrated.

ADDRESSING PATIENT'S AND PATIENT'S FAMILY CULTURAL BELIEFS AND SPIRITUAL VALUES

As alluded to above, it is important to ascertain the patient's and patient's family values and beliefs to help facilitate end-of-life decisions. Furthermore, acknowledging and supporting cultural beliefs and spiritual values have been identified as measures that can be used as indicators of providing quality end-of-life care within the ICU.[11] Cultural beliefs need to be taken into consideration when family meetings are convened to discuss end-of-life decisions. This consideration is very evident in health care centers that take care of international patients. Even patients who reside in the United States may still have a multicultural background differing from that of the treating health care provider. One must be careful in assuming that if a patient is identified as belonging to a certain ethnic group that they follow the culture beliefs of that particular ethnic group. Cultural beliefs may influence communication about end-of-life issues, decision making within the patients family, or attitudes about DNR orders.[12] A reference book that may be useful is *Culture and Clinical Care*, which gives overviews of culture or ethnic identity, spiritual or religious orientation, symptom management, family relationships, illness beliefs, and death rituals of 35 different ethnic and regional groups.[13]

Religious and spiritual values also need to be taken into consideration when discussing end-of-life decisions with patients and their families. Silvestri and colleagues[14] suggest that religious beliefs may influence medical decisions. In this study of a group of newly diagnosed, advanced lung cancer patients and their caregivers, faith in God was ranked second only to the recommendation of the oncologist in deciding between different treatment options. An assessment of the spiritual beliefs of both the patient and the patient's family should be obtained. This assessment can be performed by any member of the health care team.[15]

PATIENTS WITH CHILDREN AND AFFECT ON END-OF-LIFE DECISION MAKING

In discussing end-of-life issues, decisions may be made by the patient or patient's family based on consideration that the patient may consider more aggressive care to attempt to spend more time with their children. It is estimated that 24% of cancer patients have children less than 18 years old. A study by Nilsson and colleagues[16] concluded that patients with advanced cancer and dependent children are more likely to favor a course of treatment that would extend life rather than relieve pain and discomfort. The study also concluded that these patients had a worse quality of life during the last week of life. Based on these findings, the recommendations are to consider providing enhanced psychosocial support and that the patients may need guidance on how to discuss their illness with children.

FACILITATING A "GOOD DEATH" IN THE ICU

Since most end-of-life decisions in the ICU will involve withholding or withdrawing support, transferring a patient out of the ICU to either an inpatient palliative care unit, inpatient hospice, or home hospice may at times be difficult. In anticipation that the patient may not be transferred out of the ICU, one must be prepared for the patient to die in the ICU. The timing of a death in the ICU varies from shortly after admission to a short or prolonged stay. As much effort as goes into resuscitating a patient—if not more—should be put into ensuring that an ICU death is a good death. A statement that is often used to emphasize the effort needed to ensure quality end-of-life care is "there is no second chance to get it right."[17] Also Dame Cicely Saunders,[18,19] British physician and founder of hospice care is quoted, "How people die will remain in the memories of those who live on." An article by Beckstrand and colleagues[20] gives recommendations on how to facilitate a good death. These were derived from a survey focusing on perceptions on end-of-life care. The survey was sent to a random sample of members of the American Association of Critical Care Nurses, and the results are summarized in **Box 1**.

Some of these recommendations have already been addressed above. When considering withdrawing aggressive support, protocols should be used to facilitate this process that prevent the patient and family members from experiencing discomfort. Furthermore, some of the health care providers may be concerned that the treatments being administered to relieve suffering may also be hastening death. This concern and the importance of using protocols were discussed in an article by Kuschner and colleagues.[21] Using protocols may help avoid the ethical tensions that may arise between health care providers during the withdrawal of life support.

Kuschner and colleagues[21] also added an educational process to promote consensus building and to strengthen communication. Effective communication at the end of life is essential during the process of withdrawing life support. The communication process begins during the family meeting that is convened to discuss transitioning to palliation. The process and any anticipated changes should be discussed

---

Box 1
Measures that can facilitate a good death

Facilitators to providing a good death

Making environmental changes to promote dying with dignity

Being present

Managing patients' pain and discomfort

Knowing and following patients' wishes for end-of-life care

Promoting earlier cessation of treatment or not initiating aggressive treatment at all

Communicating effectively as a health care team

From Beckstrand RL, Callister LC, Kirchhoff KT. Providing a "good death": critical care nurses' suggestions for improving end-of-life care. Am J Crit Care 2006;15:38; with permission.

---

with the patient's family. Communication should take place between the nurse, the respiratory therapist, and the ICU physician with regard to the process of withdrawing life support. Furthermore, health care providers should be given the opportunity to voice their discomfort if they have any religious or moral objections with the process, and to move to another assignment if they choose.

PROTOCOLS FOR WITHDRAWING LIFE SUPPORT AND TRANSITIONING TO COMFORT CARE

Protocols for withdrawing life support or transitioning to comfort care should include: ensuring that DNR orders have been written, documentation in the medical record about the plan to transition to comfort care, arrangement to make the surroundings as comfortable as possible, liberal visitation periods, symptom management, ventilator or noninvasive ventilator withdrawal, and deactivation of implantable devices.

Symptom Management

Symptom management, particularly pain management, during the transition to comfort care needs to include tools to assess pain symptoms and recognition of potential barriers to providing good pain management. A concern that is commonly voiced by health care providers and patient's families is how to assess pain symptoms in a patient who may not be able to self report symptoms. This scenario is common in ICU patients since they may be on ventilator support, sedated, or unable to communicate for other reasons. In a recent article by Mularski and colleagues,[22] recommendations were made to use the Behavioral Pain Scale or the Critical-Care Pain Observation Tool, which have had the most validity testing. Another option is to "develop a brief pain-behaviors checklist that includes specific behaviors that have been noted in research that correlate with patients' self-report of pain: grimacing, rigidity, wincing, shutting of eyes, clenching of fist, verbalization, and moaning." Along with using this tool or checklist, the recommendation is to not overlook family member's estimates of the patient's pain score. In SUPPORT, "the surrogates had a 73.5% accuracy rate in estimating presence or absence of patient's pain. The tendency was for the surrogates to overestimate patient pain." Mularski and colleagues[22] further recommend using multiple proxy raters of patient pain symptoms to make a more accurate assessment of the pain symptoms.

Reviewing the above recommendations on pain management in critically ill patients at end of life, the assumption could be made that it would be easy to manage pain.

However a major barrier to providing good pain management is the concern by some health care providers of ethical or legal concerns about the escalation of opiates or other palliative measures and the hastening of death. In dealing with this concern, it is necessary for both the health care providers and patient's family to understand that in providing pain medications and other palliative measures, the intent is the relief of symptoms. This requires communication with patient's family members stressing this goal. It is also important to note that research on aggressive pain management at end of life does not shorten life but instead "may be life prolonging because it decreases the systemic effects of uncontrolled pain that can compromise vital organ functions."[22] Furthermore, in a study by Chan and colleagues[23] there was no statistically significant relationship between doses of opiates and time to death in a group of critically ill patients. Research has also demonstrated great variation in types and amounts of medications used during withdrawal of life support. Therefore it is important to include guidelines for use of opiates and benzodiazepines in the protocols, and information about patient conditions that may necessitate increasing or decreasing dosages.[22]

Deactivation of Implantable Cardioverter Defibrillators and Permanent Pacemakers

Protocols for withdrawing life support should include statements regarding deactivation of implantable cardioverter defibrillators (ICD) and permanent pacemakers (PPM.) As indications for implantation of PPMs and ICDs have increased, it can only be anticipated that some patients who receive these devices may develop cancer or have cancer that becomes terminal. Therefore one must take into consideration whether deactivation of these devices is appropriate during the transition to comfort-care-only measures. Addressing these devices separately is appropriate owing to the functions that they serve. The published literature about ICDs has demonstrated that the patient may experience pain when a shock is delivered appropriately or inappropriately at the end of life. Discussing end-of-life issues is difficult, but even more difficult when discussing when to deactivate an ICD. In a study by Goldstein and colleagues,[24] only 27% of physicians had a discussion about deactivating the ICD. The timing of this conversation in 75% of cases occurred during the last few days of life and, at times, in the last hours or even last minutes of life. Even in patients who had DNR orders, less than 45% had conversations discussing the deactivation of the ICD. The study concluded that guidelines addressing indications for implantation of ICDs should also include recommendations of when to deactivate them. However, a review of the current literature on recommendations regarding the deactivation of PPM demonstrates a disagreement on whether it is ethically permissible to deactivate a PPM in a dying patient. This disagreement is based on claims that a PPM neither prolongs the dying process nor causes discomfort.[25] In addition, in an article by Braun and colleagues,[25] the argument is made that deactivating a PPM may cause bradycardia, rate-related congested heart failure, and dyspnea resulting in increased suffering. They concluded that decisions to deactivate a PPM should be made on an individual basis and education should be provided to the patient and the patient's family to help alleviate anxiety associated with the decision of deactivation of PPM and ICD.[26] The PPM should be removed before cremation to decrease the risk of injury from explosion.

PROVIDING EMOTIONAL AND ORGANIZATIONAL SUPPORT FOR ICU CLINICIANS

Along with instituting the practices to facilitate transitioning from cure to comfort care discussed above, another issue is providing emotional and organizational support for ICU clinicians that provide care to dying patients. Addressing this issue has been identified as one of the domains that can be used to assess the quality of end-of-life care that is provided in an ICU.[11] One useful measure is convening a debriefing session after a particularly difficult case. It is useful to have someone present that can facilitate the discussion and provide the opportunity for those present to discuss their feelings about the patient's death. Ideally, the participants should come from multiple disciplines and the session should provide an opportunity to improve staff morale, enhance team work, and improve satisfaction.[27] Another measure that may be useful is to have a staff support group that meets regularly with meeting times integrated into the routine of the ICU.[11] Developing measures that will assist health care providers in coping with the care of a dying patient is important to decrease moral distress or emotional burnout. Moral distress can occur when the "practitioner feels certain of the ethical course of action but is constrained from taking that action." In a study by Hamric and Blackhall,[28] exploring the perspectives and experiences of registered nurses and physicians working together with dying patients in an ICU, the most distressing situations for both groups was feeling pressured to continue aggressive treatment when the providers felt that such treatment was not warranted. If not relieved, moral distress can potentially lead to decrease in retention of the health care providers in a workforce that is already forecasting a shortage of providers.[29]

SUMMARY

Since the majority of deaths will occur after limiting or withdrawing life support, when dealing with end-of-life issues in critically ill cancer patients focus should be given to ensuring that multidisciplinary family meetings are convened to discuss end-of-life decision making. Furthermore, throughout the process of transitioning from cure to comfort care, it is essential to support the patient and the patient's family cultural beliefs and spiritual values, and ensure good pain and symptom management. The use of protocols facilitates a smooth transition and potentially reduces variability between health care providers. Finally, integrating measures into the ICU routine that will help health care providers cope with the care of a dying patient is recommended to avoid moral distress or emotional burnout.

REFERENCES

1. Thiery G, Azoulay E, Darmon M, et al. Outcome of cancer patients considered for intensive care unit admission: a hospital-wide prospective study. J Clin Oncol 2005;23:4406.
2. Angus DC, Barnato AE, Linde-Zwirble WT, et al. Use of intensive care at the end of life in the United States: an epidemiologic study. Crit Care Med 2004;32:638.
3. Prendergast TJ, Claessens MT, Luce JM. A national survey of end-of-life care for critically ill patients. Am J Respir Crit Care Med 1998;158:1163.
4. Baile WF, Lenzi R, Parker PA, et al. Oncologists' attitudes toward and practices in giving bad news: an exploratory study. J Clin Oncol 2002;20:2189.
5. Bradley EH, Rizzo JA. Public information and private search: evaluating the Patient Self-Determination Act. J Health Polit Policy Law 1999;24:239.
6. Prendergast TJ. Advance care planning: pitfalls, progress, promise. Crit Care Med 2001;29:N34.
7. Kish SK, Martin CG, Price KJ. Advance directives in critically ill cancer patients. Crit Care Nurs Clin North Am 2000;12:373.
8. Wallace SK, Martin CG, Shaw AD, et al. Influence of an advance directive on the initiation of life support technology in critically ill cancer patients. Crit Care Med 2001;29:2294–8.

9. Mularski RA, Bascom P, Osborne ML. Educational agendas for interdisciplinary end-of-life curricula. Crit Care Med 2001;29:N16.

10. Lilly CM, De Meo DL, Sonna LA, et al. An intensive communication intervention for the critically ill. Am J Med 2000;109:469.

11. Clarke EB, Curtis JR, Luce JM, et al. Quality indicators for end-of-life care in the intensive care unit. Crit Care Med 2003;31:2255.

12. Doolen J, York NL. Cultural differences with end-of-life care in the critical care unit. Dimens Crit Care Nurs 2007;26:194.

13. Lipson JG, Dibble SL. Culture and clinical care. San Francisco (CA): UCSF Nursing Press; 2005.

14. Silvestri GA, Knittig S, Zoller JS, et al. Importance of faith on medical decisions regarding cancer care. J Clin Oncol 2003;21:1379.

15. Chambers N, Curtis J. The interface of technology and spirituality in the ICU. In: Curtis J, Rubenfeld G, editors. Managing death in the ICU: the transition from cure to comfort. New York (NY): Oxford University Press; 2001. p. 193.

16. Nilsson ME, Maciejewski PK, Zhang B, et al. Mental health, treatment preferences, advance care planning, location, and quality of death in advanced cancer patients with dependent children. Cancer 2009;115:399.

17. Ferris FD, von Gunten CF, Emanuel LL. Competency in end-of-life care: last hours of life. J Palliat Med 2003;6:605.

18. Saunders C. Pain and impending death. In: Wall PD, Melzak R, editors. Textbook of pain. New York: Churchill Livingstone; 1989. p. 621.

19. Sherman DA, Branum K. Critical care nurses' perceptions of appropriate care of the patient with orders not to resuscitate. Heart Lung 1995;24:321.

20. Beckstrand RL, Callister LC, Kirchhoff KT. Providing a "good death": critical care nurses' suggestions for improving end-of-life care. Am J Crit Care 2006;15:38.

21. Kuschner WG, Gruenewald DA, Clum N, et al. Implementation of ICU palliative care guidelines and procedures: a quality improvement initiative following an investigation of alleged euthanasia. Chest 2009;135:26.

22. Mularski RA, Puntillo K, Varkey B, et al. Pain management within the palliative and end-of-life care experience in the ICU. Chest 2009;135:1360.

23. Chan JD, Treece PD, Engelberg RA, et al. Narcotic and benzodiazepine use after withdrawal of life support. Chest 2004;126:286.

24. Goldstein NE, Lampert R, Bradley E, et al. Management of implantable cardioverter defibrillators in end-of-life care. Ann Intern Med 2004;141:835.

25. Mueller PS, Jenkins SM, Bramstedt KA, et al. Deactivating implanted cardiac devices in terminally ill patients: practices and attitudes. Pacing Clin Electrophysiol 2008;31:560.

26. Braun TC, Hagen NA, Hatfield RE, et al. Cardiac pacemakers and implantable defibrillators in terminal care. J Pain Symptom Manage 1999;18:126.

27. Block SD. Helping the clinician cope with death in the ICU. In: Curtis JR, Rubenfeld GD, editors. Managing death in the intensive care unit. New York: Oxford University Press; 2001. p. 183.

28. Hamric AB, Blackhall LJ. Nurse-physician perspectives on the care of dying patients in intensive care units: collaboration, moral distress, and ethical climate. Crit Care Med 2007;35:422.

29. Angus DC, Kelley MA, Schmitz RJ, et al. Current and projected workforce requirements for care of the critically ill and patients with pulmonary disease: can we meet the requirements of an aging population? JAMA 2000;284:2762.

Index

Note: Page numbers of article titles are in **boldface** type.

A

Abdomen, acute, in oncological surgery patients, critical care issues in, 101–102
Acquired factor VIII inhibitors, in critically ill cancer patients, 115
Acquired von Willebrand syndrome, in critically ill cancer patients, 114–115
Acute abdomen, in oncological surgery patients, critical care issues in, 101–102
Acute care nurse practitioners, in oncologic critical care, Memorial Sloan-Kettering Cancer
    Center experience, **207–217.** See also *Memorial Sloan-Kettering Cancer Center*
    experience, acute care nurse practitioners in oncologic critical care in.
Acute kidney injury
    defined, 152–153
    identification of, early, 152–153
    in critically ill cancer patients, **151–179**
        acute renal failure in, causes of, 160–170. See also *Acute renal failure, in critically ill*
            cancer patients, causes of.
        causes of, 160–170
        described, 151–152
        epidemiology of, 153–160
        incidence of, 153–158
        outcome of, 158–160
        prognostic indicators in, 158–160
        treatment of, 170–171
Acute lung injury (ALI)
    ARF in cancer patients due to, 25–26
    transfusion-related, ARF in cancer patients due to, 29
Acute renal failure, in critically ill cancer patients, causes of, 160–170
    cancer-related microangiopathy, 166–168
    contrast nephropathy, 164
    DIC, 166–167
    multiple myeloma, 169–170
    nephrotoxicity, 163–164
    sepsis, 160–162
    toxicity related to cancer treatment, 154–155
    TTP/HUS, 167–168
    tumor lysis syndrome, 165–166
    ureteral obstruction, 168–169
Acute respiratory distress syndrome (ARDS), ARF in cancer patients due to, 25–26
Acute respiratory failure (ARF)
    described, 21–22
    in cancer patients, **21–40**
        causes of, 22–31
            ALI, 25–26

Crit Care Clin 26 (2010) 229–237
doi:10.1016/S0749-0704(09)00120-1
0749-0704/09/$ – see front matter © 2010 Elsevier Inc. All rights reserved.

criticalcare.theclinics.com

Moving?

Make sure your subscription moves with you!

To notify us of your new address, find your **Clinics Account Number** (located on your mailing label above your name), and contact customer service at:

Email: journalscustomerservice-usa@elsevier.com

800-654-2452 (subscribers in the U.S. & Canada)
314-447-8871 (subscribers outside of the U.S. & Canada)

Fax number: 314-447-8029

Elsevier Health Sciences Division
Subscription Customer Service
3251 Riverport Lane
Maryland Heights, MO 63043

*To ensure uninterrupted delivery of your subscription, please notify us at least 4 weeks in advance of move.

Printed and bound by CPI Group (UK) Ltd, Croydon, CR0 4YY

03/10/2024

01040443-0008